J o
ber
s an
ss o

Dat

21.

2

29.

2

24|8

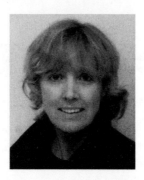

Maev-Ann Wren is an award-winning *Irish Times* journalist and commentator. A Dubliner, she graduated from University College Dublin with a degree in history and economics and a masters in economics. In her career in journalism, she has reported from Dublin, Belfast and the United States, and she has worked as a financial reporter, economics editor, columnist, editorial writer and senior newspaper editor. Her series "An Unhealthy State" won her the 2001 National Media Award for newspaper analysis and comment. She is married with two children and lives in Dublin.

MAEV-ANN WREN

UNHEALTHY
STATE
ANATOMY OF A SICK SOCIETY

**NEW
ISLAND**

UNHEALTHY STATE
First published 2003
by New Island
2 Brookside
Dundrum Road
Dublin 14

www.newisland.ie

The author has asserted her moral rights.

ISBN 1 902602 88 9   Mé   9337

British Library Cataloguing in Publication Data.
A CIP catalogue record for this book is available
from the British Library.

Typeset by New Island
Cover design by New Island
Printed in Norway by Rotanor.

10 9 8 7 6 5 4 3 2 1

*For Cormac, Claire and Sorcha with love and thanks,
for Sharon, and the many like her, who have been denied care for
far too long, and in tribute to a friend and inspiration,
the late great Dick Walsh.*

CONTENTS

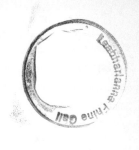

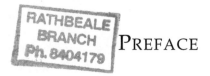
PREFACE

Without understanding, reform is impossible. My motivation in researching and writing this book was to understand how the Irish health care system had evolved, why it was so inadequate and how it might be reformed. This was no abstract enquiry. While I wrote, a good friend's wait for necessary medical treatment lengthened from four to six years.

There is a perception that the Irish health care system is so complex that remedying its problems is too daunting a task. In my research, it became apparent that the complexity is superficial, the flaws are fundamentally simple and the remedies quite achievable. This appreciation led me to travel a further path of enquiry to ask what it is about Irish society in the past and the present which has prevented reform.

This book began in a series of articles entitled "An Unhealthy State" published in *The Irish Times* in October 2000. While much broader in scope, it remains a work which owes much to the techniques of journalism. Although recent history is too close to allow for historical detachment and must be written before state papers are released, I have sought to bring to my research the objectivity and the distinction between fact and opinion to which journalism aspires even when its motivation is campaigning. My account of the early history of the health care system owes a considerable debt to the published work of others. I would particularly like to acknowledge the understanding which I gained from Ruth Barrington's *Health, Medicine and Politics in Ireland 1900–1970*, recently reprinted by the Institute of Public Administration, 15 years after the first edition, a recognition of its seminal importance.

In my investigation of the contemporary politics of health care, I benefited greatly from the 1997 Freedom of Information Act, which facilitated enquiries to illuminate conflicts in cabinet on health policy, interdepartmental arguments about spending and the role of the private sector, and the development of strategic thinking within the Department of Health. I had thought to describe this book as one of the first to benefit

1

from FOI. Now, unfortunately, it may be one of the few books to have been written in the Golden Age of FOI. Anyone who pursues the exchanges between the Ministers for Finance and Health in its pages will readily understand why the government wished to curtail FOI and why its curtailment is not in the interests of democracy.

Since the state of the health care system engenders constant controversy, I have been attempting to keep up with a moving target. Three major reports on the health service have been due for publication in 2003. I must thank the three thoughtful people who supplied me with early drafts of the Hanly, Prospectus and Brennan reports, which have contributed to my discussion of reform. How politics might affect their eventual content or publication was unclear at the time of writing. If their published content differs from the drafts discussed here, the reader will have the satisfaction of reading in these pages some of what has been suppressed. Earlier drafts tend to be braver.

The health care system is immense in its scope. I have attempted to keep my focus on the central issue of its failure to provide accessible, equitable care. Inevitably there are areas, such as the psychiatric service, care of the disabled or the development of the nursing profession, which I have been unable to explore in detail but I hope that those readers to whom they are of particular interest will perceive the pertinence of my overall analysis to their concern.

I am indebted to a great many people who have encouraged, supported and assisted me. Conor Brady, the former editor of *The Irish Times*, encouraged me to write the original series. Willy Clingan conceived the title and devotedly saw the series into print. In my research, I received generous help from many colleagues, particularly Muiris Houston, Pádraig O Moráin, Patsy McGarry and Lara Marlowe. Mary Holland insisted I investigate the doctors' strike in Saskatchewan. Noel Costello courageously volunteered to read the full book in draft. Still one of the great Irish institutions, *The Irish Times* has supported me and my efforts in very many ways and has permitted me to draw on my newspaper articles for the book.

This book might never have happened had not Fergus O'Ferrall of the Adelaide Hospital Society and my colleague Carol Coulter separately suggested it, for which I am very grateful. Fintan O'Toole helpfully directed me to New Island, who have been extraordinarily tolerant of a project which kept growing in length and gestation, and whose editors, first Ciara Considine, later Emma Dunne, have shown great professionalism, tact and skill in turning a journalist into a writer. In assembling research documents I have been assisted by many people who intrepidly explored archives on my behalf: Margaret Byrnes of the Council for Social Welfare, Paula Carey of ICTU, Maria Murphy of the IMO, Tara Buckley of the VHI, the staffs of the political parties, the Government Information Service and the Central Statistics Office and staff at many levels of the Department of Health. Barry Desmond, a former Minister for Health, gave me invaluable access to his personal papers. The staffs of the libraries of *The Irish Times*, the Institute of Public Administration, TCD and UCD have always been helpful to my pursuit of sources.

I would like to thank four former Ministers for Health for agreeing to be interviewed: Barry Desmond, Rory O'Hanlon, Brendan Howlin and Michael Noonan. This book draws on interviews with many people in politics, medicine, nursing, the Catholic Church, the trade unions, academia and in many levels of health administration. Some spoke off the record and some tolerated repeated queries over two years. This book has acquired its voice by listening to the voices of others, patients as well as professionals, who have shared their understanding and, in many cases, their determination that change should come. Since I cannot thank all of them individually, I would like to thank them collectively for their time and insights.

In my international research, I was set on the path initially by the kind help of Tim O'Sullivan of the IPA. Among those who have responded graciously to repeated enquiries were Tom Rathwell, professor of health administration at Dalhousie University, Nova Scotia, Canada; Wendy Edgar, senior policy advisor at the New Zealand Ministry of Health; Clive Gowdy, permanent secretary of the Northern Ireland Department of Health, Social Services and Public Safety; René Cacquet, former deputy Minister of Health in France; and Denis Crowley, secretary to the Social Protection Committee of the European Union.

My economic analysis has benefited greatly from the comments and work of John FitzGerald and Brian Nolan, research professors at the Economic and Social Research Institute, and their colleagues.

A mother of two does not complete a task of this magnitude without support on the home front. My heartfelt thanks to Meike Schiffko and Tina Vongrad, who kept the home fires burning over the last two years; and to my extended family, friends and neighbours, who stepped in frequently to assist me and who have been so understanding of my absences and abstractedness. My home office ran smoothly with the help of my young secretarial assistants: Louise Nicholson, Maeve Dunne, Rhys Jones and my daughter, Claire O Rourke.

When I started writing on health in 2000, it was because it was the major political and economic issue of the day. I might not have continued to find the topic of such consuming interest had I not come from a family of doctors and married into a family for so many of whom health care was of professional concern. I had grown up hearing tales of my maternal grandfather's medical career in England, pre- and post-NHS, and in a house where Michael Foot's biography of Bevan had pride of place on my father's bookshelf. My father-in-law remains outraged at the effect of the 1980s cutbacks on the service which he and his colleagues in the Department of Health had spent a lifetime building. While none of the health professionals in my extended family is responsible for either the factual accuracy or the opinions expressed in this book, and none was an interviewee, their dedication in their respective ways to the cause of better health, in Ireland and overseas, and their frustration at the inadequacies of the systems in which they have worked, has contributed hugely to my sense of the need for change.

I have been very privileged in the readers of my book. Among the people who have been kind enough to read and comment on portions of it are Martin McKee, research director at the European Observatory on Health Care Systems, John FitzGerald, Clive Gowdy and René Cacquet. Ruth Barrington and Noel Costello read the full text in a late draft, saved me from error and improved it in many ways, for which I am deeply in their debt. Throughout the entire writing of the book from its very earliest (and longest) drafts, I have been sustained by the conscientious, exacting and encouraging reading of Dale Tussing, professor of economics at Syracuse University, New York, and the author of influential studies on Irish health care. Although he has been an actor in some of the dramas described in the book, he has always understated his role. He is a true and disinterested friend of Irish health care. I remain immensely grateful for his long-distance companionship. None of these readers are responsible in any way for the content or opinions in the final text.

I could not have written this book without the support of my husband, Cormac O Rourke, and my daughters, Claire and Sorcha, who have shown such understanding and patience with an enterprise that was meant to last a summer but lasted two years. Cormac saved the book from the depredations of computer viruses, carried family life, shared my enthusiasms and doubts and encouraged me to continue believing that this was a task worth doing, wherever it led. He was, as ever, my best friend and ally.

Maev-Ann Wren
March 2003.

4

INTRODUCTION

In 2002 in one of the richest countries in the world, poor families could not afford to bring their sick children to visit a family doctor. In 2001, a woman with life-threatening cancer was forced to take court action to secure the hospital treatment prescribed by her doctor and readily available to those who could pay.

This is the Republic of Ireland at the beginning of the third millennium: a predominantly Roman Catholic state, still vocally espousing Christian values, but a state in which access to medical care is determined by income rather than need. Its most prominent politicians openly debate whether Ireland should embrace the values of the US, where health care is a commodity not a right, rather than of its European neighbours, where treatment in need is taken for granted.

Fifty years ago, Irish society was convulsed by a battle in which doctors and the Catholic Church prevented the state from introducing a Mother and Child scheme. At the heart of the scheme was a proposal for free family doctor care for all children up to the age of 16. This political goal remains to be achieved.

Today, although the poorest 30 per cent of the population receives family doctor care without charge, there are many families on very low incomes who must pay for every visit to their family doctor. The two-tier system of public hospital care discriminates between public and private patients and is characterised by such long waiting lists and, on occasion, such poor care for public patients that one in ten of the poorest 10 per cent of the population has taken out private health insurance. Health care has been underfunded for decades and, despite recent increases in spending, remains underdeveloped. Primary care is rudimentary – a patchy network of self-employed general practitioners. Much acute care is delivered by unsupervised junior doctors in small sub-standard hospitals.

How did Irish health care develop in this way? Why have Irish citizens tolerated such a poor system and such inequitable access? Why have they tolerated a widening gap between their life expectancy and the life expectancy of the average European? Why is it that, in a state where per capita income now exceeds the EU average, health spending has for decades been lower than the EU average? What are the prospects for reform, and who and what stands in its way? These are the questions which this book sets out to answer.

This is a book about the politics of health care in Ireland – at national level, at local level, in hospitals and among doctors; about how decisions about access to care and the quality of that care have been made and evaded during the life of independent Ireland; about the relationship between the medical profession and the state; about the role of the Catholic Church – for good and ill – in health care; about the politics of health spending and the location of hospitals; and about the intense debate on possible pathways to reform.

Fifty years ago, access to health care was *the* issue in Irish politics. From the year 2000, health became once again *the* issue in Irish politics. This book both records and seeks to contribute to our contemporary debate, which may prove no more than a further chapter in that sorry tale of 50 years ago or, perhaps, may be the first chapter in the happier book of the final achievement of true reform.

The structure of the book

Part One describes the condition of Irish health and health care, and explains why Ireland deserves to be described as an Unhealthy State.

Part Two reviews the politics of health care over the last six decades: from the roots of the Mother and Child scheme in the 1940s, to the convulsions of the 1950s, the lowered ambitions of the 1960s, the defeated reform of the 1970s, the cutbacks of the 1980s, the consolidation of two-tier care at the opening of the 1990s and its survival through the boom years of that decade. Themes recur but roles change: the Catholic Church develops from an immense obstacle to health care reform into the reformers' ally, yet continues to fight a rearguard action against reproductive freedom; the medical profession sets its face against many reforms but argues for others; the political parties alternately embrace and abandon reform; grand visions are succeeded by incremental change.

Chapter 2 describes the defeat of the short-lived dream of a free, national health service and the achievement of partial reform in the period to 1957. Chapter 3 relates how Fianna Fáil abandoned its support for comprehensive reform in the 1960s and how hospital consultants defeated a Labour Minister's attempt to provide universal, free hospital care in the 1970s. Chapter 4 chronicles how, in the 1980s, the granting of unlimited private practice rights to hospital consultants exacerbated the two-tier divide in care and unleashed private medicine. Chapter 5 describes the effect on care of cutbacks in spending from 1987 and the adoption in 1991 of a formal system of two-tier access to public hospitals.

Chapters 6 to 8 review the decade from 1992 to 2002, thematically as well as chronologically. Chapter 6 explores how, through shifting political coalitions and immense economic and social change, fundamental stasis prevailed in health care; how Ministers for Health were appointed in turn from each of the three major political parties but none attempted fundamental reform; and how the social partners, who had been enlisted in a consensual approach to politics, pursued an economic agenda but neglected social services like health. Chapter 7 describes how the scandal of patients' infection by contaminated blood products placed the entire system of health care under intense scrutiny and engulfed the Department of Health. Chapter 8 recounts how, despite the loss of its moral ascendancy, the Catholic Church fought to retain its institutional and legislative influence on the health care system.

Part Three dissects the Unhealthy State. Chapter 9 describes the insidious machinery of two-tier hospital care: how patients experience it; how professionals perceive it; how enmeshed it is with how doctors are employed and paid; and how the state has fostered it. Chapter 10 describes the intense politics of hospital location: how standards of care are sacrificed to satisfy the desire for an acute hospital in every locality; how politicians have abandoned the responsibility of leadership; and how the medical profession is fighting for higher standards of care. Chapter 11 describes the inaccessibility of the very first level of care – the family doctor – the efforts to reform primary care and the medical and political obstacles to free access to care.

Part Four explores options for reform. Chapter 12 untangles the facts and describes the politics of health spending, inextricably linked with the contemporary debate about tax and spending – about whether Ireland should emulate Boston or Berlin. Chapter 13 discusses the proposals for reform which have been tabled by the government and concludes that, even were they to be achieved, they would still fall far short of equitable change. This chapter also assesses the present state of medical politics and the degree to which the medical profession may still constitute a barrier to reform. Chapter 14 questions the role of the private sector in medicine, increasingly supported and advanced by the government as a solution to health care reform but permitted to operate as a parasitical offshoot of the public system. Chapter 15 assesses the proposals for a compulsory health insurance system, advanced by the major opposition parties. Chapter 16 reviews the health care systems in seven other states to see what lessons they might suggest for reform in Ireland.

Part Five concludes by looking beyond the story of the past and the lessons from other states to suggest a political path to an equitable and well-resourced health care system, of which Ireland could be proud.

PART ONE
HEALTH IN AN UNHEALTHY STATE

1

HEALTH IN AN UNHEALTHY STATE

"The experience of poor Irish people must be regarded as intolerable."
*– the state's chief medical officer, Jim Kiely, commenting
on a study of health inequality in 2001.*[1]

"The scope for 'two tiers' in terms of access to public hospitals is much
greater here than in ... our European partners."
– National Economic and Social Forum Report, 2002.[2]

We Irish are not healthy. Nor do we value our health. We do not regard
the health of our nation as an asset, or an investment, or a social goal to
be pursued.

Irish people do not live as long as the average European and the gap
between Irish and average European life expectancy is growing. Yet
Ireland is one of the wealthier European Union (EU) states and average
Irish income exceeds the EU average.[3]

Many reasons might be advanced for the earlier deaths of the Irish.
The health of populations is by no means determined simply by how
much states invest in health care or how they organise their health care
systems. Just as an individual's health may be affected by how he cares
for himself and how others care for him, by the state of his marriage, his
job, his bank balance, so too the health of a society is affected by its
wealth, its employment opportunities and, at a deeper level, its sense of
community and the value it places on the lives and health of its
members.

While in every state poorer people experience more sickness and die
younger than richer people, international experience suggests that the more
unequal a society, and the greater the degree of relative poverty and social
exclusion, the worse its overall health. Ireland has great, and growing, disparity

in income.[4] This makes Ireland an unhealthy state – metaphorically *and* literally.

In this unhealthy state, inequitable access to health care is an accepted institution. No attempt to explain ill-health and early death can ignore the inaccessibility, inequity and historical underfunding of the health care system. Most families must pay for every visit to their doctor – and the fees are significant. Consequently, preventive health care is virtually non-existent. In the state-funded hospital system, patients who can afford private insurance gain faster access and superior care; public patients – over half the population, including the vast majority of the elderly – face long waiting lists and may receive inferior care.

While educating our children is the mandatory duty of parents in Ireland, paid for and supervised by the state, caring for their health remains an option, a discretionary item of household spending, which the state funds for only the poorest. And, if a child falls seriously ill – if recurrent tonsillitis, for instance, impairs his hearing and retards the development of his speech – unless his parents have the means to purchase private care, he may wait up to a year for an operation that will place him back on the path to healthy development.[5]

Not only the state but also the health care system is unhealthy, an expression of Victorian values in which health care is a commodity to be purchased or, when it is unaffordable, to be given as a charity, never as a right. Whereas, from the late 19th century, the more progressive European states regarded a healthy population as an essential state investment and, from the mid-20th century, most European states developed universal systems in which access to care was guaranteed and regarded as an expression of social solidarity, in Ireland health care and health remain residuals, luxuries which the wealthy may purchase and the masses may access when economic conditions permit.

This rift between social values in Ireland and in the EU, of which Ireland has been a part for three decades, reflects a divergent historical experience before and during the Republic's 70 years of independence from Britain, and an emerging culture in this latest decade of boom that owes less to Europe than to the United States, where it is accepted that superior care may be purchased.

This state, this Irish society, while justifiably proud of its economic and cultural emergence in this last decade, is nonetheless an unhealthy state and a sick society: not only are Irish people sicker than they should be but Irish social values are unhealthy and foster ill-health. Irish people die younger because they tolerate an inequality between them which breeds ill-health, and they accept a health care system and a view of health care which implicitly places lesser value on the lives of those with lesser means.

Unhealthy lifestyles

One in four of us smokes. One in three adults is overweight, one in eight obese. One in four drinks too much.[6] Alcohol consumption has soared since the mid-1990s. Among EU states, only in France and Luxembourg do adults consume more alcohol than in Ireland.[7] In one study, 69 per cent of 16-year-olds reported having been drunk in the last 12 months compared to an EU average of 52 per cent. One-fifth of 16-year-olds had taken inhalants compared to an EU average of 9 per cent.[8] While the recent rise in alcohol consumption is associated with growing affluence, studies have shown that poorer Irish people are more likely to drink too much, smoke and eat unhealthily.[9]

Although for centuries the stereotype of the Irish has been as a heavy drinking race, ironically, prior to this upsurge of drinking in the mid-1990s, researchers had begun to point out that the facts did not support this stereotype and that Ireland had low rates of deaths from alcoholism and cirrhosis of the liver, low convictions for drunkenness and relatively low per capita consumption.[10] Despite this picture of relative sobriety, however, Irish society undoubtedly had an unhealthy pattern of drinking. The aggregate statistics did not capture the coexistence of large numbers of non-drinkers and a mainstream, heavy drinking pub culture. In the boom years from the mid-1990s, when Ireland for the first time retained its young people at home and in jobs, their new-found disposable income increasingly found its way into the hands of the drinks industry. Their behaviour, and its ultimate effects on their physical and mental health, became of growing concern.

The images of drunken young women lying comatose on the floors of hard-pressed hospital casualty departments, broadcast in late 2002,[11] were like a mirror held up to a society which had used its wealth to ill-effect. In the 1990s, the fruits of success had been dispersed in tax cuts, which funded conspicuous consumption and hedonistic behaviour. The public drunkenness of the young was merely the visible tip of an iceberg of excess, expressed by their affluent elders in fast, extravagant cars, multiple holidays, designer drugs and second and third homes. Meanwhile, the public sphere suffered. Ireland failed to invest in public transport, in education, in social housing programmes, in child care – and in health. Services in the very hospitals where the young women slept off the effects of over-consumption of alcohol were under threat from budgetary cutbacks.

Dying younger

At age 65, Irish men and women have the lowest life expectancy in the EU. Although Irish life expectancy has improved over the last four decades, primarily because of reduced death rates among infants and young children, failure to improve the health of the population has been reflected in a growing gap between Irish and average European life expectancy.[12] Women in France can expect to live for 82.5 years, in Sweden for 82, in Ireland for 79. Men in France can expect to live for 75 years, in Sweden for 77, in Ireland for 73.9.[13] Irish infant mortality rates still remain higher than the EU average.[14] Death rates from heart disease and cancer have consistently exceeded the EU average over the last 20 years.[15] Women, in particular, are much more likely to die of cancer in Ireland than in other European states.[16]

There is no special Irish characteristic, no lethal gene, which preordains these mortality rates. Early deaths and poor health are a consequence of how Irish society values – or fails to value – health. During the 1960s, Finnish male death rates from coronary heart disease were substantially higher than in Ireland – by the late 1990s they were lower; death rates for women were similar to Ireland's – then they fell to nearly half the Irish rate.[17] The US and Australia have also been successful in reducing death rates from cardiovascular disease, by a combination of preventive measures and surgery.[18] In Ireland, death rates at the same age from coronary heart disease vary significantly around the state. Access to services depends on location and earnings, and quality varies. There is "inconsistent implementation of internationally recognised best practice" in treatment of patients, the state's chief medical officer has pointed out.[19] Promised improvements have been slow to materialise.[20]

While the incidence of breast cancer in women is close to the EU average,[21] the death rate from the disease is above the EU average,[22] which implies that detection and care are inferior. In 2002, an organised state screening programme for breast cancer was still only offered to older women in approximately half the state.[23] The probability of receiving radiotherapy varied significantly in different health board areas.[24] While heart disease and cancer are the big killers, evidence has also been published that death rates from common conditions like chronic bronchitis, fracture of the hip, appendectomy and diabetes vary in hospitals around the state, which suggests uneven standards of care.[25]

There is abundant evidence, therefore, that the state of the health service – its underfunding, how it is organised and the quality of the medical care it offers – is relevant to early Irish deaths. Worse still, the services that are available are not allocated according to need.

Unequal health in an unequal state

The odds of dying young and experiencing ill-health are much higher if you are poorer. Unskilled and semi-skilled manual workers have over three times the mortality rate of Irish professionals of the same age.[26] The poor not only die younger, but they are also more likely to suffer chronic disabling conditions[27] or to be admitted to a psychiatric hospital.[28] Their infants are more likely to be stillborn or to die shortly after birth.[29]

Inequalities in health are not confined to Ireland but they vary in different states. Mortality differences have been less marked in egalitarian Sweden and Denmark than in other European states.[30] Reaching an understanding about why the poor die younger and suffer greater ill-health has been surprisingly controversial. At the beginning of the 19th century, it was considered desirable that sickly infants should die lest they survive to become sickly adults.[31] More recently, state authorities have tended to blame the poor for their ill-health, attributing it to their unhealthy behaviour. In 1999, Frank Fahey, Fianna Fáil Minister of State at the Department of Health, suggested that while poverty, unemployment and poor housing were threats to health, "choosing an unhealthy lifestyle" could be just as damaging. "Unhealthy behaviours" such as "smoking, poor diet, lack of exercise and alcohol and substance abuse" were "more prevalent among social classes five and six", the Minister remarked.[32]

Fahey was a Minister in a government which was exacerbating inequalities in income through its budgetary policies, and presiding over a health care system which denied equitable access to the poor. Blaming the victims was more intellectually appealing than confronting the possibility that inequalities in health flowed from poverty, inequality and inequitable access to health care.

Why are the poor more likely to be sick? A study of low-income families in 2000 and 2001 revealed that poor diet was a consequence of poverty. The families reported that they could not afford fresh fruit, vegetables or meat. The study confirmed that a low cost, nutritious diet was beyond their means. Mothers did not eat, to leave more for their children. They smoked to suppress appetite. They fed their children on high-fat convenience foods, which they knew the children would eat, because they could not afford waste. They frequently described feeling worried or depressed about trying to manage without enough money.[33]

Poverty lowers self-esteem. Chronic stress affects the cardiovascular and immune systems and increases the risk of infection and depression.[34] Even people in employment, if they are in low-status jobs which offer little control, are at increased risk of suffering coronary heart disease.[35] Depressed parents are less capable of rearing healthy children and are more likely to smoke and drink. The poor and the low paid do not "choose" unhealthy lifestyles. Their lifestyles are a consequence of their poverty.

And in Ireland's boom years, relative poverty has been growing. The proportion of the population living on incomes below half the average grew from 16–17 per cent in 1994 to 21–22 per cent in 2000.[36] While incomes generally have been rising, leading to government claims that deprivation, as conventionally understood, has been falling, income disparity has nonetheless been widening. Policies implemented by the tax-cutting government, in power from 1997 to 2002 and then re-elected, widened the gap between rich and poor.[37] The richest 20 per cent of the population received over 40 per cent of budget giveaways from 1997 to 2002, the poorest 20 per cent of the population received under 5 per cent.[38] Before this period, Ireland was already one of the more unequal states in the EU. In 1996, the richest 20 per cent of the Irish population had nearly six times the share of national income of the poorest 20 per cent. In contrast, in Denmark, the richest 20 per cent of the population had under three times the share of the poorest 20 per cent.[39]

There is growing international evidence that the more unequal a society, the worse its overall health.[40] Egalitarian societies seem to be healthier than inegalitarian ones, even if their material standards of living are relatively modest. In an inegalitarian society, the low self-esteem of the excluded may undermine their immune system and their health, cause depression and provoke self-destructive behaviour.[41] The director of Ireland's Institute of Public Health, Jane Wilde, has argued that, since income inequality is a critical determinant of a country's health status, Ireland should therefore seek to narrow the gap between rich and poor.[42]

An unequal state is by definition, therefore, an unhealthy state. Bad enough that Ireland has such inequitable incomes, bad enough that its poor have so much greater a likelihood of ill-health, but also, once they require medical treatment, their chances of receiving it are less than the rich.

"There is evidence that the less well-off in society have poorer access to health services," the state's chief medical officer, Jim Kiely, has acknowledged.[43] In the context of Ireland's already "significantly inferior" mortality rates compared to the EU, "the experience of poor Irish people must be regarded as intolerable," Kiely commented of a study of health inequality in 2001. Health inequalities, wrote this most senior doctor in the Department of Health, were "related to ... the problem of inequitable access to health services based on need."[44]

The Irish health care system – institutionalised inequity

The Irish health care system appears to be in permanent crisis. The symptoms are manifest: too few beds and staff, long waiting lists, patient care which fails to conform to the standards expected in one of Europe's wealthier countries. What is less readily apparent is that Ireland has a health care system which almost defies rational analysis. The Organisation for Economic Co-operation and Development (OECD) has diplomatically described the Irish health care system as "unique".[45] Others might consider its mix of the public and private, its state-funded institutional inequity, as bizarre.

Public health care is funded from general taxes but it is not available to everyone on the same terms. The poorest 30 per cent of the population and all over-70-year-olds qualify for medical cards, which mean they may visit their family doctor without charge and receive free medication. The remainder of the population must pay their doctor and for a sizeable amount of their medication. Private insurance has traditionally covered only a fraction of the cost of family doctor visits.[46] Families on low incomes, who do not qualify for medical cards and cannot afford private insurance, may be unable to afford a visit to their doctor or necessary medicines.[47] The state has invested little in primary care. Primary care doctors are self-employed. All manner of community services, including psychological services, are underdeveloped and inaccessible. Although the poor are more likely to suffer mental illness, mental health services are concentrated in areas of greater affluence.[48]

The state funds the public hospitals, which may be state run or under the control of voluntary groups, like Catholic religious orders. Medical card holders receive free hospital care. The remainder of the population must pay relatively limited charges. The greatest barrier to access to hospital care for people on low incomes is not these charges, however. It is that the hospital system has been so poorly resourced – in beds, in staff, in equipment – that care is rationed and the rationing is according to income, not need. While emergency cases are treated on a first-come, first-served basis, all other public hospital care is channelled through two distinct routes: a fast-track for private patients, who have private insurance, paid for by themselves or by their employers; and slow, public waiting lists for the rest. Nearly half the population subscribes to private health insurance in order to jump queues for public hospital treatment. Public patients, still the majority of the population, may wait years for treatments which private patients may receive within weeks in the same publicly funded hospital. There is a network of private hospitals, some on the same campuses as public hospitals.

This two-tier system of care is supported by the state and deeply rooted in how hospitals are organised and how doctors are employed and work. The most unusual element of the system is the manner in which it combines private and public patient care. Public hospital consultants are paid extra for every private patient they treat and, although receiving state salaries, may also work in private hospitals. They have an economic incentive to favour private patients, which contributes to public patient waiting lists and leaves much of public patient care in the hands of poorly supervised and trained junior doctors. Private medicine is booming. Never having attempted to offer equitable access to health care, Ireland has been moving inexorably to an American-style system, where money decides access, where some doctors earn very large incomes indeed from private practice and a minority may even hope to add to their earnings by becoming shareholders in state-subsidised private hospitals.

In 2002, the United Nations Committee on Economic, Social and Cultural Rights, in a critical review of Ireland's implementation of the international covenant on rights, expressed regret about the absence of a human rights framework in the government's health strategy, published in 2001, and recommended that the state revisit the strategy to remedy this, embrace the principles of "non-discrimination and equal access to health facilities and services" and introduce a common waiting list for public and private patients in public hospitals.[49]

A panel of international health care experts, who had been invited to advise the Department of Health during the drafting of the strategy, had already argued in private meetings with Department officials for "the establishment of health as a fundamental human right" as "a key starting point for the strategy", from which "full access to quality health services" would follow. They put the case that "the availability of an accessible primary care system to the whole population" was "axiomatic to a modern health system" and that "European analysis suggested there was a strong case for free primary health care".[50]

Ireland, they pointed out, should have a health status which was at least equal to the EU average, given its level of wealth and education. They suggested to the Irish administrators that investing in health could have an economic pay-off, an argument which would have been understood by the Chancellor of the German Empire in the 1880s, Count Otto von Bismarck, whose belief that military and economic efficiency would benefit from improving the health of the nation motivated him to introduce the first system of compulsory health insurance in 1883. In the political reality of Ireland in 2001, whatever the personal views of civil servants in the Department of Health, these arguments fell on stony ground. There was no reference to rights in the strategy – a working group which had stated its support for "the thrust of a rights based approach" had nonetheless rejected it, since this would allow the courts a role in deciding on health needs.[51] The strategy contained no proposal to change the 30-year-old legislation which stated that free care under the medical card system would be restricted to those for whom medical bills would cause "undue hardship". While unwilling to change this statutory basis for allocating medical cards, the Department supported greatly extending medical card eligibility, but this was one of the first political casualties of economic slowdown.

The Irish health care system – how we got here

Health systems tend to be financed in broadly three ways: by the state from general taxation, as in the UK; by the state from compulsory social insurance, as in much of continental Europe; or by private finance based on voluntary insurance, as in the United States. The level of equity and the commitment of funding within these systems vary. The US spends a great deal on a highly inequitable system. The UK system has been equitable but underfunded. The continental system of compulsory insurance, while not without its problems, has provided equitable and well-resourced health care systems, which citizens appreciate. The inequitable Irish health care system is a hybrid, the consequence of a chequered history, combining British and American elements in a unique mixture. In Ireland, three-quarters of health spending comes from the exchequer funded by tax, the remainder from individuals directly or though their private insurance coverage.

The Irish system is not a rational construct. It has evolved piecemeal. In critical conflicts, immediately prior to Ireland's independence from Britain and in the earlier decades of independence, opposition from doctors and the Catholic Church prevented the introduction of a comprehensive, equitable system, funded either through social insurance or taxation. While this failure in the 1940s and 1950s reflected the power of the Church and the medical profession, the continued failure to achieve an equitable system in the decades that followed tells a deeper tale about Irish society and politics: about a society which had for so long exported its people and its problems that, even when this ended, when in the last decade there were abundant means to address social need and inequities, it still failed to do so from an ingrained combination of fatalism and class division; about a politics, once inspired by revolutionary ideals and ambitions for a new nation-state, which then became corrupt and opportunistic, yet remained so bound up in the rhetoric and the loyalties of the national struggle that a competitive social democratic party has never yet emerged to champion causes such as equitable access to health care.

Built on political foundations rather than on any rational analysis of the health needs of the population, the health system suffered dramatic cutbacks in the 1980s. Irish public health spending fell to 57 per cent of the EU per capita average in 1989 and only eventually exceeded the EU average in 2001.[52] But the restoration of health spending took place in a rapidly growing economy, which permitted an irresponsible and inflationary combination of populist tax cuts with large (and necessary) increases in health spending. Global slowdown and the fiscal hangover after these pre-election excesses provoked new political assaults on health system funding from late 2002. Continued crisis in the health system, even after recent large increases in spending, has provoked impatient and ill-informed political scepticism about the efficacy of investing in health. Yet, it could have been predicted that, without reform of the deep-seated inequities and irrationalities of the health care system, and necessarily therefore confronting vested interests, the health system would remain in crisis.

Much poorer societies than that of the Ireland of 2002 have set out to establish comprehensive health care systems: Germany made health insurance compulsory in 1883; the UK, Denmark and France began to build their equitable health care systems after the Second World War. Ireland's failure to value health care does not so much reflect the state's slow development, as that slow development reflects its failure to value its people. In the early years of the state, influential voices argued that mass emigration was acceptable.[53] Ireland was slow to introduce free secondary education and consequently slow to exploit its potential for growth.[54] The failure to invest in health care and the many social services which are administered as part of the health care budget has been yet another brake on Irish development, defended by the conservative political establishment.

When, from the 1960s, Ireland began to dare to believe in the possibility of ending emigration and employing its citizens at home, it achieved a pathway to growth which was largely built on imported foreign capital and expertise, and replaced dependence on Britain with dependence on multinational investors, especially from the United States. Despite membership of the EEC (later EU) from 1973, despite the blunting of capitalist excess by the imposition of European social legislation, Ireland's low-tax economic model has been inimical to the development of comprehensive social services like health. Cowed by the race memory of recurrent waves of emigration, the latest as recent as the 1980s, and with only a weak, minority Left to provide an alternative analysis, the Irish body politic has attempted to be more American than the Americans. In the debate about the future direction of Irish society – summarised in 2000 as the "Boston versus Berlin" debate – politicians in power argued for low taxes and limited government intervention as superior to "the European way" of government intervention driven by "concern for social harmony and social inclusion".[55] That a low tax regime also suited businesses and the wealthy, who bankrolled the major political parties, that it suited the articulate and the influential, who were more likely to vote, assisted the argument. Poor social provision, inequality in incomes, an inaccessible health care system – these were cultural attributes which made Ireland closer to the US than Europe and which suited the Irish élite.

The Irish state can, therefore, legitimately be described as unhealthy not just because of the poor health of the Irish and because the health care system has been so underfunded and is so unfair, but also because the values espoused by its elected (and re-elected) leaders, which they defend as dictated by economic circumstances, offer little hope for a healthier future.

Powerful economic and social forces have been ranged against the argument for a comprehensive, equitable health care system. That is why it has not been achieved. Conversely, the strong and growing demand within Ireland, especially among returned emigrants, not least returned doctors, for a health care system which is comparable to those of other European states has immense subversive potential. It will not be achieved without a revolution in Irish values, an overturning of the debate in favour of Berlin rather than Boston, a willingness to demand that corporations and citizens alike contribute to the development of a civilised and more equal society, which offers not just jobs at any price but values its people and their health. That achievement would mark a coming of age of the independent Irish state.

The answer to the question "why not reform?", to the enquiry as to why the Irish health care system remains so inequitable, is rooted in Irish history. At key moments, Ireland has considered and walked away from fundamental reforms. When change has come, it has been incremental, driven by immediate political pressures rather than any grand reforming vision. Yet there *was* a time of vision. To explain how that vision was denied and died, and how Ireland came to accept inaccessible and inadequate care, requires an understanding of the turbulent history of the politics of Irish health care.

PART TWO
EVOLUTION OF AN UNHEALTHY STATE

2

Defeat of the Early Reformers

"In relation to the birth of your child and the growth of that child up to
the age of 16 years, you will have no more doctors' bills to pay."
  – *Noel Browne advertising the Mother and Child scheme on radio.*

"We shall have saved the country from advancing a long way towards
socialistic welfare."
  – *Archbishop John Charles McQuaid rallying the opposition.*

The patient was young, angry and terminally ill. One time too many he
had watched a visiting consultant treat public patients with indifference.
He confronted the doctor.

"Was it money or medicine which most motivated or concerned him?
Were his patients divided into the sick rich and the sick poor? Did he
believe that the sick poor could suffer and feel pain and separation and
even avoidable or inevitable death less than the sick rich?"

The patient, "a small, tubby, unhealthy-looking man" in sagging
pyjamas, turned on his heel. The waistcoated consultant "imperious,
tall, impeccably-coiffed", a busy man in a hurry, observed to the
hospital's manager "I would get rid of him if I were you."[1]

The patient was Harry Kennedy, an *Irish Times* journalist, who
"preferred to help others with whatever money he had" and "remained
relatively penniless". The encounter was witnessed and described by his
friend, a fellow tuberculosis sufferer and doctor, Noel Browne.

Harry Kennedy's questions were Browne's too. Kennedy died in
December 1946. Browne became the most controversial Minister for
Health in the history of the state and resigned in defeat in 1951. Still
unanswered, Harry Kennedy's questions continue to confront not just

doctors but politicians, administrators and voters – anyone who condones inequity in Irish health care.

Politics, religion and health in a post-colonial state

Harry Kennedy challenged his doctor in the third decade of the independent Irish state. Ireland's system of health care had diverged from Britain's even before independence in 1922, a consequence of Ireland's many other differences: predominantly agricultural and rural, while Britain was industrialised and urban; and with a fierce loyalty to Roman Catholicism – which centuries of religious oppression had identified with nationalism – while Britain had developed a tradition of religious dissent and secular humanism.

Before independence, the Catholic Church and elements in the medical profession, with the support of Irish parliamentarians, had successfully opposed the extension to Ireland of a medical benefit system funded by social insurance, which was introduced in the rest of the UK. When, in the 1940s, the UK's introduction of a comprehensive, free national health system provoked similar ambitions among Irish politicians and government officials, this alliance of Church and doctors re-emerged to oppose them and, in the 1950s, defeated the Mother and Child scheme, which would have offered free primary care to children and free care to mothers before and after birth. A free hospitalisation scheme was, however, achieved for the majority of the population in 1953, despite doctors' resistance.

Medical opposition to state health care was by no means unique to Ireland – in the UK, doctors mounted formidable resistance to the establishment of the National Health Service; in the Canadian province of Saskatchewan in 1962, they went on strike in opposition to the introduction of a system of compulsory health insurance. In neither state did they prevail.

Critical to the doctors' victory in Ireland was the emergence of the Catholic Church as their ally, a potent consequence of uniquely Irish circumstances. In the early 20th century, the Irish Church met much fewer challenges to its hegemony than in other states with a majority of Catholics.[2] While elsewhere in Catholic Europe anti-clerical political parties emerged from class conflict, and the most observant Catholics tended to come from the middle and upper classes, in Ireland observance remained high among all social classes. Catholicism was a badge of national identity and there was no demand for the state to take control of health care or education, which was a unique fulcrum of Church power.[3] Religious orders had played a critical role in supplying health and social services to poor Catholics. The Irish Sisters of Charity had established St Vincent's hospital in Dublin in 1834; the Sisters of Mercy followed with the Mater Misericordiae hospital in 1861. Religious orders ran special schools for the deaf and blind, asylums, industrial schools and orphanages.[4]

The Church's resistance to health care reform prior to independence reflected its identification with the interests of the propertied and ignorance of, or indifference to, the needs of workers. Post-independence, it reflected a deep suspicion of anything approaching state socialism, a desire to retain control of its health care institutions and an obsession with sexual morality, through which prism even state health care for pregnant women could be seen as a threat to public morals. This preoccupation with sexual morality, while not confined to Ireland,[5] found extreme expression in a society shaped by its unique response to the appalling famines of the 19th century: celibacy and late marriage had become widespread when farmers ceased dividing their land.[6] The Church supplied the ideology and the discipline to support this survival response, which suited the remaining farmers but, coupled with high emigration, was extinguishing the people.[7] The population of the island fell from 8.2 million in 1841 to 4.4 million in 1911.

When, after the Second World War, Catholic parties in many European states were either left-wing or prepared to ally themselves with socialists,[8] the Irish Church retained a deep suspicion of socialism and advocated that vocational groupings in society, rather than the state, should take responsibility for social organisation.[9] This combination of Church antagonism to state involvement in social provision, its desire to control morality, its traditional authoritarianism and its assumption, shared by most politicians, that the state's laws should reflect Catholic values, set the scene for the major mid-century confrontations between Church and state about reform of the health care system.

Irish political parties were ill-equipped to confront the Church in the interests of developing a welfare state or to challenge this strong national identification with Catholicism. Ireland had no tradition of social democratic politics. Whereas in other European states politics was a competition between conservative and left-wing parties, defined by 19th-century class conflicts, in Ireland the major parties had been born in the struggle for national independence and the subsequent bitter civil war over the terms on which independence was won. The retention of six northern counties under British rule ensured that nationalism remained a potent political force throughout the 20th century and, by removing the most industrialised portion of the island, split the nascent labour movement.[10] Despite great poverty in the cities, socialism was weak, the Labour Party remained in a subsidiary role and a political constituency did not develop to support egalitarian social policies, such as comprehensive, free health care. The civil war parties dominated politics. The state was initially governed by Cumann na nGaedhael, a conservative party which emerged victorious from the civil war and was subsumed into Fine Gael in 1933. Fianna Fáil, the opposing civil-war side, who rejected the treaty because it retained links with Britain, then governed continuously from 1932–1948, and, alone or in coalition, for 53 of the 80 years to 2002. Although Fianna Fáil began as a radical, popular party – which supported comprehensive health care reform – and would continue to define itself as a national movement, with an appeal transcending political class,[11] it gradually became more conservative. As Fine Gael became more liberal, the dominant parties' ideological differences blurred in their pursuit of cross-class appeal. In common with the US, where political allegiances also derived from a civil-war conflict, sustained radical politics did not emerge to give birth to a modern, European-style welfare state and health care system.[12]

1911 – How social insurance for health care was not introduced in Ireland

The significance for health care of the unique Irish relationship between religion and politics first became evident in 1911, prior to Irish independence, when the Catholic Church and elements in the medical profession opposed the extension to Ireland of a medical benefit system, funded by social insurance. At this time, many Irish people could not afford health care and the quality of care was poor. There was no shared assumption that the state should provide medical care for the population. The well-to-do avoided hospitals and paid for care at home, while the poor were treated without charge in workhouse hospitals or in voluntary hospitals in the cities, run by charities or the churches, where young doctors acquired skills for later, more lucrative use in private practice. As medical standards and the reputation of the voluntary hospitals improved, they began to offer more beds to paying private patients. Outside hospital, the poorest third of the population was treated free by local dispensary doctors; the rest paid for care or went without.

In Britain, David Lloyd George, then Chancellor of the Exchequer, introduced the National Health Insurance Bill of 1911, which provided for a scheme in which employees must and the self-employed might make contributions so that they would receive an income when unemployed, ill or disabled. Employers and the state would also contribute. Medical benefit would cover free general practitioner care and medicines.[13]

The attempt to apply the scheme in Ireland was complicated by the existence of the dispensary doctors working under contract to local authorities and receiving salaries funded from the local rates. There were also few workers' friendly societies, which were to administer the scheme in Britain. It was proposed to merge the dispensary and insurance schemes.

Only the destitute received free dispensary care. The rest must pay their doctors significant medical fees. In 1900, Irish general practitioners charged working class patients 2s 6d for a visit, one-eighth of the weekly income of a building labourer.[14] Yet the Catholic Church showed its identification with the farming class, from which it recruited most of its priests,[15] when the bishops issued a statement saying the cost of the scheme would be an undue burden on farmers and small Irish businesses and only "a mere fraction" of the population were wage earners to whom it would apply. The state then had 800,000 industrial workers and domestic servants.[16]

While a majority of doctors, many of whom worked in the dispensary service, supported medical benefit, albeit on their terms, the Irish Party which represented Ireland in the British parliament at Westminster eventually opposed grafting this new medical benefit onto the existing poor law dispensary service. They were influenced by the bishops' statement but also suggested that the doctors' demands had been "extortionate".[17] Although doctors in private practice opposed the scheme, dispensary doctors saw in the scheme an opportunity to increase their incomes, which were a source of grievance. For this brief period, a majority in the medical profession supported a state medical service, which the majority would later vehemently and consistently oppose.

When medical benefit was introduced in Britain but not in Ireland, Irish doctors who were employed by workers' friendly societies to treat their members went on strike to demand the same fees as British doctors. A committee appointed by the Chancellor eventually recommended against the extension of medical benefit to Ireland but added that the exchequer should aid the existing friendly societies pending the establishment of a state medical service[18] – which would indeed emerge in Britain but not in independent Ireland. So it was that social insurance-based medical benefit, the standard system in continental Europe and in Britain until the 1940s, was not introduced in Ireland.

The 1940s – Fianna Fáil adopts the goal of a free national health service

Health care improved in the 1930s. County and district hospitals, offering free treatment to the poor, replaced the old workhouses. With overseas funds coming into the Hospitals Sweepstakes, a kind of national lottery, the Fianna Fáil government, elected in 1932, undertook an ambitious programme of hospital building. However, by 1935 only 40 per cent of patients in the voluntary hospitals were treated free – the hospitals were perceived to favour paying patients.[19] The government made their receipt of public funds contingent on their remaining charitable institutions, ensuring that hospitals continued to treat all classes under the same roof. In the 1940s, social insurance was introduced to cover hospital treatment for workers but not their families.

Yet the health care system of the 1940s remained rudimentary. When James Deeny, a general practitioner from Lurgan in Northern Ireland, became chief medical officer in 1944, he found himself

> confronted with a crumbling neglected Poor Law system which had been very badly run-down. We had the worst tuberculosis problem in Western Europe, a chronic typhoid problem, a very high infant mortality rate with a huge number of babies dying from enteritis, a high maternal mortality rate, workhouse hospitals, few medical specialists outside Dublin, decaying dispensaries, low standards and the senior medical establishment more concerned with sport, gracious living and style than professional excellence.[20]

Elsewhere, the 1940s was a decade of reform in health care. The UK established its NHS in 1948. The French established their social security system in 1945, building on occupational health insurance schemes introduced in the 1920s. Further afield, the Canadian province of Saskatchewan introduced health insurance to cover hospital care in 1946.

Ireland was governed by Fianna Fáil, under Éamon de Valera's leadership, from 1932–1948. Radical in the 1920s, in government in the 1930s, Fianna Fáil not only built hospitals but introduced a programme of slum clearance, house building and unemployment assistance, and sought to develop native industry by protectionism. Like the populist movements of Latin America, which grew as a response to colonialism, Fianna Fáil sought to merge class differences in an ideology of national development, which promised gains to all classes.[21] The small Labour Party, which supported Fianna Fáil in 1932, found it difficult to compete. Although de Valera recognised the special position of the Roman Catholic Church as the majority church in the Constitution of 1937, and

Fianna Fáil became progressively more conservative through its years in power, up to the 1950s its initiatives in the politics of health care showed a radicalism which would later depart the party.

In the 1940s, influenced by the Beveridge Report (1942) which laid the foundation for the UK's NHS, Fianna Fáil and health officials began to aspire to the goal of a free national health service. There was no separate Department of Health. Since the 1930s, health care had been the responsibility of Conor Ward, a parliamentary secretary at the Department of Local Government and Public Health. A senior IRA man during the War of Independence, Ward was a dispensary doctor, a highly intelligent but abrasive man,[22] who had alienated the medical profession by his interventionist approach to the development of the hospital service and his readiness to discipline doctors who abused their positions. The profession no longer supported a state medical service.[23]

Ward appointed a committee of civil servants, including Deeny, to propose reforms. The 1945 *Report of the Departmental Committee on Health Services*, "probably the most radical document ever" on Irish health care,[24] proposed that a free national health service should be introduced for the whole population on a phased basis. GPs would be district medical officers and private practice would become peripheral.

"Influenced by current thinking we looked forward to the entire population being covered gradually by a service without charge, as in New Zealand,[25] the UK and elsewhere. The development was to be approached in stages and was to be, as in Canada, partly financed by insurance contribution and partly by state funds both central and local," Deeny later wrote.[26]

The unpublished report formed the basis for a White Paper, published in 1947. But in the meantime the Irish Medical Association (IMA) had claimed its first scalp, with the resignation of Conor Ward in 1946. Further alienated by Ward's refusal to consult the association on proposed public health legislation, the profession revealed its muscle. A former president of the IMA, Patrick McCarvill, made a wide series of allegations against Ward, only one of which (inadequate tax returns on his business) was upheld, but that was sufficient to ensure his political demise.[27]

Seán MacEntee, the Minister for Local Government, took over responsibility for health. MacEntee was a former Minister for Finance, a tough Northerner who had fought in the 1916 rebellion, and "a first-class orator, caustic and articulate".[28] He continued to promote the cause of a national health service, provoking an overtly ideological objection from the Department of Finance that his proposals would amount to "the socialisation of medicine" and would cause the disappearance of private practice.[29]

Health became a department in its own right in 1947 and yet another doctor, James Ryan, its first Minister. With the ultimate medical revolutionary credential – he had been a medical officer in the General Post Office during the 1916 Rising – he was now a career politician, who had not practised as a doctor for over 20 years.[30] A better tactician than Ward, he shepherded through the Health Act of 1947, which incorporated Ward's public health measures. Most controversially, the Act provided for the free treatment of mothers before and after birth and for children during their school years.

These measures were driven by necessity not ideology. Many women were dying in childbirth because of inadequate care, the infant mortality rate was high and chronic untreated conditions in childhood were causing lifelong disability.[31] The White Paper made clear that the 1947 Act was only a first step and that the department's preferred long-term goal was a free national health service.[32] Working on the new measures for the treatment of women and children, Deeny hit on a name for the scheme: "We'll call it the Mother and Child Service, no one could oppose a scheme with a name like that."[33] But they could and they did.

Fine Gael strongly opposed passage of the Act on the grounds that general practitioners' incomes would suffer and that it went against Catholic social teaching. Deputy Tom O'Higgins, the chief medical officer for Meath, said general practitioners in private practice would be "completely wiped out" since they made between 70 and 80 per cent of their income from looking after young children.[34]

James McPolin, chief medical officer in County Limerick, supplied the rhetoric for the doctors' extra-parliamentary opposition to the Act. Having had a brush with the Department of Health, which considered suspending him because health services in Limerick were a "black spot", McPolin had emerged as an ardent opponent of state medicine, although state salaried himself. In a series of articles he argued that state medicine contravened the moral law. It was a father's duty to provide medical care for his dependants and the role of the family doctor and the Church, not the state, to educate mothers and children about health.[35] The central council of the IMA passed a resolution opposing the White Paper proposals for "state control".

Most ominously, the Catholic bishops sent a private protest to the government about the Act, the first formal protest from the hierarchy to an Irish government about legislation,[36] which echoed McPolin's concerns. The rights of the family and the Church in education were infringed by the power given to health authorities to educate women about motherhood and children about health. The Church had two concerns: that a state medical service would ultimately include sex education and information about contraception and abortion;[37] and that the state might take control of Catholic hospitals. The British national health service was then being extended to Northern Ireland, threatening Church control of the Mater, the largest Catholic hospital in Belfast.[38]

Implementation of the 1947 Health Act was delayed by a subsequently unsuccessful constitutional challenge and de Valera deferred answering the bishops' letter. Then, in 1948, Fianna Fáil lost power.[39]

The defeat of the Mother and Child scheme

Fianna Fáil had begun to lose its radical appeal in the 1940s. Alienated voters supported Labour and new parties: the republican and socially reformist Clann na Poblachta, to which Noel Browne belonged, and Clann na Talmhan, which had small-farmer support. These three parties coalesced with Fine Gael in 1948 to form the first inter-party government, in which Noel Browne was Minister for Health.

Browne could have been a tool made for the purpose of challenging medical complacency in the face of the suffering of the poor. He had seen his family destroyed by illness, his parents unable to afford care for the tuberculosis which killed them and many of his siblings. Eventually, he too was infected. After his father's death, his dying mother brought the family to England. By luck, Browne received the patronage of a wealthy family, which turned this Roman Catholic emigrant orphan into a Trinity College Dublin educated doctor, a politician and the man who eliminated tuberculosis in Ireland. When appointed Minister for Health at the age of 32, he believed he had at best one or two years to live.[40] With no history of revolutionary politics, on his first day in Dáil Éireann, Browne inherited the task of unravelling the complex medical and church politics surrounding the 1947 Health Act.

Browne came to politics as a doctor campaigning for the provision of sanatoria – essentially isolated hospitals where patients with TB could be nursed and avoid passing on their infection. Between 1942 and 1945, 16,186 people died of TB.[41] Not until the mid-1940s was there provision for free treatment in sanatoria irrespective of income.[42] As Minister for Health, Browne approached the eradication of tuberculosis like a war. On his wall was a large chart on which the progress in building every hospital, sanatorium or clinic was regularly updated like the advance of armies in a battle.[43]

"The young people throughout the country thought he was

wonderful, as indeed he was. He also had complete medical support at this time," James Deeny later wrote of Browne's early days in health.[44] Under the preceding government, Deeny had been the author of plans for the provision of sanatoria.[45] Browne was the Minister who made his plans a political reality.

Between 1948 and 1953, 2,000 additional beds became available to TB patients,[46] an achievement which eclipsed the targets of the 2001 government health strategy – 3,000 acute hospital beds over 10 years – envisaged as the "largest ever concentrated expansion of acute hospital capacity in Ireland".[47] The death rate from TB dropped from 12.5 per 10,000 population in 1945 to 5.4 in 1952. With BCG vaccination of children, there was an 82 per cent drop in childhood deaths from TB in Dublin between 1948 and 1953.[48] Later critics argued that the new drug streptomycin eradicated TB and that Browne's sanatoria were white elephants, but streptomycin was of limited value to older patients, costly and unobtainable for many years, while sanatoria strengthened patients' resistance to the disease and reduced its spread.[49]

Deeny described Browne as "a very clever man", "very kind indeed to the patients who adored him", likeable, compassionate but also intolerant and "a magnificent destructive critic". Their relationship foundered when Browne went to war with the medical profession and Deeny was eventually moved sideways.[50]

A doctor who believed himself dying, from a background of disease and death, Browne brought to his ministry inevitable prejudgements about his profession. Early in his medical career he had acquired a distaste for private practice – "I have always found the cash nexus between the patient and doctor indefensible."[51] In Britain during the second world war, he saw "consultants who were among the world's leading physicians and surgeons and yet worked for state salaries. They worked ceaselessly, conscientiously, and with complete satisfaction in their profession."[52]

Through his long medical career (Browne eventually died at the age of 81 in 1997), he opted where he could for salaried jobs and declined private practice.[53] He later reflected how in Ireland

unlike the salaried postman, who is trusted to deliver every single letter given to him, the doctor cannot be trusted to work conscientiously for a salary like everyone else. Together with his colleagues in the law, the doctor must have a sweetener in the form of a fee every time he serves each individual in the community ... One of the results of the fee-for-service medical practice system here has been an enormous growth in the cost of the health services without a significant increase in their efficiency.[54]

The neophyte Minister for Health was faced with the necessity to amend the 1947 Health Act to meet the concerns of the bishops, the doctors and Fine Gael members of his own cabinet. Unlike Aneurin Bevan, who in 1948 established the NHS with the support of his Labour colleagues, Browne was a member of a motley coalition cabinet, which included opponents of the Act such as Fine Gael's Tom O'Higgins – an officer of the IMA. The Taoiseach, John A. Costello, later explained that he agreed with the bishops' condemnation of the Mother and Child scheme[55] and opposed socialised medicine.[56]

By far the most formidable of Browne's opponents was the Catholic Archbishop of Dublin, John Charles McQuaid, who, through his chairmanship of Dublin's Mater hospital and control over the appointment of consultants to Catholic voluntary hospitals, was a powerful force in health care. The son of a dispensary doctor, McQuaid had formed a close and politically significant bond with the Fianna Fáil leader, Éamon de Valera, who discreetly campaigned for McQuaid's appointment[57] and with whom he communicated constantly during de Valera's drafting of the 1937 Constitution, in a partially successful effort to ensure that it would enshrine Catholic teaching.[58]

McQuaid believed that bishops and priests "must interfere in politics, as by Divine right to guide the Faithful, not of course in mere politics where no moral issues are threatened, but whenever political or social or economic programmes are at variance with Divine Law".[59]

He developed close links with the medical profession through the doctors' Guild of St Luke and the Knights of St Columbanus. He inspected lists of hospital personnel to ascertain religious affiliations, convinced of the need for more Catholic appointments.[60] On his own terms, McQuaid was a social reformer. He persuaded Catholic voluntary hospitals to open clinics for venereal disease, organised the building of Our Lady's Hospital for Sick Children in Crumlin and initiated the Catholic Social Services Conference which provided food and clothing for the poor.[61] But he also continued to campaign against Protestantism and for the organisation of society on what he regarded as Catholic principles. He effectively prevented the formation of a National Anti-Tuberculosis League because he was concerned that it might be controlled by Protestants.[62]

As a Catholic graduate of the Protestant Trinity College, Browne was automatically suspect to McQuaid. In 1944 the archbishop had announced that any Catholic who attended Trinity College Dublin without his permission would be guilty of mortal sin.[63] Minister and bishop were soon at odds when Browne unsuccessfully attempted to bring the new Crumlin children's hospital under local authority control. A later offer to refund the development cost of the Catholic Bon Secours hospital in Dublin, provided it was open to the public under Corporation control, met "a look of mystified pain" from the Reverend Mother, who intended its exclusive use by the middle and upper classes.[64]

Browne wanted democratic control of voluntary hospitals not only to ensure access to all but so that medical appointments would be made on merit, rather than on "hereditary or sectarian religious grounds". He also found the then Protestant-dominated Meath hospital "notoriously bigoted".[65]

He later attributed the slow development of state initiatives in medicine to Church control of the leading hospitals. Governments dared not seek to improve "the overall primitive level of care … for fear of political reprisals by the Church".[66] While in later life Browne's experiences could make him appear paranoid about Church influence, it was only with the establishment of the Eastern Regional Health Authority in 1999 that any serious attempt was made to bring Dublin's essentially state-funded voluntary hospitals under state control.[67]

In June 1950, Browne produced his proposals to amend the 1947 Health Act to introduce what became known as the Mother and Child scheme. Dispensary doctors would become district medical officers and would provide a free medical service for children up to the age of 16, for which they would be paid by capitation, an annual amount for each patient. In Dublin, the maternity hospitals would care for mothers before and after birth and for infants up to six weeks; outside the cities this service would eventually be provided by the district medical officers only. Compulsory medical inspection of school children, which had been the subject of constitutional challenge, would be abandoned.[68]

Whereas Bevan managed to keep the doctors divided in their opinions, Browne lacked Bevan's political sophistication and united them in opposition. Although dispensary doctors stood to gain by the scheme, Browne alienated them by announcing that local authorities should inform him of complaints about their services. Private general practitioners faced an effective threat to their entire practice. Browne had antagonised the powerful Dublin consultants by funding his programme of local-authority hospital building from the Hospital

Sweepstakes, which had originally been established to finance the voluntary hospitals.[69] He made no secret of his support for a salaried profession.

In early 1950 he wrote to his sister in the United States: "By the time I have finished being Minister for Health I shall have so few friends in the medical profession that my chances of earning my living here will become more and more remote. As you know they are a pretty vicious bunch and are daily becoming more and more hostile."[70]

He had adopted a confrontational approach to his profession from his appointment, refusing consultations with the IMA in 1948, apparently assuming it would be impossible to gain their agreement. The IMA had been observing the establishment of the NHS and feared the eventual development of a state-controlled and salaried medical service. The association wrote to Browne objecting to "the provision of free medical treatment to non-necessitous persons".[71]

The IMA saw Browne's eventual scheme as the first step to the introduction of a full-time, salaried medical service under central bureaucracy which would mean the end of the private practitioner.[72] After receiving details of the scheme, the IMA polled its members asking if they would work for a scheme which "includes free treatment for people who are able to pay for their own medical care". Only 54 per cent of the membership responded and, of the 994 replies, 78 per cent were negative. Up to 500 doctors were not in the IMA. So despite the negative poll, there was unexplored potential for Browne to find support within his profession.[73]

When the IMA came to believe that Browne had been the author of an anonymous political pamphlet that attributed the doctors' objections to the fact that their incomes would now be taxed, this did not help his relations with them or other members of cabinet. The pamphlet asked: "Isn't it about time we started to find out what they are actually 'making', especially the ones in the 'Squares' and the 'Crescents'? ... We all agree that the doctor must get a fair wage and we will give it to him but he will get a fair wage, not the profit of a black marketeer."[74]

Browne was now fighting on two fronts. At a meeting with McQuaid and his fellow bishops, they stated their objections to his scheme: that the right to provide for the health of children belonged to parents, not to the state which should not "deprive 90 per cent of parents of their rights because of 10 per cent necessitous or negligent parents"; that "education in regard to motherhood includes instructions in regard to sex relations, chastity and marriage. The State has no competence to give instruction in such matters"; and, in an apparent reference to Trinity College, that doctors trained in "institutions in which we have no confidence" might deliver gynaecological care which in other countries included "birth limitation and abortion".[75] The bishops were apparently ill-informed about the extent of poverty, since about one-third of the population was then thought to be receiving free medical care from dispensary doctors.[76]

Although there is a consensus that the Mother and Child controversy was a critical confrontation between Church and state, in which the Catholic Church clearly overstepped its role in society, it was later argued that the medical profession drew the Church into the battle.[77] One of the bishops, Donal Herlihy of Ferns, reflected "We allowed ourselves to be used by the doctors, but it won't happen again."[78]

Predictably, McQuaid saw the confrontation differently. He urged his fellow bishops, to reject the scheme because "we shall have saved the country from advancing a long way towards socialistic welfare. In particular we shall have checked the efforts of Leftist and Labour elements, which are approaching the point of publicly ordering the Church to stay out of social life."[79] Later, Catholic justification for the hierarchy's rejection of the scheme would also cite the dangers of giving the state a role in sex education.[80]

Despite the opposition of both bishops and doctors, Browne proceeded to introduce his scheme, sending pamphlets announcing it to the hierarchy and writing to all doctors inviting them to participate. In a radio broadcast, he announced that the only change that people would see would be "in relation to the birth of your child and the growth of that child up to the age of 16 years, you will have no more doctors' bills to pay".[81]

However, he had lost the support of the Taoiseach. Costello famously told him "whatever about fighting the doctors, I am not going to fight the Bishops, and whatever about fighting the Bishops, I am not going to fight the doctors and the Bishops".[82]

Browne met McQuaid at his own request and, incredibly to a modern reader, agreed to accept the Church's teaching, once the hierarchy had made an authoritative ruling. He apparently pinned his hopes on a distinction between Catholic social and moral teaching, considering himself bound by the latter but not the former. He had consulted, in utmost secrecy, Frank Cremin, a priest and Professor of Theology at Maynooth University, who agreed that since Catholics in Northern Ireland could use the NHS without moral danger and, since the hierarchy had not claimed that the Mother and Child scheme was contrary to Catholic moral teaching, Catholic politicians could conscientiously agree to implement it.[83] McQuaid had no problem seeing off this challenge. Catholic social teaching was simply Catholic moral teaching on social matters, he told Costello.[84]

In a letter which Costello read to a cabinet meeting in April 1951, the bishops added the further objection that taxation to fund the scheme would morally compel citizens to avail of it. The cabinet, right across the political spectrum, accepted that the scheme should conform to Catholic social teaching and have a means test – it would then no longer be regarded as "socialistic". Browne insisted on asking each cabinet member in turn "Do you accept?"[85]

Within days, he resigned at the request of his party leader and ensured that the controversy would become a *cause célèbre* by publishing the correspondence between the Church and government. The government soon fell over an unrelated issue. Browne resigned from Clann na Poblachta and fought an election, dominated by health issues, as an independent. Fianna Fáil returned with Éamon de Valera as Taoiseach, elected by one vote with Browne's support. Seán Lemass, a future Fianna Fáil Taoiseach, had met Browne secretly and promised "there's no bargain, no deal, but we'll try to give you a good health service".[86]

Browne would later join Fianna Fáil, then the Labour Party, then the Socialist Labour Party. He remained an outsider in Irish political life. James Deeny, author of the ill-fated scheme, concluded that "the real tragedy of the débâcle was that it set back public health in the country for years".[87]

Free hospital care for the majority – an eventual compromise

Once again Minister for Health, Fianna Fáil's James Ryan found the foxes in charge of the chicken coop when he returned to the Department. Costello had been briefly Minister for Health after Browne's resignation and had set up a joint committee of the Department and the IMA, which Ryan immediately disbanded, telling the association members "'to get out' – in a polite way".[88]

Fianna Fáil had promised to implement the 1947 Act. The government's eventual reforms were far-reaching but differed from the 1947 formula. The 1953 Health Bill proposed a major extension of entitlements to free hospital services but watered down the mother and child proposals. The Mother and Child scheme now only offered free care for mothers before and after birth, for infants up to six weeks and treatment in health clinics for children up to six years old. Free general practitioner care for all children up to the age of 16 had been abandoned. Like Browne, Ryan removed compulsory inspection of children from the legislation and, to placate the bishops, deleted the reference to the "education of women in respect of motherhood".[89]

While the primary care proposals had been significantly diluted, the politically popular expansion of free hospital services to over 80 per cent of the population threatened the private income of hospital consultants. It would mean "the birth of your children in public maternity wards", the IMA argued in an appeal to the middle classes to maintain the distinction between public and private fee-paying patients.[90] The IMA instead sought a voluntary health insurance scheme[91] – the germ of the private health insurance industry which Ireland has today.

McQuaid shared the IMA's concerns. However, he now faced an experienced minister, a united government and a much more radical party than Costello's Fine Gael. Despite his formerly close relations with de Valera, McQuaid had come to respect him as an adversary. De Valera was and would remain the dominant leader of independent Ireland. Adored and abhorred by the respective civil-war sides, pragmatist and idealist, he had "a genuine, if paternalistic, compassion for the poor".[92] "The inner spirit of sympathetic and open collaboration with the Hierarchy will be missing from a Fianna Fáil government … a definite liberalism is always present," McQuaid observed.[93]

When McQuaid expressed concern about the no-means-test aspect of the Mother and Child scheme, Ryan conceded a token £1 charge for upper-income women. He proceeded with the Bill and on a collision course with the medical profession, whose "mischief makers" he described as "deadly in their opposition and unscrupulous in their methods".[94] A general meeting of the IMA rejected the Bill unanimously and the association lobbied the hierarchy with immediate effect. The bishops sent a statement to the national papers, arguing the Bill infringed the rights of fathers to provide for the health of their families by giving the state responsibility for treating mothers in childbirth and extending hospital services to the majority of the population. This would lower the "sense of personal responsibility and seriously weaken the moral fibre of the people".[95]

The bishops were now fighting a rearguard action to maintain the independence and influence of their Catholic voluntary hospitals. The massive public hospital building programme, which would result in over 7,000 new beds between 1949 and 1956, had produced a new generation of publicly employed consultants working for local authority hospitals and appointed by the Local Appointments Commission. The extension of hospital services to the majority of the population at nominal or no charge, with local authorities paying voluntary hospitals and consultants for their treatment, would increase the voluntary hospitals' dependence on public funding.[96]

De Valera responded with alacrity to avoid another public confrontation between Church and state. He achieved the withdrawal of the bishops' statement and agreed a number of concessions: to increase the charge for upper-income women for the Mother and Child scheme; limit the power of local authorities to run post-graduate medical schools; restrict the medical inspection of school children to primary schools; and open the public hospitals to clinical teaching by appointees of the university medical schools, thus ensuring Catholic influence in the public hospitals through the medical schools of the Catholic National University.[97]

The bishops accepted the amendments, although stating this "is not to be construed as positive approval to the Bill".[98] The medical profession was dismayed at the loss of the bishops' muscle on their side – "like losing one's best troops", the Dublin surgeon Bob O'Connell later said. McQuaid advised the doctors to operate the Bill, which the bishops would not support them in resisting. He asked if they were going to fight the Bill "by taking to the mountains with guns?"[99] With this dissolution of the alliance of bishops and doctors, the doctors ended their resistance to the Bill's enactment.

The 1953 Health Act achieved the kernel of the Mother and Child scheme: the provision of free post- and ante-natal care for women. However, it left GP services unchanged, free medical care for children was limited to infants up to six weeks and treatment in health clinics up to six years. The free hospital and specialist services, which in 1945 the Department of Health had wanted to extend to the whole population, were now only available to those on lower and middle incomes. This was certainly a major advance in access to services but the principle of means testing, of differentiating between classes of patient remained. Consultants and GPs had protected their private-fee income. The majority of the population – children and adults – must still pay to see their family doctor. And, in hospital, consultants would have an incentive to devote greater attention to their fee-paying patients.

A general election in 1954, and the return of an inter-party government with Costello at the helm, nearly derailed the legislation again. Presciently, Ryan had rushed through regulations covering the details of the Act just three days before the election. His successor as Minister for Health was a lawyer, Tom O'Higgins, son of the former

Minister for Defence, who had retained his IMA loyalties in the previous inter-party government. The younger O'Higgins's appointment was "timely" and "a welcome relief" for the medical profession.[100] O'Higgins sought to change the regulations introduced by Ryan but found he could only do so by a new Act, which he had difficulty convincing his Labour Party cabinet colleagues to accept.[101] Ultimately, he introduced legislation which had the effect of postponing the extension of hospital services to the middle income group until 1956 and preventing the extension of free mother and infant care to the upper income group.[102] With this sympathetic incumbent, the profession achieved a reduction in ministerial control over the medical registration council and permission for county surgeons to engage in private practice outside local authority hospitals.[103] The IMA's crowning achievement in this period was the introduction of its favoured solution to the funding of the health services – a voluntary health insurance scheme. O'Higgins introduced legislation to establish the Voluntary Health Insurance Board (VHI) in 1957. Since higher income groups could now insure themselves for medical treatment, this was also in effect insurance for the medical profession that their private income would be secured.

The years between the internal departmental committee's proposal of a comprehensive state health service in 1945 and the eventual passage of the 1953 Health Act, while marked by a sequence of titanic battles between bishops, doctors and politicians, were nonetheless years of advance in the provision of state health services: of greatly increased access to free hospital care, of improved care for mothers and infants, of massive hospital building, of new specialist appointments and of the virtual conquest of tuberculosis. The medical profession may have opposed change but it was not monolithic. Four doctors attempted to reform the health system – Conor Ward, Noel Browne and James Ryan, through the medium of politics, and James Deeny, as chief medical officer. Had the momentum of those years and the vision of the 1940s been maintained, Ireland might have developed an equitable and accessible health service, like its European neighbours.

However, despite these achievements, the opponents of reform had won a critical battle. The blueprint for comprehensive reform advanced by health officials in 1945 had been abandoned. Health care would not be delivered as a right. Means testing remained. This met the Church's concern, driven by its fear of socialism, to limit state responsibility for health, and also met the doctors' concern, driven by their fear of state employment and wages, to maintain the distinction between those who paid for their doctor and those who did not. For patients, this meant that all but the poorest must pay to see a family doctor. For the health service, the investment in accessible hospital services, combined with the reformers' abandonment of the cause of accessible primary care for all, meant that health care would now be biased towards the most expensive and complex responses to ill-health.

This victory for reaction did not have to be for all time. The nature of Irish society and of the Catholic Church was about to undergo massive change.

3

CONSULTANTS OBSTRUCT FREE HOSPITAL CARE

"The vast majority of people were against socialised medicine. Those who could pay should pay."
— *Fianna Fáil's Donogh O'Malley.*

"Representatives of the medical consultants opposed the introduction of my scheme until such time as they decided the population should have free hospital and medical services."
— *Labour's Brendan Corish.*

The politics of Irish health care metamorphosed in the 1960s. This was a time of immense change in society, in the economy and within Fianna Fáil, which was in government from 1957 to 1973. The erstwhile revolutionaries became the new establishment. Fianna Fáil abandoned its radical ambitions for comprehensive access to health care and Fine Gael began to adopt a reforming stance. The Catholic Church was no longer a barrier to reform: the Second Vatican Council had revolutionised church attitudes to social change. Catholic bishops supported a socialist Minister's attempts to extend free hospitalisation in the 1970s. However, sexual liberation opened up a new front for battle between Church and state. And the winds of change did not end the power nor shake the reactionary politics of the medical profession, who defeated the free hospitalisation scheme.

Fianna Fáil's retreat from radicalism

When Seán Lemass replaced Éamon de Valera as Taoiseach and leader of Fianna Fáil in 1959, his overriding concern was economic development following a decade of economic crisis and emigration.

Under Lemass, Ireland abandoned protectionism and opened up to foreign investment. Successful economic planning increased faith in state intervention. Economic growth brought social revolution in its wake.[1] By the late 1970s, the formerly ageing and declining population was now rising and had the youngest average age in Europe. The marriage rate rose sharply; age at marriage dropped. In 1969, for the first time, more people were employed in industry than in agriculture.[2] In 1962, the national television station went on air. By the late 1960s, a native women's liberation movement had developed. In 1973, Ireland joined the European Economic Community (the precursor to the EU). This more youthful, more urban society was therefore exposed to much wider influences than before and, although religious observance remained high, the ability of Catholics to discriminate between their personal faith and their individual political convictions had matured. The emergence of a protest movement seeking civil rights for Catholics in Northern Ireland in the late 1960s, followed by the development of violent conflict there, raised awareness in the Republic of the sectarian bias in its Constitution, which in 1972 the electorate voted to amend to remove recognition of the special position of the Catholic Church.

Despite this new climate of openness and liberalism, a comprehensive, free health service was no longer a Fianna Fáil objective. Seán MacEntee, who had formerly championed a national health service, now as Minister for Health from 1957 to 1965, introduced outpatient charges for people on middle incomes, rationalising that it was "only right, just, fair and equitable" that those who could afford to contribute should do so.[3] Initially hostile to the VHI, he then welcomed its contribution to health funding.

His successor, Donogh O'Malley believed that "the vast majority of people were against socialised medicine. Those who could pay should pay."[4] O'Malley published a White Paper on the development of the health services which stated that "the Government did not accept the proposition that the State had a duty to provide unconditionally all ... health services free of cost for everyone". It defended selective provision of free services as a more effective use of state resources than "a comprehensive free-for-all national health service".

"General medical services have remained available only to about thirty per cent of the population, because it is considered that the expenses arising from attending a general practitioner are not normally an undue strain on families in the middle income group."

Eligibility for hospital services had been extended to a wider group because they were "likely to be much more costly".[5]

Subsequently, O'Malley applied an entirely different approach when, as Minister for Education, he introduced free secondary education in 1967, reflecting a belated recognition by the Irish state of the value of investing in education. This was to have immense consequences for the economy and society, and eventually contributed to the extraordinary growth of the 1990s.[6] However, the proposition that free health care might equally benefit society no longer convinced Fianna Fáil. The party's advocacy of a comprehensive health service now appeared to be written out of history. O'Malley's successor, Seán Flanagan, saw no reason why it should be the duty of the state to provide health services for all, any more than it had a duty to organise free transport or free bread for all. "Our health policy has been, is and will be based on a different philosophy and one I think which is more in accord with our national tradition."[7]

It was left to the opposition parties to urge fundamental reform of the health services. In 1959, the Labour Party proposed a free service financed from taxation and insurance contributions. Fine Gael favoured a comprehensive health service for 85 per cent of the population, providing access to free GP and hospital services, funded by social insurance contributions from employees, employers and the self-employed. Since the contributions would not be proportional to income, this would have been a regressive scheme bearing more heavily on lower earners. Tom O'Higgins, the former Fine Gael Minister for Health, rejected a redistributive scheme funded from taxation on the grounds that "that means that you tax the few to provide a service for the majority", which was "state paternalism" and "foreign to our temperament". "Most of our people far prefer to pay their own way in so far as they can." O'Higgins nonetheless considered it a "glaring omission and one which renders the entire [health] service absurd" that a person "must first prove himself to be a pauper" to avail of the dispensary doctor's service and, otherwise, received "no medical service outside hospital".[8] Fine Gael retained its commitment to the social insurance approach in its 1965 election platform, *Winning through to a Just Society*.

The retreat from radicalism of Ireland's dominant political party was of critical significance for the future of the health service. Fianna Fáil's stance was doubtless influenced by the rising cost of the service, reflecting the great growth in hospital bed numbers in the early 1950s, the extension of free hospital services to a majority of the population and rapidly rising wage rates in the 1960s. However, the party was also changing. Although Lemass was a reader of Beveridge, the father of the British welfare state,[9] and a defender of state intervention, he famously believed that "a rising tide lifts all the boats".[10] No one could fault him for his commitment to ensuring that the tide would indeed rise. The limitation of this philosophy was that, despite growing wealth and employment, inequality persisted. It was, nonetheless, a convenient stance for this populist party which, having set out to build a native capitalist class, by the 1960s had succeeded and was increasingly beholden to that class. Lemass accepted the party's first large business donation.[11] Never again would Fianna Fáil espouse a comprehensive, free health service. It would, instead, introduce incremental improvements in access to and in the organisation of the service. These tended to be driven by immediate crises, pressure from lobby groups such as the trade union movement, which this corporatist party believed in keeping an ally, or electoral concerns, rather than by any grand vision for the service. Health became another service to be distributed in pork barrel politics rather than an investment in the future.

The birth of the General Medical Services scheme and the health boards

Following its antagonism to Fianna Fáil reforms in the 1940s and 1950s, the medical profession had strained relations with MacEntee at the beginning of the 1960s but, by the end of the decade, was gaining the ear of Fianna Fáil ministers. At MacEntee's insistence, in 1962 the IMA was forced to establish a separate body, the Irish Medical Union (IMU), which would have the right under trade union legislation to negotiate for the profession and soon acquired a distinct identity. Doctors on public sector salaries – dispensary doctors, local authority consultants and junior hospital doctors – had the greater interest in joining the union. Consultants in the voluntary hospitals in Dublin, the *crème de la crème* of the profession, whose earnings came chiefly from private practice, considered trade union membership beneath them and remained attached to the IMA, as did some Dublin general practitioners with large private earnings. The Minister then inconsistently extended to the IMA a limited right to negotiate.

The IMA had offices in Fitzwilliam Square conveniently close to the Dublin consultants' "rooms". Cormac MacNamara, a Waterford City general practitioner and influential medical politician, who was instrumental in engineering the subsequent merger between the IMA and IMU, recalled:

> They could drift in to meetings from their rooms. The Medical Union was in a more egalitarian location on the corner of Harcourt Street. It was the

equivalent of Fine Gael versus Fianna Fáil, silk hats versus soft hats. The IMA had a dress dance. The Medical Union had no evening dress at their dinner. It was quite a thing when they eventually decided to do that.[12]

Some doctors found it advantageous to be members of both organisations. "With which of the forks of your tongue are you speaking this evening?" one such ecumenist was challenged.[13]

Not until the 1970 Health Act did Fianna Fáil again sponsor significant change in the health service – and this was administrative change, rather than improved access, and on terms that suited the profession. The Act replaced the old dispensary system for the poor with the new General Medical Services (GMS) scheme,[14] in which patients could choose their doctor. It established health boards to administer the health service instead of the local authorities,[15] and Comhairle na nOspidéal[16] to regulate consultant posts, with a majority of consultants among its members. The Act included only one significant extension of eligibility: expenditure on drugs above a certain threshold would be refunded by the health boards, irrespective of income.

O'Malley's White Paper had proposed that, following the dismantling of the salaried dispensary system, doctors should ideally now be paid by capitation – that is, by an annual sum for each of their GMS patients rather than by a fee for each visit. However, the profession lobbied for fee payment, which they achieved under O'Malley's successor, Seán Flanagan. Now the state had ceded any control over general practice, which was to remain the domain of, in effect, private entrepreneurs. Although the dispensary system was mourned by neither patients nor doctors because of its Poor Law connotations, this salaried local authority service, which might have been used as the basis for a modern state service, had disappeared. The bringing together of former dispensary patients – now holders of medical cards – and private patients into the same doctors' waiting rooms, to receive treatment which would not discriminate between them, was regarded as an advance. Some doctors continued to discriminate informally but these appeared to be the exception rather than the rule.[17] It still remained the case, however, that the majority of patients, some on very low incomes, must pay from their own pockets for their treatment. Only those who were unable to arrange GP care "without undue hardship"[18] would be eligible for free care.

A central motivation in the establishment of the health boards was to liberate local health authorities from the burden of funding health service improvements from local rates, an increasingly heavy and unpopular local property tax.[19] The members of the boards would include a majority of local councillors, with representatives of medical and other professions. Although it was envisaged that a proportion of the boards' funding would continue to come from the local rates, with additional income from central government (a health levy was imposed on middle and upper income groups in 1971), the health charge on the rates was so unpopular that it was phased out by the Fine Gael/Labour coalition, elected in 1973 and committed to funding all health costs centrally. Consequently, local health boards now had power without responsibility – "local control without local taxation"[20] – which meant that it was always easier to vote for more services than to take hard decisions about their optimal location. The publication of the FitzGerald Report in 1968, which recommended the rationalisation of local hospital networks, had provoked enormously hostile local reaction and would continue to reverberate in local and health politics. Named after its chairman, Patrick FitzGerald, professor of surgery at University College Dublin and a voluntary hospital consultant, the report of this government-appointed council recommended there should be just 4 regional and 12 general hospitals, each with at least 600 and 300 beds respectively and a catchment area with a population of at least 120,000. Other county hospitals would become community health centres.[21]

The 1970 Health Act was passed during the tenure of Erskine Childers as Minister for Health. The Cambridge-educated Minister, later a much-respected President of Ireland, was earnest, verging on the eccentric. He once proposed research on whether ugly people were more likely to become insane than the good-looking but "dropped the idea when the difficulties in establishing an objective prescription for ugliness were put to him".[22] Although a member of the Protestant Church of Ireland, Childers made significant concessions to the Catholic Church in the Act. He permitted the powerful Dublin voluntary hospitals to retain control of consultant appointments, subject to Comhairle's approval of their posts. The objective of Noel Browne and other democratic reformers that the state should control appointments to the voluntary hospitals had been defeated. The Local Appointments Commission would be restricted solely to appointing health board consultants. In 1971, Childers accepted "as a principle" that the voluntary hospitals should control their day-to-day administration and selection of staff,[23] despite their dependence on state funding. The following year, he attempted to revisit the issue, requesting Comhairle to suggest common selection procedures, which would be "acceptable to all the interests concerned"[24] but neither he nor subsequent Ministers achieved a common procedure. Hospitals run by the Catholic Church had been reassured that they could insist on Catholic ethics in medical practice, whatever the religious affiliation of members of staff or patients. The Church's former hostility to increased eligibility for state health services had now disappeared, however. The Act made provision for changing eligibility for health services by ministerial regulation, without provoking opposition from either the Church or doctors.[25]

A further significant amendment to the Act afforded consultants in health board hospitals greater opportunity for private practice, since the hospitals might now offer private and semi-private accommodation.[26] The 1970 Act therefore permitted the medical profession greater opportunities to earn private fees and discriminate in favour of fee-paying patients in local hospitals and opened up for general practitioners a whole new market for fees from state-funded GMS patients.

Defeat of a socialist Minister's free hospitalisation scheme

When appointed Minister for Health and Tanaiste in 1973, Brendan Corish of the Labour Party made the first significant attempt to extend eligibility for health services since the introduction of free hospitalisation for the majority of the population 20 years previously. He sought to extend free hospitalisation to the entire population. Leader of the Labour Party since 1960, Corish told its annual conference in 1969 that the seventies would be socialist. He had not always been so radical, had like the rest of his party failed to support Browne at the time of the mother-and-child confrontation in 1951 but would later change the Labour Party into a socialist party affiliated to the Socialist International. The son of a TD and labour leader, he was a trade unionist, who represented the rural county of Wexford. This well-liked man proved no match for the opposition of organised medicine.[27]

The 1969 Labour Party conference had restated its support for "a free comprehensive health service" which would "absorb the private sector into the public services and thereby eliminate the two-tier system", an early reference to the two-tier care which was to remain a feature of the health service. Capital investment in health care would be funded from general taxation and current health spending would be funded from social insurance to be levied as a percentage of earnings.[28]

Within six months of his appointment, Corish announced that by April 1974 hospital services would be available free to all. He proposed to fund the scheme by a weekly flat-rate contribution from all employees. Corish was in part responding to trade union lobbying. Income eligibility limits for free hospital care discriminated between different categories of worker and had not kept pace with rising wages. Whereas in 1953, it was envisaged that over 80 per cent of the population would qualify for free hospital care, by 1973 this had dropped to 74 per cent.[29] Corish met immediate opposition from the IMA and the IMU. Hospital consultants threatened industrial action. Bereft of their ecclesiastical allies, for the bishops supported Corish's scheme, the medical profession were revealed in their true colours as trade unionists as willing as any other powerful group to defend their incomes by withdrawing their labour.

Hospital consultants could now potentially lose their entire private practice income. If the population as a whole decided to avail of free hospital care, they would become salaried employees. The profession would not agree to a salaried service and demanded to be paid on a fee-for-service basis. Corish was forced to postpone implementation on his planned date – April 1st 1974 – when consultants said they would not cooperate with the scheme in the absence of agreement on payment.[30] They refused to define non-cooperation, but implied that, while they would undertake emergency cases, "vital services" would be withdrawn.[31] Although Corish continued to describe the government's decision to introduce the scheme as "irrevocable", it disappeared into the limbo of a review group on consultants' remuneration, which was boycotted by the medical organisations.[32]

Announcing the postponement of his scheme to the Dáil, Corish made clear that its democratic will and the policy of the government had been thwarted by the consultants' threatened industrial action.

> To my intense regret I have received neither the understanding nor the co-operation which I could have expected as Minister for Health charged with the responsibility of implementing a policy decided upon by the Government elected by this Parliament. Instead representatives of the medical consultants opposed the introduction of my scheme until such time as they decided the population should have free hospital and medical services.

Corish explained that he had decided to postpone the introduction of the scheme

> for a limited period in order to avoid any danger to human life and to avoid confrontation with the consultants on this occasion in the hope that they will reconsider their general attitude ... if they propose to

restrict admissions to hospitals, then human health and even life could be placed at risk. I am not prepared to take such a risk.

Corish said he had not intended to abolish private practice for consultants or to end private wards but to offer everyone the option of free treatment in a public ward. He had thought consultants favoured a salaried, pensionable contract but they had then sought fee-for-service, which "could lead to bad medical organisation" and was "very difficult to cost".[33]

This view was shared by his officials, one of whom later described how the IMA annual congress had been "inspired" by an address by the president of the Canadian Medical Association "extolling the Canadian system of payment by way of fee per item of service" and "a state of euphoria for such a method of payment swept through the profession and the medical negotiators were mandated to go for this and for nothing else". The official, Dermot Condon, a future secretary of the Department, then visited Canada and obtained copies of the fee schedules for up to 6,000 different procedures and consultations. "To introduce it here would have been a licence to print money," he concluded.

Reflecting on Corish's defeat in a memorandum to the next Labour Minister nine years later, Condon wrote that Department officials had been put "in a very difficult negotiating position" by decisions by the Minister and "I think perhaps the Cabinet of the day" that "firstly, there should be universal eligibility for all the population for hospital and consultant services and, more damaging still, that the new arrangements would come into operation on a pre-determined date".[34]

In opposition, Fianna Fáil was not supportive to the Minister or his objectives. The party rejected free hospitalisation for all[35] and suggested that Corish should have extended eligibility for the GMS rather than free hospital care to the better-off.[36] This was a tenable proposition, on grounds of equity, but appeared motivated by political opportunism. Although Fianna Fáil's health spokesman, Charles Haughey, advocated greatly increased GMS eligibility, "urgently needed to alleviate widespread worry and hardship",[37] the proportion of medical card holders grew during the lifetime of this government, reflecting growing unemployment, and declined when Fianna Fáil returned to power with Haughey as Minister for Health. Haughey was equally opportunistic in response to Corish's published plan to rationalise rural hospitals, a partial response to the FitzGerald Report which would have reduced the number of general hospitals from 54 to a maximum of 33. Fianna Fáil made an issue of local hospitals in the 1977 election and much of the plan was not implemented.

Corish was a member of an increasingly embattled government. An oil crisis in 1973 caused spiralling inflation. GDP fell in Ireland and most of western Europe in 1975.[38] The government borrowed to fund public spending but began to cut back in 1976 and 1977. Corish had to impose restrictions on spending in the health service and, like other incumbents before and after him, became preoccupied with value for money.[39]

The Catholic Church finds a new adversary – sexual liberation

The dog that didn't bark when Brendan Corish proposed to remove the income limit for free hospital services was the hierarchy. Unlike their predecessors in the 1950s, the Catholic bishops of the 1970s no longer believed that state provision would weaken the moral fibre of the people or that state maternity care posed a threat to morality. When the majority of the population had been eligible for free hospitalisation for nearly 20 years, to extend free hospital, maternity and infant welfare services to the excluded upper income group was no longer at odds with the social or moral teaching of post-Vatican Two Catholicism. Corish was able to claim in the Dáil that the hierarchy's advisory Council for Social Welfare welcomed his scheme.[40]

Thinking in the Irish Church reflected international developments. Now the excesses of capitalism were of at least equal concern as the excesses of socialism. In the 1960s, Pope John XXIII had urged greater state intervention in the economy to "prevent the emergence of mass unemployment"[41] and described health care as a fundamental human right.[42] While the Second Vatican Council's (1962–5) openness was not shared by the Irish hierarchy, more complacent than their colleagues in more heterogeneous societies,[43] Cardinal Conway conceded that some Church fears about state control "now appear to have been exaggerated."[44] Although still too wedded to its institutional role in health care and education to share the militant solidarity with the poor espoused by liberation theologians in Latin America,[45] by the 1970s the Irish Church had begun to offer a left-wing critique of government social policy. The Council for Social Welfare believed that social policy should aim "to reduce gross inequalities within the community", which would require "massive redistribution of income".[46] By 1977, the bishops themselves were arguing for higher taxes, redistribution of wealth and a national programme to eliminate poverty, including "better access of the poor to health care, particularly for expectant mothers and for children, if necessary".[47]

This newfound radicalism came in tandem with a reawakening of church anxiety about sexual morality, provoked by the sexual climate of the 1960s and reinforced by the 1968 encyclical *Humanae Vitae*, which restated the Church's traditional ban on artificial contraception. However, obstructing state health care was no longer to be the route to controlling morality. The Church lobbied instead for legislative imposition of Catholic morals and relied on its traditional control in Catholic hospitals and influence in health board hospitals to prevent medical practice that it considered contrary to Catholic moral teaching.

Thus, following publication of *Humanae Vitae*, Kieran O'Driscoll, the Master of Holles Street maternity hospital, announced that the contraceptive "pill" would no longer be prescribed by the hospital. Holles Street had been running a family-planning clinic, in the expectation that the papacy would lift the traditional ban, and since 1967 had offered the pill to "couples who felt in conscience able to take it" – about half of whom did so, according the hospital's 1967 Clinical Report.[48] In the mid-1960s, an estimated 15,000 women were using the pill, which circumvented the legal ban on the import of contraceptives since it was ostensibly a "cycle regulator".[49] However, John Charles McQuaid was both chairman of the board of governors and parish priest for Holles Street. Shortly before he retired in 1971, he announced that:

> Any contraceptive act is always wrong in itself. To speak, then, of a right to contraception, on the part of an individual, be he Christian or non-Christian or atheist, or on the part of a minority or of a majority, is to speak of a right that cannot even exist.[50]

Following his retirement, the bishops moderated their approach, conceding that the state was not bound to prohibit contraceptives, in response to an attempt to liberalise contraceptive legislation: "There are many things which the Catholic Church holds to be morally wrong and no one has ever suggested, least of all the Church herself, that they should be prohibited by the State."[51] However, a Fine Gael/Labour government Bill to provide for the import of contraceptives was defeated in 1974, when Fianna Fáil was joined in voting down the Bill by the Taoiseach, a conservative Catholic, and other members of the government parties, notwithstanding a Supreme Court judgment that the import ban had invaded the privacy of a woman whose next pregnancy could be fatal.[52]

Fianna Fáil's metamorphosis into an establishment party in the 1960s buried the ambitions of the 1940s for a comprehensive national health service. Despite the hopes of Labour, industrialisation and urbanisation did not mean that the seventies were socialist and did not translate into mass support for social democratic politics. Labour's participation in government with the conservatives of Fine Gael at a time of global recession merely paved the way for Fianna Fáil's return in 1977. The medical profession exerted a growing influence over Fianna Fáil – manifest in the introduction of fee payment for GPs in the GMS and of greater opportunities for private practice for consultants in health board hospitals. Brendan Corish's failure to deliver free hospital care for all spoke eloquently of the profession's continued power, even when shorn of its ecclesiastical allies. Although former dispensary patients benefited from the introduction of a choice of doctor, eligibility for free primary care remained extremely limited and the system of care remained undeveloped. The bias in the health care system towards hospital care was exacerbated by the abolition of a local revenue base for health, so that health boards had no incentive to take decisions about the optimal allocation of local hospital services and resisted the recommendations of the FitzGerald Report. In this they were encouraged by Fianna Fáil, who fomented anxieties about local hospitals in their push to regain power. Fianna Fáil's abandonment of an encompassing vision of a comprehensive health service free to all gave way to piecemeal reform and unplanned investment, driven more by electoral concerns than the rational development of the service.

4

THE UNLEASHING OF PRIVATE MEDICINE

"It is not intended that there should be an exact measurement of the time spent by you in discharging your contract."
            – wording of consultants' common contract, 1981.

"I think health is a bit like housing. People are entitled to different levels of housing."
    – Jimmy Sheehan, orthopaedic surgeon and founder of the private Blackrock Clinic.

Fianna Fáil's triumphant return to power with its largest ever majority in 1977 set the health system on a roller-coaster of rapidly rising investment followed by gradual retrenchment. Despite its former advocacy of an expanded GMS, the party's unplanned and politically opportunist investment in health care in the late 1970s addressed neither the deficiencies of primary care, the most glaring obstacle to access, nor the need to rationalise the local hospital network to provide superior care in fewer, bigger acute hospitals. Although Fine Gael and Labour were again partners in government in the 1980s, their 1970s convergence on health care reform disappeared when, following the Fianna Fáil excesses of the late 1970s, Fine Gael's overriding concern became fiscal rectitude. Labour's support for a comprehensive free system did not translate into political initiatives.

A Fianna Fáil Minister, Charles Haughey, extended access to free hospital care in 1979, achieving part of Corish's objective. The entire population became eligible for free accommodation in hospital but, significantly, the highest 17 per cent of earners was still obliged to pay consultants' fees. A new contract for hospital consultants, agreed by a

Haughey government, gave them the best of all worlds – state salaried, pensionable posts, with the right to unlimited private practice in or outside public hospitals. This consultants' contract turned heavily state subsidised, private medicine into a growth industry, encouraged the development of private hospitals staffed by consultants on state salaries and consolidated the two-tier system of preferential access for private patients in public hospitals. A Labour Minister, Barry Desmond, fought a rearguard action against the rising tide of private medicine in the 1980s but, with constrained public health spending, there was an inevitable increase in demand for private health insurance to buy more rapid access to superior care.

The post-Vatican-Two liberalism within the Catholic Church began to wane and the hierarchy's interest in dictating public morality, through legislation and its control of hospitals, continued to limit availability of contraception and curtail medical practice, while the passage of a constitutional amendment intended to outlaw abortion would have far-reaching consequences for women's health.

A munificent Haughey – health spending doubles

Charles Haughey towers over recent Irish history, a complex and controversial figure whom the young have known only as an ailing, elderly man, emerging, escorted by lawyers, from tribunals of inquiry into the murky interrelationship of his business and political affairs. In 1977, he cut an entirely different figure. The new Minister for Health had been resurrected after he was sacked from cabinet in 1970 and then tried and acquitted of charges of conspiring to import arms for the use of Catholics in Northern Ireland. He returned to the Fianna Fáil front bench as health spokesman in 1975 with one goal – and it was not health care reform. His ambition was to win the leadership of Fianna Fáil and the position of Taoiseach, which he achieved in 1979.

Haughey was an accountant, upwardly mobile from relatively modest roots and married to a daughter of Seán Lemass. His invisibly acquired wealth remained a topic of idle speculation until Ireland developed a taste for deeper enquiry in the 1990s. As Minister for Health, he was generous with the state's resources. Eager to woo his backbench colleagues, he capitulated to local demands with a rapid and unplanned expansion of the health services which, as Taoiseach, he would later dismantle in an equally unplanned way. He became a born again clean-liver, a crusader against smoking and excess, who cleared away the ashtrays from the top table at a Fianna Fáil Ard Fheis and gave interviews with a cup of tea in his hand. By 1979, he had an "astonishing" 75 per cent approval rating, two points ahead of the Taoiseach, Jack Lynch.[1]

Health spending more than doubled between 1977 and 1980, benefiting from the government's attempts to deliver on promised full employment by kick-starting the economy through increases in public spending, funded by rising borrowing. Despite high inflation, spending on hospital services rose by 50 per cent, when adjusted for rising prices.[2] Overall health spending rose to 7.8 per cent of national income in 1980 compared to under 4 per cent in 1971.[3] Public health spending per capita was 82 per cent of the EU average in 1980, a level not again attained until 1997.[4]

A munificent Haughey announced plans for new hospitals in Tallaght and Beaumont to the west and north of Dublin and, ignoring the recommendations of the FitzGerald Report, elevated preserving "the role of the county hospital" to a principle. When, on a tour of County Clare, he was shown plans for a new obstetrical unit at a small local hospital, he "produced a pen and signed his sanction" on the spot. A pipe band later led him through cheering crowds.[5]

Free hospital care but unlimited private practice for consultants

The Irish Congress of Trade Unions had continued to campaign for the extension of free hospital care following Corish's defeat. The galloping inflation of the 1970s had inevitably placed more people on incomes above the eligibility level for free hospital care and facing significant hospital bills.[6] Haughey's solution was to extend free hospital maintenance to the entire population and to restore eligibility limits for free consultant services to a level that should cover 83 per cent of the population but would continue to ensure that the highest income group should pay consultants' fees.[7] By protecting private practice, he avoided repeating Corish's confrontation with the profession over the introduction of a salaried service. Haughey's scheme became operative in April 1979 and was funded by a health contribution of 1 per cent of gross income.

Haughey's approach was typical of Fianna Fáil pragmatism. It kept the trade unions quiescent, although ICTU protested that the consultants had exercised a "veto".[8] It passed muster with the medical profession, although the Medical Union's approval hung in the balance during a lively debate, in which one speaker described the scheme as "a national health service by stealth" and proposed that the clock should be turned back 25 years to limit free hospital treatment to medical card holders. Cormac MacNamara, the Waterford general practitioner, swung the meeting when he pointed out that, had the Minister consulted doctors in advance, he would have been accused of giving in to them; that patients' access to hospital beds was still under the doctors' control; and that, given the high cost of maintenance in hospitals, the union must "utterly reject any suggestion of moving against the Irish people in the matter of free maintenance in hospital care".[9]

Haughey was adept at maintaining good relations with the medical profession, among whom MacNamara became particularly influential. MacNamara was president of the Medical Union when it voted to accept the consultants' common contract in 1980; a key figure in its merger with the IMA to form the Irish Medical Organisation (IMO) in 1984; and IMO president when the consultants' contract was revised in 1991. In the late 1970s, he was an unusually articulate, leather-jacketed young doctor. In 2002, he would remain an *éminence grise* of the IMO. Then in his fifties, managing partner of the largest general practice in the state, employing 45 people, a businessman as much as a doctor, he had become a dapper figure in expensive suits and a chauffeur-driven car. Unusual in medicine because of his overt Fianna Fáil sympathies, MacNamara still retained the aura of a Fianna Fáil-er of the 1970s: of a man who had made his own way and had scant sympathy for the pampered establishment of the Dublin voluntary hospital consultant. He genially challenged his professional colleagues about their traditional contempt for administrators: "These fellas had to do competitive exams to get in to the civil service at a time when you only needed the matric to get into medical school."[10] He would surprise younger, more radical doctors when, in 2002, he supported a free, state GP service.[11]

If MacNamara was to prove a useful Fianna Fáil ally in the Medical Union and among general practitioners, Haughey also had his friends in the IMA and among hospital consultants, most notably Bryan Alton, a physician at Dublin's Mater – the Fianna Fáil northside hospital in permanent rivalry with the southside and Fine Gael St Vincent's. The media came to describe Alton as Haughey's "personal physician" but he had also treated Eamon de Valera, Erskine Childers and Seán Lemass – "physician to the nation", a colleague suggested. Although the Sisters of Mercy owned the Mater, its true locus of power was the consultant hierarchy and at its apex was Alton, "a medical wheeler-dealer, a messenger between the nuns, the Archbishop and the politicians – and always to the benefit of his colleagues". Larger than life, assured, amiable, wealthy, the corpulent Alton drove a Rolls Royce, chain-smoked cigars and sported a goatee beard.[12] He was elected to the Senate to represent the National University of Ireland and was influential in the IMA's campaign against capitation payments for GPs before the introduction of the GMS.[13]

When Haughey was elected Taoiseach in 1979, his successor, Michael Woods, a mild-mannered horticultural scientist in the shadow of his leader, took over negotiations on a common contract for consultants at health board and voluntary hospitals, which had been recommended since the FitzGerald Report. Consultants in health board hospitals were usually salaried, pensionable state employees, with very limited rights to private practice,[14] whereas consultants in the voluntary hospitals generally received no salary and earned most of their income from private patients, who paid them directly. The non-fee-paying patients of voluntary hospitals had originally been charity cases. After the introduction of free hospital care for the majority of patients in 1953, the health authorities paid the hospital a daily capitation rate for each public patient, from which a sum was allocated to a "pool" to be divided among the consultants,[15] some of whom continued to regard their non-fee-paying patients as recipients of charity.

In place of these diverse arrangements, the new common contract provided for a salary to be paid to consultants in both health board and voluntary hospitals for a basic 33-hour working week.[16] On top of this, consultants could engage in unlimited private practice, for which they would be paid on a fee-for-service basis. This was an immense change for consultants in the local authority hospitals, who could now pursue private practice like their voluntary hospital colleagues, while consultants in the voluntary hospitals had gained the security of pensionable state employment without ceding their private practice rights.[17]

The contract came into force in April 1981, having been accepted a year earlier by the Medical Union, whose president was now MacNamara. His negotiating skills and understanding of his unruly constituency won the respect of officials, battle-weary from their attempts to reach agreement with representatives of the IMA and IMU, between whom they had discovered there was "no love lost".[18]

The IMA initially voted against the contract. While some voluntary hospital consultants argued it might erode their professional freedom and independence,[19] the overriding fear was erosion of private-fee income. The contract stated that admissions should be governed by "medical need", so that a hospital might limit facilities for non-urgent "fee-paying patients of a consultant".[20] The IMA was persuaded to permit its members to accept the contract only after the Department of Health made "the manner of fulfilling a consultant's service commitment [to public patients] less time restrictive".[21] The contract stated "it is not intended that there should be an exact measurement of the time spent by you in discharging your contract",[22] with the result that officials reported in 1984, "there is no precise information available on the extent of private practice in public hospitals".[23]

Haughey and Woods had offered a sweetheart deal and, by 1983, the majority of consultants had signed the contract.[24] The allure of pensionable and secure state employment, with effectively unmonitored private practice rights, proved stronger than championing professional independence against an illusory threat from the state. In this consolidated two-tier system, consultants would receive a state salary to treat the majority of patients, yet they retained a financial incentive – payment of extra fees – to devote more time to the treatment of private patients than to their unmonitored public commitments. Private patients could now receive consultants' personal care while lying in a public ward in the next bed to a public patient who could be treated by the consultant's junior. So imprecise was the contract in what it required of consultants for their state salaries that the Department urged its review, almost before the ink was dry.

"We have never been satisfied that the contract reflects in any reasonably adequate manner the high standard of professionalism which should be the hallmark of a consultant. The IMA must shoulder much of the blame for this," the secretary, Dermot Condon, informed his new Minister, Barry Desmond, in 1983.[25]

The Catholic Church and medicine – controlling medical ethics

Negotiation of the contract reawakened the Catholic Church's interest in medical politics. The six Catholic-controlled voluntary hospitals in Dublin objected that it contained no clause to give the hospitals ethical control over consultants. Although Woods argued that the contract recognised the hospital authorities' rights to "safeguard" their "ethical principles",[26] for over a year the hospitals refused to offer the contract to consultants. While the hospitals sought to have their ethical codes included in the body of the contract, the Medical Union insisted on their location in an appendix – an obstructionist position but hardly a campaigning stance for professional independence.[27] The hospitals conceded the point and achieved their objective: consultants working in Catholic hospitals would be bound by Catholic ethics.

A consultant might now have to sign a contract of employment that stated "I acknowledge and undertake that it will be part of my duty as a consultant to observe and safeguard the principles embodied in the ethical code of the [employing hospital]" and that, in the event of a conflict between the consultant's contractual "right to the exercise of independent judgement in medical and ethical matters" and the hospital's ethical code, "insofar as matters of ethical principle are concerned, the rights of the [employing hospital] shall take precedence."[28]

Faced with the demands of the Catholic Church for a controlling say in the treatment of patients, the profession was willing to surrender its professional independence, now exposed as no immutable principle, no more than a banner to wave when the Department or hospital managers might wish to monitor the priority accorded to public patients. The agreement of this "Archbishop's Contract"[29] strengthened Church control of treatment in these hospitals, already circumscribed by the publication of an ethical code by the Archbishop of Dublin in 1978.

McQuaid's successor, Dermot Ryan, had recommended the establishment of hospital committees "to set out more clearly ethical policy, both for the day-to-day running of the hospital and for the problem cases".[30] In the battle against sexual liberation, he found allies among militant lay Catholics such as the obstetrician John Bonnar, who had urged the establishment of ethics committees.[31] Earlier in 1978, Dermot MacDonald, the Master of Holles Street, performed a sterilisation for a woman with "a combination of medical and social problems", despite opposition from the hospital's Matron and a warning from Ryan, the chairman of the board. He only subsequently managed to see off pressures for his resignation by threatening to call a press conference. The hospital established an ethics committee, whose members included a theologian appointed by the Archbishop. MacDonald's successor opposed sterilisation and "the need for the ethics committee declined".[32] The bishops explicitly banned sterilisation in 1985: "Catholic hospitals may not provide facilities for such operations. Catholic medical personnel may not co-operate with them."[33]

Although the Primate of Ireland, Tomás Ó Fiaich, had called for a separation of Church and state in 1977 and said that churchmen should not "bring pressure to bear on legislators",[34] when Haughey attempted to find a formula to legalise contraception, on which the preceding government could not agree, the bishops sought its restriction to the married.[35] By 1978, some 48,000 women were using the pill, of whom

13,000 received it free under the GMS as a "cycle regulator".[36] Haughey described his 1979 legislation, another characteristic pragmatic compromise, as "an Irish solution to an Irish problem": contraceptives including condoms would be available only on a doctor's prescription, for "*bona fide* family planning purposes" and sold only by chemists.[37] The IMA recommended to doctors that they should not prescribe non-medical contraceptives.[38]

Fiscal crisis, health cuts and the submergence of a reform agenda

In 18 months between 1981 and 1982, three elections brought three changes of government against a backdrop of crisis in Northern Ireland, mounting public debt and popular unrest about high taxation. Eileen Desmond of the Labour Party was Minister for Health for the brief eight-month life of a Fine Gael/Labour coalition. A respected political veteran and activist on women's issues, she had little opportunity to make an impact. This government cut spending in a supplementary Budget: current health spending fell by over 3 per cent in real terms, and hospital spending by 4 per cent, in 1981.[39] The Department of Finance even contemplated a sharp cut in medical card numbers so that only 25 per cent of the population would receive free general practitioner care.[40]

When Fianna Fáil returned with Michael Woods again in Health, he introduced some outpatient charges and reduced the range of medicines which might be prescribed free to medical card holders. Although overall current health spending rose by nearly 3 per cent in real terms in 1982, spending on the hospital services was cut by over 2 per cent.[41] This Haughey government was plagued by scandal, lasted under a year and was succeeded by a further Fine Gael/Labour coalition, which survived until 1987 with Labour's Barry Desmond as Minister for Health. As the coalition struggled to respond to the aftermath of the Fianna Fáil borrowing binge of the late 1970s, Desmond was fated to be remembered as the Labour Party Minister who closed hospitals.

A small, balding man with a background in trade unionism, whose father had been a Labour Party senator and Lord Mayor of Cork, Desmond represented the atypically liberal south Dublin constituency of Dun Laoghaire. He brought to politics an appetite for confrontation and the sonorous phrases of a trade union orator. He immediately announced his support for "a full comprehensive health service available to all, with priorities based on people's medical needs rather than on their ability to pay for services", to be funded by a national health insurance system which would incorporate the

VHI.[42] This European-style model of health care he described as "basic democratic socialism applied to our health services".[43]

He never pursued such radical reform. Although he found the Taoiseach, Garret FitzGerald of Fine Gael, "ideologically in favour", the rest of the cabinet did not support this "social democratic ethos". While Desmond argued that it need not mean higher taxation, the Departments of Finance and Agriculture and his Labour Party colleagues feared he was wrong.[44] Desmond's promised green paper outlining his proposals was never published, but drafts reveal that the Department of Health shared this general pessimism about the affordability of reform, saw "no likelihood of additional funds being made available for the purpose of broadening eligibility" and anticipated "pressure to contract public health expenditure", now at 8 per cent of national income for three years.[45] The paper explored how eligibility might be limited, subsidies reduced or charges increased.

The draft paper included a description of the role of the state in health care, which the Department would still balk at adopting publicly when it prepared its 2001 health strategy: "Health is perceived in the modern state as a basic human right, the protection of which is accepted as a valid function of the State."[46] Although not openly advocating a rights-based approach to health care, under Desmond the Department was evidently concerned about the inequity of the emerging system. Private patients now gained faster admission, consultants' personal attention and "better amenities", "at a relatively small cost" because of state subsidies to private care, such as tax relief on VHI premiums and below-cost hospital bed charges. State funds should instead be concentrated on "ensuring a minimum acceptable standard of care for all citizens" and those who chose private hospital care "should do so at their own expense". The Department nonetheless advised that to charge private patients the full cost of their maintenance in public hospitals would cause "a substantial increase in VHI premia, a dramatic reduction in the demand for private care and a consequent outcry from the medical profession".[47] A more circumspect "consultative statement on health policy", published in 1986, advocated abolishing or modifying income tax relief on VHI premiums and deploying the revenue saved to primary and preventive care.[48]

The Department was evidently still smarting from Corish's public defeat at the hands of the consultants ten years previously. The draft green paper's conservatism about extending eligibility was not just a response to fiscal crisis, but also reflected an assessment of the power of the medical profession. Extending eligibility for hospital services, in effect giving all patients free hospital medical care, would require changing the consultants' common contract: "Strong opposition could be anticipated from the consultants who would probably see a threat to their incomes from private practice. There is no reason to believe that the attitudes of the medical profession towards such a change would be materially different from the stance adopted in 1974 when a similar change was successfully opposed."[49]

Reform of the health care system, or even extended eligibility, was never on this government's agenda. "For a thing like that to happen, you are talking about legislation and you really have to come into government in the first month with the bill almost drafted," Desmond would later reflect.[50] The government – and Desmond – rapidly became embattled. "Events overtook the ideology. It was just fire brigade stuff all over the place."

Alarmed by rising borrowing, the FitzGerald government attempted to stabilise the national debt[51] by cutting spending and raising taxes. Between 1982 and 1986, current public health spending stayed static in real terms but spending on hospitals fell by 1.5 per cent.[52] Desmond is remembered, in the medical profession in particular, as the man who savaged the health service. In relative terms, the charge does not stick. Much worse was to come under the government elected in 1987.

Desmond defended some cutbacks, others he fought. He withdrew eligibility for medical cards from students whose parents' incomes exceeded the eligibility limits, provoking student protests and the jailing of Joe Duffy, President of the Union of Students of Ireland, and other student leaders for contempt of court. Desmond successfully overturned Finance's refusal to sanction increased income eligibility for medical cards in line with inflation[53] but failed to win funding for a state pension scheme for GPs, intended as part of a package of reforms to improve general practice and reduce pressures on the acute hospital system.[54]

In 1986 he announced the closure of eight hospitals, including two psychiatric hospitals, which he defended as required by hospital rationalisation rather than cost-cutting.[55] He had consistently argued for a shift from hospital to primary and community care, particularly in the psychiatric services.[56] Ireland's hospitalisation rate for mental illness was double England's[57] and the influential 1984 report *Planning for the Future* had advocated movement from institutional- to community-based services for the mentally ill and disabled.[58] In the general hospital services, Desmond could claim the support of the FitzGerald Report and mainstream medical opinion for concentrating resources in larger centres and had already attempted without success to rationalise services in Cavan and Monaghan. His closures were incomparably more modest than the National Planning Board's recommended cut of 5,000 beds over two years,[59] a 26 per cent reduction which the Department thought likely to cause "irreparable harm to the hospital system",[60] and which presupposed that Ireland's bed numbers should fall to UK levels, although both were below the EU average.[61]

The political and practical weakness in Desmond's position was that he was closing hospitals at a time of constrained public spending, when there was little evidence that funding would emerge for alternative facilities. Although unplanned expansion of the hospital services, in response to local pressures, without regard for optimal care or allocation of resources and at the expense of investment in primary care, undoubtedly needed to be addressed, and although there was a good case for replacing outdated facilities with superior care in modern hospitals or in the community, there was general scepticism that affording patients access to superior medical care was the motivation for the closures.[62] Shortly after the announcement of the closures, FitzGerald decided to reshuffle his cabinet and attempted to remove Desmond from Health, which Desmond successfully resisted.[63] A year later, when Labour's withdrawal from government over further proposed budgetary cuts in health and social welfare provoked a general election,[64] fiscal stringency had not solved the crisis of public indebtedness and not since the 1950s had there been such pessimism about the economy.

The rising tide of private medicine

With the introduction of the common contract, salaried consultants in public and voluntary hospitals pursued their right to private practice and private medicine boomed. The Voluntary Health Insurance Board had responded to the extension of free hospital services in 1979 by marketing new plans, such as maternity cover, to retain and attract members. Membership jumped from 20.7 per cent of the population to nearly 25 per cent in 1980 and 29 per cent by 1986.[65] In 1986, two new private hospitals opened in Dublin: the Blackrock Clinic and the Mater. As a believer in equal access to medical care, Desmond played the Canute-like role of attempting to stem the rising tide of private medicine. He engaged in battle on three fronts: preventing consultants in the new Beaumont hospital on Dublin's northside from building a private hospital on the site; insisting on separate insurance plans to cover the Blackrock Clinic and the Mater; and attempting to ensure that consultants in public hospitals paid for the use of facilities for their private patients. He was frequently at odds with the medical profession, now represented by the Irish Medical Organisation (IMO) following a merger between the IMA and the IMU in 1984.

Prior to the 1980s, private hospitals had been generally run by religious orders. "Nursing homes" provided genteel care in elegant surroundings. They were not equipped to undertake complex medical procedures, which took place in the public or voluntary hospitals. "In some instances it was recognised that the spiritual needs of the wealthier required particular attention and some orders concentrated their work in a paid capacity, using the profits generated to further other charitable works in the community." So Jimmy Sheehan, the founder of the Blackrock Clinic and successor to the religious in developing private medicine, interpreted their motivation.[66] This "particular attention" to the spiritual needs of the wealthy was accompanied by particular attention to their physical needs – access to superior nursing and medical care. Where religious orders developed private nursing homes beside public hospitals, they justified their involvement in the care of the wealthy as a means of retaining the services of consultants for the poor.

Under Desmond, the Department was hostile to the "new departure" of "hospitals being established as business entities, in which their owners' sole motivation is the generation of commercial profit", the draft green paper reveals. Potential "objectionable" consequences included: creating a "two-tier system of hospital care with the wealthy being treated in different hospitals, by different staff and with a higher standard of care than the less well off"; drawing scarce skills to the private sector; making it difficult to ensure that the costs of private medicine were borne by its beneficiaries; and leading to over-investment in fragmented hospital services rather than community services.[67]

Beaumont was a public hospital, built in Haughey's north-east Dublin constituency and merging the staffs of two established city centre hospitals: Jervis Street and the Richmond. The consultants believed that Michael Woods had ceded to them the right to their own private hospital on the site,[68] like the private hospital at the Sisters-of-Charity-owned hospital, Vincent's, on the southside. Yet Vincent's was a voluntary hospital, whereas Beaumont was a public hospital and Desmond was determined to prevent its resources and staff being siphoned off into private medicine. "For as long as I'm Minister for Health, I'll refuse to allow the construction of private hospitals in Beaumont, James' and Tallaght. There's no need for these private clinics and hospitals."[69]

Desmond argued that keeping public and private practice within the same hospital meant that the public hospital would benefit from the VHI payments for private beds. Permitting the consultants to build a for-profit hospital would remove that income from the public hospital and result in consultants spending more time in the private facility.[70] As investors in the hospital, they would have a double incentive to increase their private practice at the expense of their public patients. During a stand-off in negotiations, the newly constructed public hospital remained idle for two years before it was opened in 1987. Fianna Fáil then reversed Desmond's stance but the consultants' interest had waned and did not revive until 2001.[71]

The Blackrock Clinic was different, an entirely private enterprise, albeit staffed largely by consultants with public contracts in other hospitals. It was the brainchild of Jimmy Sheehan, an orthopaedic surgeon, who nearly 20 years later remained a tenacious lobbyist for private hospitals and was promoting plans for a network of private hospitals across the state. Sheehan would become a unique outcropping on the Irish medical landscape: a medical entrepreneur, who expressed disdain for the profit motive; a defender of professional independence, who imposed Catholic ethics in his hospital; and a critic of state provision of health care, who would prove adept at securing state aid for his later ventures. Even his antagonists in health politics described him as "a Renaissance man". He added a degree in bioengineering and a doctorate in mechanical engineering to his medical qualifications and patented his own designs for artificial knee and hip joints. He combined a soft-spoken, almost tentative demeanour with forthright expression of unusually conservative views.

Sheehan had found himself "semi-redundant" in his post as a consultant at St Vincent's during the cutbacks of the early 1980s, constrained to perform fewer operations when he had a five-year waiting list. He declined the opportunity to become an employee on a state-funded salary and never signed a common contract, which he considered "unprofessional" because "the essence of a professional person is the freedom of practice". His own account of his motivation for establishing the Blackrock Clinic was to provide care for people who could afford private insurance, which would reduce their demands on the state sector. "If the public services had been able to cope with the situation, Blackrock would never, ever have arisen."[72] When Blackrock opened, he resigned his Vincent's post, unusually committing himself fully to private medicine.

As he developed into the foremost proponent of private medicine, Sheehan eventually enunciated a philosophy of health care as a commodity, which people should work to purchase unless they were "needy", in which case the state should provide for them – although he believed state care would be inevitably behind the times. While it was "immoral" for private patients to gain preferential access to public hospitals, multiple tiers of care might exist within a private system.

> The state cannot provide for everyone. That is what they tried to do in the Communist states and they failed miserably. I think health is a bit like housing. People are entitled to different levels of housing. If they want to put their effort into providing for better housing, they have to work very hard for it and people have forgotten about that in relation to their own health.[73]

Sheehan enlisted his brother Joe, a doctor in the US; Maurice Neligan, a cardio-thoracic surgeon; and George Duffy, a physician, as shareholders in the new hospital. Initially, he hoped to involve the VHI and the Department of Health as investors. The Department had no interest and the VHI, though well-disposed, was prevented by government from participation, so he went into partnership with the hospitals subsidiary of BUPA, a British provident society with a significant health insurance business. BUPA started with a 56 per cent stake and grew in influence when it invested more in a preference shareholding.[74] Although BUPA Hospitals' parent company was a not-for-profit provident society, this investment in Irish health care would provide revenues for the parent company. Sheehan would later regret its involvement. Blackrock became a commercial concern and "not the leading edge facility that it was 20 years ago." He also changed his general view of insurers as investors. "Health insurers shouldn't be involved in owning hospitals. They have a conflict of interest. They may end up dictating some aspects of care. I don't think you should have any third party involved between the doctor and the patient."

Sheehan's medical partners shared some but not all of his motivations. Maurice Neligan had found himself underemployed in the crowded Mater public hospital, where he had "nowhere to go" when he was not operating. The idea of working and earning more, in a better environment, of developing private practice "without the opprobrium of people saying I was doing so in a public hospital" won him to Sheehan's venture. Neligan, however, retained his public contract and commitment to the public sector. His was the traditional stance of Dublin voluntary hospital consultants: "you made your money in private practice but you looked after the underprivileged". While

Sheehan believed Blackrock should be run "along strictly Catholic lines" so that procedures like sterilisations were out of the question, Neligan did not agree. Neligan eventually sold his shareholding to Sheehan.[75]

Although Barry Desmond accepted that philanthropy was a partial motivation for these medical entrepreneurs, who also wanted to control "their money and their centre of excellence", and to offer treatments which were rationed in the underfunded public system, the Minister could not justify state support for the development of Blackrock, with its superior tier of care for private patients provided largely by salaried public hospital staff and funded by VHI subscribers, whom the state heavily subsidised through tax relief. Blackrock and the Mater private hospital, established by the Sisters of Mercy to replace a more modest private establishment, offered high-tech medicine at high-tech prices, with daily bed charges at double the rate of the existing private hospitals.[76]

Having prevented the VHI from investing in Blackrock, Desmond insisted that it introduce higher insurance premiums to cover treatment in the new hospitals, with no cross-subsidisation from other subscribers. Since the hospitals could not draw on the full pool of VHI members, they struggled financially and their image became more élitist than their founders intended. "Barry made the hospitals élitist. We were trying to get VHI patients out of the public hospitals. There is no doubt that in so doing we have made money for ourselves and for our colleagues but that was not our primary motivation," Neligan would maintain, while, for Sheehan, the image of Blackrock as "a fancy hospital for the élite has at all times been an irritant".

In his third major battle with the medical profession over private medicine, Desmond sought to require that consultants should pay for the use of public facilities in private practice, which had been the case in some specialties up to 1979, when Haughey conceded that consultants might keep all their private fee income.[77] The IMO refused to engage in discussions with local health boards on how this might be implemented. Eventually the Minister proceeded by diktat and the Department reduced its allocations to health board and voluntary hospitals by an amount which the hospitals were required to recover from consultants. The effectiveness of this arrangement varied and it was later dropped.[78]

The Catholic Church and medicine – family planning, sterilisation and abortion

Despite the apparent willingness of some Catholic Church figures to separate Church and state in the 1970s, after Pope John Paul II sought to turn back the tide of post-Vatican-Two liberalism the Catholic Church and some of its laity fought secularisation with increased ferocity. The Fine Gael leader, Garret FitzGerald, who had reinvigorated the party with his liberal politics, had launched a "constitutional crusade" to remove the Catholic ethos in legislation and the Constitution[79] and supported Desmond's substitution of a more liberal regime for Haughey's family planning legislation. The legalisation in 1985 of the sale of non-medical contraceptives to anyone over 18 without a doctor's prescription, by chemists and in family planning clinics and maternity hospitals,[80] was contemporaneously viewed as "the first victory of politicians against the Church in matters of public morality"[81] and later described as "of epoch-making importance" by the dissident Swiss Catholic theologian, Hans Küng.[82] While the government parties forced their deputies to vote in favour, Fianna Fáil enforced its deputies' opposition, provoking the expulsion from the party of Desmond O'Malley, who voted with the government and later founded the Progressive Democrats.

Although the IMA had lobbied for a change in the law so that doctors could cease to be moral arbiters,[83] some prominent hospital consultants opposed the passage of the Act as did increasingly politicised and militant Catholic lay groups, such as the newly formed Family Solidarity. Kevin McNamara, the Archbishop of Dublin and a defender of orthodoxy,[84] called the legislation a "turning point in Ireland's history", which confronted politicians with moral problems "of the gravest kind". Sexual morality should not be left to the individual conscience.[85] The Bishop of Limerick, Jeremiah Newman, reminded politicians "who profess to be Catholics that they have a duty to follow the guidance of their Church in areas where the interests of Church and State overlap".[86]

Desmond's contraceptive legislation did not refer to sterilisation,[87] although he accepted that access to tubal ligation was "most inadequate", because of ethical committees and conservatism in the medical and nursing professions.[88] The Irish Nurses Organisation voted in 1985 against a proposal in favour of making sterilisation "readily available".[89] Desmond refused to issue a list of public hospitals which offered sterilisation, in case this prompted the establishment of ethical committees. He acknowledged that, despite state funding, the elected government could not control the availability of services. "I cannot force hospitals to disband ethical committees where they're in existence."[90]

Eamon Casey, the Bishop of Galway, wrote to doctors in his area in 1985 stating his opposition to the performance of sterilisations in Galway Regional Hospital. It would emerge that Casey had privately enjoyed the sexual liberation which he publicly sought to curtail, having fathered a child by a young American woman. In 1992, *The Irish Times* revealed that he had used diocesan funds to pay a settlement to the child and his mother, a key moment in the cascade of events which would erode the authority of the Catholic Church over the next decade.

This Fine Gael/Labour government twice met defeat by the forces of Catholic reaction. A referendum to legalise divorce was defeated in 1986 following influential church opposition[91] and, in 1983, a constitutional ban on abortion, which equated the right to life of a mother with that of her unborn child, was adopted with the bishops' support and despite the government's opposition to its wording. Although all Irish abortions were performed in England, the Taoiseach, Garret FitzGerald, was committed to amending the constitution to prevent a court challenge legalising abortion. He first accepted a wording proposed by Fianna Fáil,[92] which he later attempted to replace[93] when he realised it presented problems of interpretation. The original wording prevailed when some government deputies voted with Fianna Fáil, and it was then put to the people and accepted in a referendum. While both Fine Gael and Fianna Fáil were committed to maintaining a ban on abortion in Ireland, this constitutional amendment went further. It threatened existing medical practice to protect a woman's life and provided legal grounds to prevent women obtaining information on abortion and, ultimately, to prevent travel for an abortion.

Fianna Fáil populism, coupled with Charles Haughey's opportunist approach to politics, delivered some reform in the 1970s – universal free maintenance in hospital, which liberated higher earners from bills for hospital accommodation – but the introduction in 1981 of the consultants' common contract was a seminal moment in the consolidation of two-tier access to hospital care. By extending unlimited private practice rights to all consultants, the contract established a framework for continued discrimination between classes of patients, which would survive subsequent revisions to last into the next century. Lacking any uniting philosophy or vision of health care, no longer an egalitarian party yet still seeking cross-class support, Fianna Fáil strove simultaneously to satisfy trade union demands for extended eligibility, doctors' self-interest and its wealthier supporters' requirements for continued privileged access and care. The consequence was a contradictory package of reforms and the growth of private medicine, further boosted by the Fine Gael/Labour government's curtailment of public spending on health.

Fine Gael's former advocacy of health care reform was forgotten in government in the 1980s and Labour's policy was never seriously entertained. At a time of retrenchment, there is an even stronger argument for ensuring that state spending on health is concentrated on those with greater need, but it is also a time when reform will result in some losers, and these would have been Fine Gael's middle class electorate. Desmond's resistance to the growth of private medicine, a justified defence of the public system, might have been better understood had he pursued a system of equitable access.

5

THE ERA OF THE CUTS

"A two-tier system ... has been the position since the foundation of the State and this system, with its integrated mix of public and private care, has served the nation well."
– *Fianna Fáil Minister for Health, Rory O'Hanlon.*

"The Minister is enshrining in our system a permanent separation, a fast lane for those who can afford and a slow lane for those who cannot."
– *Fine Gael's Richard Bruton.*

"Health cuts hurt the old, the sick and the handicapped," read the Fianna Fáil billboards on the walls of the cities and towns of Ireland in the 1987 election campaign. Once in government, as part of its emergency programme to confront economic crisis, Fianna Fáil implemented far larger cutbacks than the Fine Gael/Labour coalition. The effect on the health services was catastrophic and longlasting. The health cuts deepened the two-tier divide. Public patients faced lengthening waiting lists and deteriorating care, while the middle class fled from the impoverished public health system into the welcoming arms of state-subsidised private care delivered in public or private hospitals, largely staffed by doctors on state-salaried public hospital contracts. Free hospital maintenance, extended to the entire population in 1979, was now compromised with the introduction of hospital charges for all but medical-card holders.

Intense debate developed about the effect of the cutbacks on access to health care, about hospital consultants' terms of employment and the accentuation of the two-tier system. The many voices demanding greater equity included the government-appointed Commission on

Health Funding, the Catholic Church, the trade union movement, officials in the Department of Health and the political parties. Hospital consultants established the combative Irish Hospital Consultants' Association (IHCA) in response to popular criticism and government underfunding. Although health care provoked and dominated a general election in 1989, a reform package, introduced by the Fianna Fáil/Progressive Democrat government in 1991 with the support of the social partners, neither stemmed the rising tide of private medicine nor brought equity into the public system. The government extended free public hospital care to the entire population provoking little resistance from hospital consultants, who now no longer saw it as a threat to their private-fee income because patients were flocking to insure themselves to pay private fees. The introduction of a system to identify public and private beds in public hospitals, which was ostensibly intended to protect access for public patients, had the effect of institutionalising preferential access to public hospitals for private, fee-paying patients and further increased the attractiveness of private health insurance to those who could afford it.

Fianna Fáil continued in power until 1994, with Charles Haughey as leader until 1992. Its social radicalism a distant memory, the party was now chiefly defined by its pragmatism, its ability to adopt whatever policy or strategy would secure power and retain the most powerful and wealthy interests among its supporters. Although Fianna Fáil's vote was declining and not since 1977 had it commanded a majority of seats in Dáil Éireann, the fragmentation of politics with the emergence of the Progressive Democrats (PDs) on the right and the Workers' Party on the left, presented the party with a window of opportunity. Fianna Fáil abandoned its resistance to coalition and governed in coalition with the PDs from 1989 and with Labour from 1992.

1987 – the health cuts

In the 1980s, emigration and unemployment soared; population and national income fell. As other states emerged from their worst recession of the post-war years, Ireland remained submerged. Despite growth in employment in 1986, the 1987 general election was dominated by debate about the economy and the national debt and produced, in effect, national government, when Fine Gael's leader, Alan Dukes, supported the efforts of the minority Fianna Fáil government to restore fiscal stability by cutting spending. The government also had the support of the social partners – employers, farmers and trade unionists – who agreed a programme[1] of moderate wage increases in return for income tax reductions, which meant that spending must fall. In the first two years of this government, public current health spending was cut by nearly 7 per cent in real terms and spending on hospitals by 7.5 per cent.[2] By 1989, public spending on health had fallen to 6.7 per cent of national income, having remained close to 8 per cent from 1980 to 1986.[3] The EU states were now spending on average almost twice as much as Ireland on the health of each citizen. Irish per capita public spending on health fell to 57 per cent of the EU average in 1989.[4] Not until the 1990s' revelations of widespread tax evasion did the view gain support that some of these cutbacks might have been avoided had tax compliance been enforced or the tax base been enlarged to levy higher taxes on wealth, profit and property.

The Minister for Health from 1987 to 1991 was Rory O'Hanlon, a well-liked general practitioner from the border county of Monaghan. Through three generations, the O'Hanlon family would show a gift for identifying with the Irish *Zeitgeist* – from revolution through public service to media irreverence. As a young man, the Minister's father had been handpicked by the revolutionary leader Michael Collins to assassinate suspected British spies.[5] The Minister's son, Ardal O'Hanlon, would become a popular comedian, playing the wonderfully absurd Father Dougal in the television comedy *Father Ted*.

The first doctor in Health since Jim Ryan in the 1950s, and the first practising doctor since Noel Browne, Rory O'Hanlon had been a member of the IMU central council and the North-Eastern Health Board. He expressed no radical reform ambitions, although he later declared his commitment to a "comprehensive, equitable and efficient health care system".[6] He parked the task of developing a blueprint for reform with the Commission on Health Funding in 1987. It was evident that, as a doctor, he would rather have developed than reduced services, and even the opposition parties, when proposing a motion of no confidence in him in 1990, did so more in sorrow than in anger, conceding that he had implemented collective cabinet decisions.[7] He managed to preside over extraordinary cutbacks without attracting the retrospective odium that the medical profession reserved for the blunt Barry Desmond.

The cutbacks were savage. Hospitals closed. In Desmond's era, notorious for its hospital closures, 704 acute hospital beds had been cut, a 4 per cent reduction. In O'Hanlon's first term, between 1987 and 1989, 3,244 acute beds were cut, a 19 per cent reduction. A further 13 per cent reduction took place under Fianna Fáil Ministers up to 1993.[8] In the Eastern region around Dublin, there was a 29 per cent reduction in bed numbers.[9] Beds also went in other institutions, such as psychiatric hospitals and geriatric homes. Between 1980 and 1986, there had been an overall drop in all beds of 985, or 2 per cent. From the beginning of 1987 to 1990, overall bed numbers fell by 6,377, a drop of nearly 15 per cent.[10]

The government's implementation of the cutbacks was elusive. O'Hanlon announced reduced allocations not closures, although hospitals would close as a consequence. Brendan Howlin of the Labour Party charged "I find it incredible that this Minister is prepared to close hospitals but not prepared to admit it", when he elicited from the Minister that 19 hospitals "had changed roles".[11]

The government placed an embargo on recruitment in the health service and introduced hospital charges. In Fianna Fáil's expansionary phase, between 1977 and 1981, employment in the public health services rose by 30 per cent, from 50,611 to 66,060. By 1988, nearly 10,000 of those 15,000 new jobs had disappeared again.[12] The free hospital service, which had been introduced for the majority of the population in 1953 and extended to the entire population in 1979, was no more. Patients without medical cards must pay a £10 daily charge for inpatient care and a once-off £10 charge for outpatient care. The principle that services should be free at the point of delivery – central to the UK's NHS – had never been strongly rooted in Ireland but it had been progressively extended in the hospital services, if not in primary care. Now it was unceremoniously abandoned. Howlin reported that charitable organisations had "given money to people who need it to pay for casualty treatment".[13]

The level of public outrage at the health cuts shook political consensus. The Irish Congress of Trade Unions backed a half-day work stoppage by health service unions and thousands marched throughout the country. Junior hospital doctors, represented by the IMO, went on strike for ten days in protest at threatened job losses and increases in their already excessive working hours.[14] Within days of the settlement of their dispute and on the eve of the work stoppage, Fine Gael decided to vote against the government's health estimates, arguing that, although the party had supported cutbacks in public spending, it would have achieved the same result in "a more compassionate and humane way".[15] Haughey called Fine Gael's bluff. He threatened to call an election if the health estimates were defeated, which would bring his administration to an end after only three and a half months. Fine Gael abstained on the vote in what was generally regarded as a humiliating setback for the Fine Gael leader, Alan Dukes. "Game, set and match to Mr Haughey," observed a government spokesman.[16]

The effect of the cuts

Ireland now had a manifestly underfunded public health care system, in which growing waiting lists and deteriorating public care were accelerating the flight to private care. The cuts were in public, not private care. Of the one in six acute hospital beds closed in the greater Dublin area in 1987 and 1988, virtually all were public.[17] Like consultants, hospitals responded to their financial incentive to admit private patients and converted public wards into private wards to gain extra revenues, a strategy they were actively encouraged in by the Department of Health, which even insisted on the designation of private beds in Crumlin children's hospital. Whereas in 1972 around 10 per cent of public hospital beds were supplied to private patients, by 1987 this had risen to approximately 20 per cent.[18] State subsidy of private care continued – tax relief on VHI premiums was worth £43.8 million in 1987, up from £6.5 million in 1980.[19] Fear of public waiting lists[20] increased membership of the VHI to over 36 per cent of the population in 1993. By 2001, an estimated 46 per cent of the population would have private health insurance.[21]

The cuts were also unplanned. Beds stayed in rural hospitals, where votes depended upon them. Dublin, the greatest centre of population, suffered most. In 1990 the government gave "undertakings" about the future of two hospitals in County Roscommon to secure the support of an independent deputy, Tom Foxe, when facing a motion of confidence.[22]

Reputable international opinion supported a change of emphasis from hospital to primary care but, in these cutbacks, primary care suffered as well as the hospital service. Dale Tussing, the American author of an influential study of Irish health care that had recommended such a gradual shift in emphasis, to be encouraged by the simultaneous introduction of hospital charges and a free general practitioner service,[23] now accused the government of "unplanned cuts" following "years of unplanned growth, which was never guided by a vision of what kind of health service the country wants".[24] An economist from Syracuse University, who had been a research professor at Dublin's Economic and Social Research Institute (ESRI), Tussing pointed out that, while public health services were being cut, private care continued to benefit from state subsidies – a policy of privatisation by stealth. "If there is fiscal stringency," he argued, "it is only sensible that no public money goes to the private sector."[25]

The deepening public/private divide in hospital care was mirrored in primary care. The government negotiated a scheme with general practitioners which paid them by capitation – a fixed pre-paid annual amount – for their GMS patients, while they continued to receive a fee for each private patient's visit. Tussing had suggested that, in a free GP service, GPs should be paid by capitation because fees encouraged doctors to over-treat, but he had warned that to pay GPs by capitation for some patients and not others could create two classes of care.[26] Now, as John McManus, a general practitioner and Workers' Party health spokesman, pointed out, doctors would have an incentive "to discourage public patients by referring them on to more costly services such as consultants or hospitals".[27]

This discrimination was exacerbated by the introduction of measures to reduce the cost of medication for GMS patients but not for private patients, although private patients' spending on medication was partially reimbursed by the state. In 1992, the government agreed to fund the development of general practice by permitting GPs to retain for re-investment in their practices half their savings from prescribing below an "indicative drug budget" for medical card patients. A Department working group later observed that the indicative drug-prescribing scheme worked against the prescription of preventive medications.[28] Although GPs gained a state contribution to their pensions and to the cost of employing secretaries and practice nurses, hospital closures increased their workload and primary care remained underdeveloped. Not only did patients face charges for attendance at hospital casualty departments but also more patients had to pay for primary care: GMS membership dropped from 37.4 per cent of the population in 1986 to 34.9 per cent in 1990.

The aftermath of the cuts in national and medical politics

The health cuts came home to roost in the 1989 election, precipitated by health spending. Labour had sought an increased allocation of state funds to compensate haemophiliacs, who had been infected with HIV by blood products supplied by the health service. This issue would return to haunt successive and, indeed, preceding ministers.[29] When the government suffered defeat on the Labour Party's motion, Haughey described it as an attempt to undermine the government's financial authority and went to the country.

A late poll disclosed that 86 per cent of the electorate viewed health cuts as the primary election issue.[30] Fianna Fáil fared badly in the election and, with fewer seats, was forced to enter coalition with the Progressive

Democrats. During the campaign, Haughey revealed how out of touch he was with public feeling on health cutbacks when he confessed in a radio phone-in: "I personally wasn't aware of the full extent of the problems and difficulties and hardships."[31]

Haughey promised to address public waiting lists and to allocate additional resources to health. In 1990, his government increased public current health spending by over 5 per cent in real terms and spending on hospitals by over 9 per cent, but the number of acute public hospital beds continued to decline. Following his re-appointment, O'Hanlon faced a "winter flu" crisis, which illustrated that the hospitals had insufficient beds and provoked a motion of no confidence in him in February 1990. For weeks, 30 patients on average spent the night on corridors in Galway Regional Hospital. A geriatrician, Michael Hyland, said that poor management had resulted in the deaths of elderly people.[32]

Hospital consultants found their working practices subject to unaccustomed criticism as intense debate developed about the deepening of the two-tier divide. The Voluntary Health Insurance Board disclosed that in 1988 the average consultant received £24,000 annually for treating private patients, in addition to a public salary of £33,000. While many consultants had relatively small private practices "due to location or personal preference", others could "gross double or, in some cases, three or four times the average figure".[33] The average male industrial worker that year earned £18,000.[34] The VHI payments by no means expressed consultants' total private earnings, since consultants frequently charged more than the VHI covered, a practice which contributed to public hostility. The VHI's chief executive, Tom Ryan, openly criticised rising professional fees and urged members to ask consultants how much they would charge before treatment began.[35]

The flight to private care and cost of treatment in the new private hospitals precipitated a financial crisis for the VHI, which reported losses in 1987 and 1988, was forced to increase premiums and reduce benefits[36] and refused to cover further private hospitals.[37] In 1991, the VHI agreed increased fees for consultants who did not bill above this agreed amount,[38] which most consultants eventually accepted. The insurance company could now negotiate a ceiling for professional fees, while insured patients were covered for the full cost of private inpatient treatment, although outpatient visits to consultants remained only covered in part.

In 1988, consultants responded to the more hostile environment by breaking away from the IMO to form the Irish Hospital Consultants' Association (IHCA), under the leadership of the abrasive John Fielding, professor of medicine at the Royal College of Surgeons in Ireland (RCSI) and a consultant gastro-enterologist at Beaumont Hospital. The merging of the interests of consultants and other doctors in the IMO had only lasted for four years. Fielding remained president of the IHCA until 1992. Although the rules of the RCSI prevented him from earning private fees, the IHCA was committed to the defence of private practice. Fielding's penchant for controversy eventually led to his resignation from both his positions in 1996 at the age of 58. The college suspended him after an inquiry exonerated a colleague against whom he had made allegations.[39] Fielding moved into private practice in the Mater Private Hospital.

Fielding answered the consultants' need to be heard. "A strong guy when the profession needed one", he was good at supplying media soundbites. If he sometimes went a bit further than the rank-and-file desired, "they were happy that something was being said loud and clear" and supported his dogged defence of their rights and prerogatives.[40] When he died in 2002, 87 per cent of practising consultants were IHCA members, although a minority continued to prefer the more conventional trade unionism of the IMO.[41]

Fielding turned the IHCA into a powerful political lobby group. He said at the association's formation that it would never go on strike but would effect change through the reasonableness and strength of its arguments.[42] The junior doctors' strike had contributed to consultants' sense of alienation in the IMO. However, in pursuit of a pay deal in 1997, the IHCA would threaten to withdraw cooperation with hospital administration and warned that this could cause administrative chaos.[43]

Within six months of the IHCA's foundation, Fielding had recruited fellow Corkman, Finbarr Fitzpatrick, as secretary-general of the association. Fitzpatrick had been a highly effective general secretary of Fine Gael during its resurgence under Garret FitzGerald. Following Fine Gael's loss of power in 1987, he had briefly returned to his original profession of teaching as principal of a vocational school in County Cork. Fitzpatrick was a heavy smoker and a pugnacious debater, whose style combined political nous, sardonic asides and conversational pepperings of Latin. He rapidly acquired a mastery of the intricacies of medical politics, which often gave him the upper hand in confrontations with less well-informed antagonists. Well-versed in national politics, he complemented the patrician and academic Fielding. He became so much the identified voice of the association that members of the public would address him as "Dr Fitzpatrick" at public meetings. Into a second decade, Fitzpatrick would retain the loyalty and trust of the majority of the state's consultants, whose conviction of the existence of an "anti-consultant agenda"[44] never persuaded their spokesman that a more open and conciliatory approach to politics might better advance their interests. The IHCA made a virtue of confrontation. Whereas the IMO represented all classes of doctors, was a member of the Irish Congress of Trade Unions and took a wider view of the future of the health service, the IHCA preferred megaphone diplomacy to the search for consensus. That its bellicosity did not enhance the public image of consultants was a matter of indifference to Fitzpatrick, who believed that consultants might as well be confrontational, since they would never be liked. "We have always made it clear that we are not in the popularity stakes but what one would hope is that there is a measure of confidence in hospital consultants and their ability and skill." After all, he observed, "the general populace" also disliked bank managers, journalists and politicians. "I wouldn't wish it to be otherwise other than to be regarded with a degree of suspicion from health board cum management cum department side. I feel, if cordiality prevails, you'll be sold down the drain by the Government department of the day."[45]

The IHCA was founded at a meeting attended by some 350 consultants, one-third of their number,[46] and promised to campaign on public waiting lists. While consultants were concerned about the effect of the cutbacks, they were also exercised about the introduction of a withholding tax on their payments from the VHI.[47] This required that they would now be paid directly by the insurance company rather than by their patients, characterised by consultants as an intrusion into the doctor-patient relationship, a revealing argument which suggested that they had no relationship with their public patients for whose care they were paid by the state.

The IHCA acquired a licence to negotiate from the Haughey government, "a disastrous decision" in the opinion of a future Minister for Health, Brendan Howlin, who discovered "you then had two competing organisations bidding for members by who could be the most macho with the Department".[48]

Pressure for reform

In this turbulent period, it was evident that the health care system was inequitable and poorly run, that decisions about the allocation of resources were being dictated by local politics not optimal care, that cutbacks in the hospital service were impinging more on the weakest and that primary care was deficient. Divergent groups, within and outside Dáil Éireann, united in arguing for reform.

Reporting in 1989, the government-appointed Commission on Health Funding confirmed the public perception of a growing apartheid in health care, of a "rationing system" based "on ability to pay", and recommended common waiting lists for public and private patients and a more tightly policed contract for consultants.[49] While very many consultants might well fulfil their responsibilities to public patients, given their unmonitored public commitment and ability to earn private fees "it is generally accepted, however, that, as a result of the incentive structure, some consultants do not".[50]

The Commission recommended fixed-term contracts for consultants, with a monitored public commitment, a much more cut-and dried arrangement than the loosely worded common contract which had so dissatisfied its Departmental negotiators. The Commission's chairwoman, Miriam Hederman O'Brien, a lawyer by training, had been influenced by the more rigorous terms of employment of consultants in the United States, whose teaching, research, public and private commitments were clearly delineated and monitored by their head of department.[51]

In key respects, the Commission supported the status quo: the public/private mix in hospital care; charges for general practitioner services; and tax-based funding of the system. The Commission did not consider it inequitable for private patients to gain more rapid access to care in the private sector, provided the public sector delivered care "within a reasonable period of time".[52] However, the Commission insisted that, within public hospitals, while private insurance might secure private accommodation it should not buy more rapid access. Private care should cease to be subsidised by the state through tax relief on health insurance premiums or below-cost charges.[53]

The Commission ducked the critical issue of how much the health services should cost on the grounds of insufficient data.[54] Its members held divergent views on many issues, so that its majority recommendations were not always consistent. While recommending the extension of free consultant care to all, a majority nonetheless favoured modest hospital charges. The trade unionist Phil Flynn was alone in opposing user charges for hospital services and supporting free general practitioner care for all.[55] The Commission listed impressive arguments for excluding private practice from public hospitals, yet nonetheless recommended its retention. Despite acknowledging the possibility that: some consultants neglected public patients to concentrate on private patients, their financial interest in private patients worked against equitable admissions, their demands for priority for private patients prevented a team approach to treatment, and, since they needed the public sector to attain professional recognition, they would not leave public hospitals if denied private practice, the Commission was ultimately convinced by the counter-argument that this denial could result in the loss of "talented consultants", "articulate patients" and revenue from private accommodation.[56]

The central problem in the health service, the Commission concluded, was the system of administration not the system of funding. "The simple question 'who is in charge?' cannot easily be answered for the Irish health services."[57] It recommended that a national Health Services Executive Authority should replace the health boards, which would become health councils with the power to delay but not veto decisions on local health services. "Board members, who are either local politicians or representatives of medical and related professions, tend to be influenced by considerations other than the best delivery of the health services."[58]

The report was shelved. Had some key recommendations been implemented – common waiting lists, a fixed-term contract for consultants, the end of tax subsidies for VHI premiums, the effective abolition of the health boards – they could have turned the rising tide of demand for private medicine and rationalised the organisation of health services. Although the report had predictably provoked the ire of the IHCA, which recommended its shredding,[59] the power of the consultants was not "an insuperable barrier" to its implementation, Hederman O'Brien later reflected. "Some of them favour change and other groups have been taken on by the governments of the day." In her view, the report was not implemented because the government feared upsetting

an unknown number of people – not only consultants but also local councillors, administrators and maybe the general public. Implementation would have taken three to five years, which in our political system has become almost impossible. The political system is one of the barriers to reform, if not the major one.[60]

The Commission reported at a time of widespread disquiet about the effect of the cutbacks on the health care system and near universal agreement on the unacceptability of inequitable access to care, which united politicians of all parties, the Department of Health, the Catholic Church, the trade unions and members of the medical profession.

O'Hanlon said that for paying patients to receive priority admission "could not be tolerated"[61] and expressed support for a common waiting list.[62] The Fine Gael leader, Alan Dukes, sought "equality of access".[63]

The Progressive Democrat leader, Desmond O'Malley, thought two-tier care "particularly obnoxious".[64] His colleague, Bobby Molloy, accused some consultants of "ripping off the system for their own gain".[65] Labour described access to health services as "a fundamental human right",[66] while Pat Rabbitte of the Workers' Party was "appalled" that public and private patients were not treated equally.[67] The Catholic bishops' Council for Social Welfare argued that "equity should be a core value in health policy".[68] The Irish Congress of Trade Unions (ICTU) sought an end to private practice in public hospitals.[69]

If inequity was so universally regarded as unacceptable, how then should an equitable system be constructed? Here opinions diverged. Fundamental reform of the health care system from its traditional tax-based funding to an insurance-funded system as in France or Germany, although rejected by a majority on the Commission, nonetheless had a growing number of proponents. It was variously advocated as a route to greater equity, to ensuring a consistent stream of income for health care and to educating the public on health care costs.

Prior to entering coalition with Fianna Fáil in 1989, the Progressive Democrats advocated a National Health Insurance Scheme to cover hospital services and abolish distinctions between public and private patients. Most people would pay premiums in proportion to their incomes, while the state would pay contributions for those on the lowest incomes.[70] The subsequent programme for government with Fianna Fáil made no allusion to this policy and contained only the vaguest reference to "examining systems which will achieve equality of access to basic health care".[71] Gerry McCartney, an assistant secretary in the Department of Health, argued publicly for a similar "compulsory health insurance levy", which "should be considered as ear-marked taxation which establishes entitlement to a comprehensive health service". Failure to reform, he suggested, would be "disastrous both in terms of the level of services and equity of access".[72]

Pat Rabbitte of the Workers' Party was, unusually, in agreement with the Progressive Democrat free-marketeers when he suggested that consultants' economic interest in providing superior services for private patients should be removed by channelling their salaries for treating public patients through the VHI, which would pay them fees for all patients[73] – effectively an insurance-based system of funding hospital care. Cormac MacNamara, now incoming president of the IMO and a member of the Commission on Health Funding, dissented from its majority view and argued for health care to be funded by earmarked taxation or insurance contributions to raise public consciousness of its cost.[74]

The Catholic bishops' Council for Social Welfare, which had promoted awareness of poverty and supported Corish's attempts to extend free hospital care in the 1970s, now proposed a comprehensive public health system, funded by social insurance, and an end to state subsidies to private care.[75] The Church did not pursue its advocacy of social reform with the same insistence as its strictures on sexual morality, even though the council's membership included Jeremiah Newman, the bishop of Limerick, who had advised Barry Desmond that he had a duty to follow his Church's guidance, when he was liberalising access to contraceptives.

The Church did not speak with a united voice, reflecting the conflict between its expressed belief in equity and its ownership of private hospitals. The conflict became overt when Gemma Byrne, a Sister of Mercy, chief executive of the Mater Private Hospital and a member of the Commission on Health Funding, dissented from the majority view, shared by the bishops' Council for Social Welfare, that VHI tax relief should be phased out.[76] Hers was a consistent stance for the owner of a private hospital. The Catholic bishops and the superiors of religious orders subsequently published a joint health care statement which argued that to deny "the principle of equity" was to take the view that "some lives are worth saving more than others", and, while defending the role of the Church-run voluntary hospitals, suggested that their owners "must be able to show that they are providing for the real needs of the poor".[77]

When the Progressive Democrats dropped their advocacy of an insurance-based system on entering government with Fianna Fáil in 1989, the prospects for such a fundamental change receded. It was of course also possible to achieve equity by reforming the existing tax-based system, the approach favoured by the Commission on Health Funding, by ICTU and apparently also by Labour, who supported "a comprehensive national health service" but in 1989 dropped any reference to funding from social insurance, advocated by the party in 1969 and later by Barry Desmond.[78] In government in the 1990s, neither Labour nor Fine Gael, whose focus was on administrative change,[79] would pursue equitable reform. Reforms adopted in 1991 by the Fianna Fáil/Progressive Democrat government were to become the template for the next decade.

Reform institutionalises inequity

In a formula agreed with the social partners, negotiated with the medical profession and backed by legislation, Haughey's government ostensibly addressed equity but in effect ensured that the two-tier system would survive for the next decade and into the next millennium. Not only did two-tier health care remain, but O'Hanlon also defended it in the Dáil:

> Deputies opposite have said that we have a two-tier system and suggested that this is a new development but it is not. That has been the position since the foundation of the State and this system, with its integrated mix of public and private care, has served the nation well.[80]

The government's reform package had three central components: extension of eligibility for free consultant care to the entire population; an attempt to control the public/private mix in hospitals by legislation and ministerial regulation; and a revision of the consultants' contract. There would, however, be no common waiting list. State subsidy of private care – in effect, state promotion of the two-tier system – would continue.

The measures to extend eligibility and control the public/private mix had been endorsed by the social partners, with whom the government had just agreed a new three-year programme, designed to further the still tentative process of economic recovery.[81] Although ICTU aspired to a comprehensive national health service free at the point of use, with free primary care as its priority,[82] it nonetheless accepted a programme which contained no reference to the extension of eligibility for free GP care and stated the government's commitment to "maintaining the position of private practice both within and outside the public hospital system".[83] With unemployment at 13.4 per cent and recent high emigration, trade unionists valued economic benefits for their members – lower taxes, job security, a wage deal – above equitable access to health care. A growing number of trade unionists were now VHI members, beneficiaries of preferential access whose interests ICTU represented in meetings with the insurance board.[84]

Although O'Hanlon had earlier expressed distaste for private patients' preferential access, his rationale for his defence of two-tier care was the traditional one: permitting private practice in the public system guaranteed better care for public patients. "Everybody receives the highest standard of medical and nursing skills in hospitals under the Irish health system."[85] His faith in the quality of care offered to public patients – by "the very best consultants"[86] – suggested ignorance of the medical profession's view, expressed by the IMA in 1975, that public patients were treated "less well" by junior doctors who "may not be competent",[87] a state of affairs which persisted into the 1990s, as a study group established by O'Hanlon would report in 1993.[88]

Permitting consultants private practice in the public system was not necessarily incompatible with introducing a common waiting list, which the government nonetheless rejected. O'Hanlon implied that it was the government's view and that of the social partners that hospital consultants could not be trusted to administer a common waiting list fairly. The National Economic and Social Council (NESC), a forum of the social partners, which supported a common waiting list, had questioned the effectiveness of a list administered by consultants with a financial incentive to admit private patients,[89] a reservation which provided an escape route for a government with little apparent desire to promote equitable access to care.

A common waiting list "could place the public patient at a disadvantage", O'Hanlon told the Dáil. The decision to admit a patient must always rest with the consultant, "who would have responsibility to draw up the common waiting list and decide where a patient should be placed on that list." Consequently, the government and the social partners believed "that the public patient would be best protected by ensuring that for non-emergency treatment, public beds are available exclusively to public patients".[90]

The Health (Amendment) Act 1991 provided for hospitals to designate a proportion of their beds as public and a proportion as private, subject to the Minister's approval.[91] While the legislation stipulated no explicit ratio, the split of beds in effect stayed close to its existing level – the proportion of designated private beds rose from 19 per cent in 1991 to 20 per cent in 1993[92] and remained at that level in 2002.[93] The so-called "80:20 split" became the policy tool to protect public patients' access to public hospitals. Long waiting lists for public patients would bear witness to its inefficacy and the proportion of private patients treated would far exceed 20 per cent.[94]

The new legislation obliged patients who opted for consultants' private care to pay for private accommodation. Formerly, a patient could jump public queues by opting to pay a consultant privately, while occupying a bed in a public ward. Consultants' private patients could theoretically fill every bed in the hospital which had not been occupied by an emergency case. The Commission on Health Funding had recommended that private patients should be limited to private beds, for which they should pay the full cost, but crucially had intended that a common waiting list would ensure patients were treated according to need, with public patients, if necessary, accommodated in private beds.[95] By omitting a common waiting list, the government's legislation was providing private patients with designated private beds, which they could occupy even if public patients were in greater medical need. It offered public patients equitable access to public beds rather than equitable access to care.

This unsatisfactory attempt to address the two-tier system reflected the Minister's consumerist philosophy of health care, his belief in the right of the individual (who could afford it) to purchase superior health care, so that public and private medicine should continue to co-exist in the public system. "I believe in Ireland that if people want to pay for their own medical treatment out of their own disposable income, that is their right," he later elaborated. It followed that private patients had a right to buy faster access, provided their bed was a private bed. "If people want to pay for faster access, as long as they are not impinging on public patients, well then I don't have a problem with that."[96]

Although he was notionally extending eligibility for free professional treatment to the entire population, O'Hanlon openly admitted that he did not expect this to reduce the demand for private medicine.[97] He argued that increased demand for private care could be met by expanding the number of private beds in public hospitals, which would be "self-financing".[98] This logic collapsed in the real world of the public/private mix because private patients were not charged the full cost of their care. Private beds remained a state-subsidised vehicle for queue-jumping by private patients.

O'Hanlon's philosophy of health care as a commodity, apparently shared by his cabinet colleagues, left no room for the egalitarian notion that consultants and public hospitals might receive the same payment for each patient to remove any motivation for discrimination. If, as he believed, private patients must be allowed the right to purchase superior care, then there was a certain inevitability about his defeatist view of consultants' behaviour: that they would either manipulate a common waiting list to favour their fee-paying patients or, if they could not do so, would absent themselves to treat those patients elsewhere.

The Minister's most astute critic was Fine Gael's health spokesman, Richard Bruton, who pointed out that the legislation never mentioned equity. While it provided for the identification of public and private beds, it did not provide for fair access or "equal waiting times".

"We will now have private waiting lists and public waiting lists. The Minister is institutionalising queue-jumping. We will live to regret this move," Bruton prophetically charged. "The Minister is enshrining in our system a permanent separation, a fast lane for those who can afford and a slow lane for those who cannot."[99]

For the next decade, the policing of bed designations would absorb administrative and research energies and distract from the issue of equity. There would remain two waiting lists, one fast, one very much slower – and this was the intent of the 1991 legislation. Implicit in O'Hanlon's speeches was this rationale: the public/private mix was best for public patients because it retained the best consultants in public hospitals; to retain them they must be permitted private practice; private patients would only pay private fees if they gained faster access; ergo faster access must continue. Only later did he append the more telling motive – private patients had a right to buy faster access.

O'Hanlon and Bruton had a brief exchange that revealed the Alice-in-Wonderland nature of a logic which could equate two-track access with equity. The Minister was explaining that a patient who paid to see a consultant privately for an outpatient consultation, and then opted to be treated as a public patient, would be allowed no advantage over a public patient awaiting an outpatient consultation. He was unwilling to recognise the queue-jumping which payment of the fee had achieved.

O'Hanlon: "His place on the waiting list will be the same as if he had waited for a public consultation at the out-patient department ..."

Bruton: "That is nonsense."

O'Hanlon: "That is the way it is going to be."

Bruton: "That does not make it right."

O'Hanlon: "It does make it right. He will have the same place in the queue as if he had waited for the public appointment."

Bruton: "That is not possible because the other person is not even in the queue yet."[100]

Haughey and the consultants' common contract – round two

The final act of this drama occurred off-stage in negotiations with the medical organisations on a revised contract for consultants. Consultants now faced the extension of their services free to the entire population, a *fait accompli* which had been agreed with the social partners and could potentially remove their entire private fee income. There could be no more eloquent evidence of the growth of private medicine and the decline of the public system than consultants' relatively supine attitude to this extension of eligibility, compared to their trenchant opposition to Brendan Corish's free hospitalisation scheme in the 1970s – a stance which the Department had anticipated would remain equally strong in the 1980s.[101] With a guaranteed right to private practice on and off the hospital site and with the public signing up for private insurance in increasing numbers every year, there was now no risk that they would become salaried servants of the state. Indeed, a subsequent review of consultants' pay would conclude that there was "no justification for the payment of compensation" to consultants for the extension of eligibility, since no evidence was available that it had affected private practice income.[102]

Although the IHCA walked out of negotiations on this issue, this was purely in protest that they had not shared the inside track with the IMO, who, as members of ICTU, had been aware that universal eligibility was to be included in the impending social partnership agreement. The IHCA returned to the negotiating table, taking the view, according to Finbarr Fitzpatrick, that "at the end of the day, the government of the day decides health policy and within that, health entitlements. We couldn't negate or turn back the decision with regard to eligibility."[103]

The real battle in the negotiations was over the Department's desire to tighten up the terms of the consultants' contract. A report on consultants' pay, from a review body chaired by the senior counsel, Dermot Gleeson, had recommended that the contract provide for oversight of the mix of public and private patients, to ensure that admissions were governed by medical need. If a hospital authority thought it necessary, facilities for consultants' non-urgent private patients should be limited or their right to off-site private practice withdrawn. Some consultants should become "medical managers", with "a critical role to play in reviewing with individual consultants the impact of private practice on their public commitment". Although the review body was "not concerned with ideological questions as to the desirability or otherwise of private practice", it observed that the practical integration of public and private medicine was "fraught with all kinds of complications"[104] and there was "confusion as to the extent of the commitment" required of consultants.[105]

The Department of Health's vehicle to make consultants more accountable to hospital managements was to be the introduction of "practice plans". In place of the original contract's assurance that "it is not intended that there should be exact measurement of the time spent by you discharging your contract",[106] the revised contract would provide for a plan to be negotiated between individual consultants and their employers that included their projected activity and scheduled time commitment.[107] The negotiation would involve a review of the previous year's activity: the number of patients treated, their length of stay, the number of patients on the waiting list, the notional time it would take to clear the list, the number of public and fee-paying patients and "variations in the nature or extent of a consultant's work as between his public and private practices".[108] Although the practice plans offered a means to control consultants' private practice, the contract did not state that their salaried hours should be devoted to public patients and contained a revealing omission: unlike its predecessor, it did not state that medical need should govern admissions to public hospitals. Here was confirmation that this was not the intent of the new system of bed designation, despite the recommendations of Gleeson and the Commission.

The IHCA greeted the proposed contract with distaste, insisting that it threatened clinical independence.[109] O'Hanlon responded hotly that this was "a gross distortion" of his position. "The rights of a consultant to clinical independence in the treatment of individual patients is explicitly guaranteed and strengthened in the proposals." The IMO's chief executive, Michael McCann, said the IHCA's assertion was "an absolute, utter and bloody lie".[110] Relations between the rival organisations were strained. Cormac MacNamara, then IMO president, regarded the IHCA as "passengers, who sat in another room, shouting 'professional independence'".[111] The IHCA's Finbarr Fitzpatrick countered that MacNamara was "like a fish out of water, as the only GP present with consultants and professional negotiators".[112]

"On actual policy issues there was no real difference between the two bodies," MacNamara later observed.

> For those relying on the contract, it was essential that the terms were beneficial. For those whose incomes depended on private practice, flexibility to pursue private practice was a core value. It was shrouded with descriptions of threats to professional autonomy. There was never any real threat to the professional autonomy of doctors. The ongoing threat to all doctors is less resources. No administration has seriously sought to interfere with professional autonomy.[113]

The IHCA's defence of clinical independence did not extend to challenging the ethical codes appended to the contract by the owners of Catholic voluntary hospitals. The consultants would do battle with the state on their terms and conditions but not with their Catholic employers.

Practice plans were incorporated in the 1991 revised contract but five years later, a further review of consultants' pay reported that "almost no progress has been made with these plans", which had provoked "industrial confrontation".[114] Opinion would differ as to why the plans had failed. O'Hanlon attributed it to the nature of hospital management:

"Clinical independence of the doctor is obviously very important but, if you apply that to its logical end, the consultant decides what patient goes in, how long the patient stays, what procedures are adopted for the patient. Effectively they are managing."[115] George McNeice, the IMO's chief executive from 1992, maintained the plans "were allowed to die quietly by the management side" because, if consultants produced plans, they could itemise their requirements for beds and staff "and management would have to fund all those, so management never wanted to pursue them".[116]

The failure of the plans reflected an inconsistency at the heart of state policy on private practice: while the Department wanted to police the public/private mix, it also wanted consultants to continue treating private patients, so that hospitals might earn income from private charges, and, at the highest level, the government believed in private patients' right to purchase superior care. Hospital managers were aware of the *realpolitik*: that the political will did not exist to confront hospital consultants on the issue of how their working practices impinged on the care of public patients. The contradictions in the state's position were exposed later in the 1990s, when the state withdrew the option of a full-time, salaried post for consultants who wanted an exclusive commitment to a public hospital. This had been introduced in the 1991 contract, on the recommendation of the Gleeson review. Some consultants had sought it because they had either little opportunity for private practice, or wanted to devote more time to research or teaching, or wished "to concentrate on the public health care services".[117] The post was dropped in 1997 because of "the new emphasis within public hospitals on private beds as a source of additional revenue".[118] This was the climate in which practice plans failed.

In the Dáil, Richard Bruton maintained that, had the consultants' terms of employment been regulated to the degree that Gleeson recommended, then consultants could have been trusted to administer a common waiting list.[119] He proposed an amendment to "state clearly that the basis of allocation between public and private beds is to ensure fair waiting times between the two".[120] For a government who believed that hospitals should sell preferential access, which patients had a right to buy, such an amendment made no sense.

From the 1987 cutbacks to the institutionalisation of two-tier access to public hospitals in 1991, this four-year period determined the shape of the health service for the next decade. Despite wide-ranging debate about reform, primary care would remain undeveloped and inaccessible and public hospitals would afford preferential access to private patients. Fianna Fáil had become the voice and the vehicle for this influential and growing minority, whose "right" to spend their income on private care, expressed by Rory O'Hanlon, would now be defended by the state, while public patients bore the brunt of the extraordinary cutbacks in public health spending. This catch-all party had so turned its back on its past that it had become the defender of privileged access. Despite the forensic dissection of Fianna Fáil's approach by Fine Gael's Richard Bruton, his party offered no coherent alternative, while Labour had become more focused on the effect of the cutbacks than the inequity of the new system. Consequently, these parties were ill-prepared to dismantle this new edifice of privilege when they found themselves in government and at the helm in Health during the 1990s.

6

NO BEDS IN THE BOOM

"In negotiations with the medical profession, it was always seen that you couldn't touch private practice."

— *Department of Health official.*

"The government ... really required the public system to be inferior. Why else, if it was first rate, would people pay for a private system?"

— *Labour Minister, Brendan Howlin.*

Two-tier hospital care remained unassailed in the 1990s, despite the participation in government of all major and some minor political parties. Although Fianna Fáil, Fine Gael and Labour each had incumbent Ministers in the Department of Health, the system of preferential access for private patients, institutionalised in 1991, survived to be incorporated into the 2001 health strategy of a further Fianna Fáil/Progressive Democrat government. The desirability of maintaining a mixed system of public and private care in public hospitals became a sacred cow of official policy, supported by political consensus. Access to primary care worsened since rising incomes left fewer people eligible for medical cards – 31 per cent of the population in 2000 compared to 35 per cent in 1990.

This heady decade of economic recovery and progress towards peace in the North saw an explosion of creativity and enterprise, as the beneficiaries of free secondary education reached their prime. Multinational corporations, particularly from the US, were attracted to Ireland by low corporate taxes, the completion of the EU single market and the availability of a youthful, skilled labour force. Per capita national income rose from two-thirds of the EU average in 1990 to exceed it in 2001.[1] Emigration reversed, unemployment fell, employment grew astonishingly, by over 50 per cent between 1991 and 2002, and the population increased by 11 per cent.[2]

Yet the number of acute hospital beds remained virtually static from 1993 to 2001. Only slowly through the 1990s did public health spending climb back from its nadir – 57 per cent of the EU per capita average in 1989. While elsewhere in Europe, trade unions had achieved the development of the welfare state as a return for wage moderation, Ireland's social partnership agreements delivered reduced personal taxation instead[3] and, despite trade union militancy about health professionals' pay and conditions, overlooked the needs of the health service. Not until 2001, when the legacy of neglect had begun to impinge on popular and political consciousness, did public health spending reach and exceed the EU average.[4]

The Department of Health had scarcely recovered from the trauma of the cutbacks, when it became engulfed in the scandals of infection by blood products, which diverted policy-makers' attention from the overstressed and inequitable system. The Catholic Church's reforming voice on social issues was disregarded, while revelations about clerical sexual abuse undermined its authority and its efforts to impose Catholic morality. Despite declining numbers and influence, Catholic religious retained their ethical hold in the major voluntary hospitals, their final redoubt in a state which had embraced secular mores.

In a decade of shifting coalitions, Fianna Fáil refined its chameleon qualities, coalescing with Labour on the left, following the Progressive Democrats on the right and only ceded power for three years to the Rainbow coalition of Fine Gael, Labour and Democratic Left. In 1997, Fianna Fáil re-entered coalition with the Progressive Democrats to form a minority government with the support of independents. In 2002, this coalition was the first government to be re-elected since 1969, when both parties gained seats and together commanded a majority.

Overlapping coalitions and the durable social partnership consensus blurred ideological differences and buried the issue of health care reform, which a shaken Department of Health seemed incapable of championing. Not until two years before the general election of 2002 did this silent issue re-emerge in a renewed explosion of debate.

Cross-party acceptance of the two-tier system

Between 1991 and 2002 every Minister for Health accepted the two-tier system of hospital bed designation. O'Hanlon was succeeded briefly by

Mary O'Rourke in 1991 and, in 1992, by John O'Connell – appointed by the new Taoiseach, Albert Reynolds, after allegations of corruption finally provoked Haughey's resignation. The 62-year-old O'Connell lasted under a year in the ministry, appointment to which had been his lifelong ambition. A general practitioner and self-made man, O'Connell had survived an impoverished childhood to become the wealthy founder and publisher of the *Irish Medical Times*. He was a political maverick, a former Labour Party TD who left following an internal row and joined Fianna Fáil. Had O'Connell achieved his ambition earlier in his career, and as a member of the Labour Party, he might have pursued radical reform. "I would have taken it on like a bloody crusade," he reportedly said when, to his chagrin, the Health portfolio went to Labour leader, Brendan Corish, in 1973.[5] Now, nearly 20 years later, he promised much but delivered little.

O'Connell's tenure as Minister ended following the 1992 general election, which was dominated by economic concerns – a currency crisis and persistent high unemployment[6] — although 80 per cent of the electorate considered health a "very important" political issue.[7] Only Democratic Left, which had evolved from the Workers' Party, campaigned for comprehensive health care and an end to discrimination between public and private patients on waiting lists.[8] Labour's approach was as anodyne as the other major parties'. The party abandoned its earlier advocacy of a comprehensive national health service, offered no blueprint for reform and warned that "'tax and spend' policies will not solve our problems now".[9]

In the aftermath of the Haughey years, Labour didn't need to advocate radical health care reform to more than double its representation. Floating voters supported Dick Spring, the Labour leader and outstanding parliamentary critic of the Haughey regime, who then brought Labour into coalition with Fianna Fáil. The new Minister for Health was Labour's Brendan Howlin, whose father had been Brendan Corish's local director of elections. Short, bearded, a 36-year-old former teacher and adept debater, "Wexford's cherub with the iron fist"[10] had acquired a reputation for toughness in local politics. He appointed Tim Collins, a militant leader of the junior doctors' 1987 strike, as his adviser.

Howlin accepted in its entirety the two-tier system of access institutionalised in 1991. He published a health strategy, *Shaping a Healthier Future*, in 1994 which stated the government's commitment "to maintaining the position of private practice within the well established public/private mix".[11] Equitable access would be protected by the designation of public and private beds, "close monitoring" of accessibility and undefined "remedial action where necessary".[12] The formula determined in 1991 would remain, with all its shortcomings. Furthermore, the hitherto implicit government desire to promote private practice was now openly expressed policy. The strategy argued if "the market for private practice is to be sustained, it is essential that the current level of voluntary health insurance coverage is maintained".[13] Obliged by an EU directive to open the private health insurance market to competition, the Department of Health had now apparently developed a greater interest in maintaining a healthy market for insurance, than in considering how that market was distorting access to health care.[14] Paradoxically, the European states which insisted on this free competition had quite different health systems in which insurance was generally not a route to privileged access.

Although he came from a party that had supported a comprehensive national health service and would later, following its merger with Democratic Left, advocate compulsory health insurance, Howlin became in effect a proponent of Fianna Fáil health care policy. The programme for government, agreed between Fianna Fáil and Labour, never once mentioned equity in health care nor referred to health in its principal objectives, which were overridingly economic.[15] Against a backdrop of international recession and currency crisis, "you couldn't go in and start afresh" with health care reform, Howlin believed. In truth, he did not appreciate the need for reform.

"Prior to going into office, I never had thought out a structured way to abolish the public/private clash," he later confessed.

> I actually intrinsically didn't understand how incompatible their existence was with absolute equity. I was content to feel that we could provide a first class public health system, without realising that if we did that, there would be no reasons for sustaining a private system.[16]

Howlin worked energetically to improve public health care in his 22 months in office. He introduced a waiting list initiative that, by negotiating with hospitals and paying their staff to work overtime, cut the number of public patients waiting for care by 38 per cent, from over 40,000 to under 25,000, in six months. When some specialists proved resistant to this push, the Minister responded by chartering a helicopter to fly patients from Cork to the Royal Victoria Hospital in Belfast. Howlin saw the initiative as short term. "We needed a parallel permanent increase in capacity." The initiative remained; the capacity did not materialise.

Public waiting lists, he came to see, reflected the "constant pressure for the public system to be less than the best":

> The government wanted a chunk of the population – 30 per cent or thereabouts – to pay for private health insurance but, in order for that to happen, they really required the public system to be inferior. Why else, if it was first rate, would people pay for a private system?[17]

His strategy launched a four-year action plan with precise targets to reduce mortality in areas such as cardio-vascular disease and cancer but lacked a framework for implementation. It adopted equity, quality and accountability as key principles and, while its failure to deliver equity was an inevitable consequence of its acceptance of the 1991 bed designation formula, it also failed to achieve clinical accountability, still "almost non-existent" in 2001, according to a subsequent critique.[18]

After the collapse of the Fianna Fáil/Labour government in 1994, the Rainbow coalition endorsed Howlin's strategy in its programme for government.[19] With 37 Labour and Democratic Left deputies to Fine Gael's 45, this was nominally the most left-wing government in the history of the state but radical health care reform did not rank among its priorities. Although the new Taoiseach, Fine Gael's John Bruton, had formerly spoken of a need to "abolish the distinction between public and private patients",[20] and his brother Richard had so ably analysed the shortcomings of the 1991 Health Act, the government was committed to perpetuating the two-tier system, "a fundamental plank" of the Howlin strategy, as understood by the new Minister for Health, Michael Noonan of Fine Gael.[21] Noonan, like Howlin, believed that the primary problem of the public health service was under-resourcing and, furthermore, that maintaining private practice would raise more resources for health because the insured "would pay their way", a popular misconception, which failed to recognise the degree of state subsidy for private care and the fractional contribution of insurance to the overall health budget.[22] Later he too became an out-of-office convert to reform, when he observed how the health system failed to respond to increased investment. As leader of Fine Gael, he sought an end to the "outrageous form of apartheid in our two-tier health service".[23]

Noonan was a particularly embattled Minister for Health, whose achievements were eclipsed by his handling of the hepatitis C scandal. Intelligent, with an acerbic wit, his flat Limerick accent a mimic's delight, this schoolteacher and experienced former Minister found Health a "rough ride".[24] As effectively the first Fine Gael Minister for

Health for nearly 40 years, he had the traditional Fine Gael suspicion that the civil service served Fianna Fáil and he complained that the Department was resistant to new ideas.[25] He won respect for his successful introduction of legislation on abortion information, reformed access to sterilisation and contraception, managed to avert a nurses' strike and initiated a national cancer strategy.

The continuity in health policy remained unbroken when Fianna Fáil returned in 1997 in coalition with the Progressive Democrats. Fianna Fáil's Brian Cowen published a White Paper on private health insurance in 1999, which made clear that, despite "drawbacks to the mixed model of care delivery",[26] the public/private mix would stay, as would the system of bed designation. Private practice provided an "additional income stream" to public hospitals.[27] "Concerns about equity" would be addressed by "targeted initiatives" such as "more rigorous enforcement by hospital management of the bed designation arrangements" and of "the extent of private practice by individual doctors".[28] The White Paper showed some appreciation of the degree of state subsidy for private care, proposing that economic pricing of private beds in public hospitals should be introduced over five to seven years, but tax relief on insurance premiums, reduced by the previous government, would continue.[29] A sequel to the earlier EU-driven deregulation of the private insurance market, the White Paper proposed that the status of the VHI should be changed to increase its commercial freedom and enable third-party investment in the company, or privatisation "if deemed desirable".[30]

Politics was now dominated by the elusive leadership of the Teflon Taoiseach, Bertie Ahern. From 1997 to 2002, Ahern presided over a booming economy, inflated by tax cuts introduced by his increasingly self-congratulatory government. Health slid into further crisis until its re-emergence as an issue of pressing public interest forced the government to publish a new health strategy just six months before the end of its term. Only 7 per cent of the electorate had considered health one of the main issues in the 1997 general election.[31] Unemployment of over 10 per cent was then of greater concern. Democratic Left was alone in committing itself to the eventual aim of providing free health care for the entire population.[32] The Labour Party, which again endorsed the Howlin strategy,[33] was the notable casualty of the election. Political commentators concluded that voters had objected to its coalition with Fianna Fáil, but Labour's move to the centre, not least on health policy, may well have contributed to its loss of appeal.

In the new coalition's programme for government, health did not rate in a list of "Seven Key Concerns of the Irish people".[34] Fianna Fáil had wooed the electorate with promises of a tax-cutting bonanza, while public spending should be tightly controlled – leaving little scope to invest in hospital beds or staff.[35] Brian Cowen, as Minister for Health from 1997 to 2000, described his new brief as "Angola" because it was littered with land-mines, on which an unsuspecting Minister might tread. This burly, aggressive former solicitor, already an experienced Minister at 37, decided that discretion was the better part of valour after Noonan's purgatory and disappeared into his department. When he gave his first major interview 17 months later, he explained, "Health needed to catch its breath." Challenged with the popular perception that he could not wait to get out, he responded "That's crap, nonsense. I'm working hard ... I love the job ... The idea that we are skulking and sulking around about jobs is ridiculous."[36]

Cowen did not court popularity. Prior to his White Paper's publication, he announced increased charges for private patients in public hospitals, arguing against subsidised private health care "as a matter of social justice", when confronted by Fine Gael's Alan Shatter.[37] Shatter's defence of this subsidy was inconsistent with his colleague Richard Bruton's earlier assault on two-tier medicine, as indeed Cowen's concern for social justice was incompatible with his endorsement of continued two-tier access: familiar contradictions in a politics dominated by two catch-all parties, whose ostentatious disavowal of ideology and desire to attract voters with competing interests – private and public patients – made consistency a challenge.

The continuity in health policy during the 1990s was reflected not just in the parties' stances on two-tier access and the development of the private insurance market but also in their approach to health administration and the consultants' contract. The Eastern Regional Health Authority (ERHA) was established under Cowen in 1999 to integrate the administration of services in the east and bring the dominant voluntary hospitals under greater state control.[38] This had been recommended in 1991, promised in Howlin's 1994 strategy[39] and pursued by a taskforce under Noonan. The ERHA differed from the health boards: it commissioned but did not deliver care and was statutorily required to monitor and evaluate services.

Negotiations on a further revision of the consultants' contract began under Noonan and concluded early in Cowen's term. The option of a public-only contract was removed, although 90 out of 1,064 consultants had availed of it in 1996. This reflected the recommendation of the latest review group on consultants' pay, chaired by financier and former civil servant Michael Buckley, which found the public-only contract incompatible with "the new emphasis within public hospitals on private beds as a source of additional revenue".[40] This was a critical development. While consultants had in the past fought for private practice rights when threatened by state medicine, now consultants who wished to eschew those rights were to be denied the opportunity of a full-time commitment to the public sector because of the belief, in the Department and the Rainbow government, that two-tier access and the fees it generated were essential to the maintenance of the system. Both the IMO and IHCA supported the option of a public-only contract and subsequently lobbied for its restoration.

A half-century after officials in Health had proposed the goal of a free national health service for all, their successors now recited the "public/private mix" like a "mantra", according to a dissenter. "In negotiations with the medical profession, it was always seen that you couldn't touch private practice." Not only could you not touch it but, it seems, the Department now wished to impose it, in line with the policy enunciated in the Howlin strategy of support for "the market for private practice" and private health insurance, which virtually everyone of influence now purchased.

The Department attempted to reconcile this enhanced interest in private practice with a concern that consultants should not pursue it "at the expense of, or neglect of, their commitments to public patients", the Buckley review recorded. The Department believed this could be achieved by controlling the number of designated private beds "and ensuring that unacceptably long waiting times for consultation or treatment in the public system were not used to generate private practice". The review group was openly sceptical – "We are not entirely convinced of the merits of the current system" – but recommended its continuation since it had been "agreed by all parties in 1991" and was still supported by both the Department and the IHCA.[41] The Department abandoned its unimplemented practice plans but proposed that consultants on public contracts should inform hospital management of their whereabouts when not in the hospital, which provoked an IHCA walk-out. Peter Kelly, a consultant pathologist who chaired the IHCA's negotiating committee, said such demands were "intrusive, oppressive and clearly an interference with an individual's right to privacy". He said there was no evidence consultants were not fulfilling their contracts and the majority of consultants would be willing to forgo pay rises rather than accept such working conditions.[42]

The medical organisations flexed their muscles to effect during these negotiations. The IHCA had rejected the Buckley pay proposals[43] and, while not threatening to strike, later suggested that, in the event of an unsatisfactory outcome, consultants would consider withdrawing their cooperation with hospital policy-making and administration, which would result in administrative and planning chaos.[44] The IMO was prepared to threaten a consultants' strike. Industrial action could be "on the agenda" if negotiations were unsatisfactory, warned its president, Hugh Bredin.[45] "It won't be of benefit to the Minister, politically or otherwise, particularly with an election coming up, to have senior medics in the country's hospitals frustrated and unhappy," Finbarr Fitzpatrick warned Noonan.[46]

In the contract agreed with Cowen, consultants were required to give advance notice in writing of planned absences and provide a weekly agreed schedule. The contract stipulated that the proportion of a consultant's on-site practice accounted for by private patients should reflect the proportion of designated private beds in the hospital but still did not require that the consultants' state-salaried hours should be devoted to public patients.[47] Its provisions to balance the interests of public and private patients were less precise than the abandoned practice plans and would prove equally ineffective in ensuring equitable access. The contract was a victory for the IHCA and, like its predecessors, would soon provoke critical review. Within months, Cowen established a forum on medical manpower to address emigration by young doctors, which eventually exposed the issue of how hospital doctors worked to much wider scrutiny.

The cross-party acceptance of the two-tier system was shared and endorsed by the powerful social partnership institutions for much of the 1990s.[48] Although ICTU continued to support free health care[49] and equal access,[50] pursuit of health system reform gave way to a more sectional defence of the interests of health care workers. "It was a much narrower agenda because pay and conditions became intolerable. It is very hard to argue for everyone to come into a system if you know that the system can't take it," a trade union negotiator of the period recalled.[51] By 2000, there had been 12 industrial disputes in the health service in 4 years, including the first national nurses' strike, which lasted 9 days in 1999 and secured significant improvement in pay and conditions. A year earlier, Cowen had admitted that there was a shortage of nurses[52] and a Commission on Nursing had urged action on outstanding pay issues, recognition of nurses' growing professionalism and the development of a more formal career path with greater promotional opportunities.[53] When Labour Court conciliation failed to satisfy the nursing unions, they took to the picket line to general public support.

By 1996, social-partnership agreements had forgotten health completely. The Rainbow government negotiated an agreement in which access to health care did not merit a mention in an entire chapter on "action for greater social inclusion".[54] The National Economic and Social Council, the further voice of the social partners, shared this amnesia, although in 1993 it suggested a review of income eligibility for medical cards "to remove obstacles to rapid employment growth",[55] motivated by concern that denial of free health care to the low paid might deter the unemployed from seeking work, not that the low paid and their families might suffer untreated illness. Not until 2000, when the crisis in the health care system could no longer be ignored and voluntary groups were making their voices heard in negotiations, did partnership evince concern about medical card eligibility levels and hospital bed capacity.[56]

Peter Cassells, ICTU's secretary-general from 1987 to 2001, acknowledged that for trade unionists equitable access to health care had not arisen as a serious issue in partnership negotiations. Since many workers were VHI members, this would "obviously colour people's views". Trade unions pursued the interests of health care workers and extended eligibility for services, not equity. Patients and the general public were not represented in partnership.[57]

Health spending recovers – health crisis deepens

It would be hard to overstate the effect on Irish health care of the 1980s cutbacks. While Ireland was cutting its health spending, other countries were increasing theirs. An OECD review over the period 1980–1993 found that in Ireland the share of national income devoted to health had dropped by 23 per cent, when in 13 other OECD countries there had been a 24 per cent increase.[58]

Recovery was slow in the 1990s. NESC baldly concluded in 1990 that "it is difficult to make the case that overall increases in health expenditure are justified".[59] This ostrich-like consensus that Ireland could survive on little over half average European health spending took time to shift. Public current health spending rose in real terms[60] in every year of the decade although it took until 1997 before per capita health spending was restored to its 1980 level, relative to the EU, and not until 2001 did it exceed the EU average. Capital investment in health remained at a very low level in the early years of the decade and only began to climb significantly in 1994.[61] Although employment in the public health service rose each year, rapid expansion only began from

1999.[62] Symptomatic of the lowered ambitions for health care in the early 1990s was a study of nursing personnel, commissioned by the Department of Health in 1990, which concluded in its final report in 1995 that there was an over-supply of nurses and recommended a gradual reduction in the number of student places, even though from 1994 student nurses had begun to withdraw from ward duties to undertake degree courses.[63]

The Fianna Fáil/Progressive Democrat coalition, formed in 1989, increased public current health spending by an annual average of close to 5 per cent in real terms and spending on hospitals by over 6 per cent.[64] By 1992, per capita public health spending had climbed back to 72 per cent of the EU average compared to 57 per cent in 1989. However, the number of acute hospital beds continued to fall until 1993. The Fianna Fáil/Labour coalition in power for 1993 and 1994 increased real public current health spending by a somewhat lower annual average of 3.5 per cent and spending on hospitals by under 3 per cent on average. Howlin raised hospital charges but later ceased levying an outpatient charge on patients who had been referred to hospital by a GP. He secured a significant increase in capital investment in 1994, which Noonan rivalled in 1995, the first year of the Rainbow Coalition. This government increased current health spending by an average of over 4 per cent and hospital spending by close to 5 per cent on average, but most of this was achieved in its final, pre-election year. Both the Fianna Fáil/Labour and Rainbow coalitions reduced the number of funded training places for nurses so that, by 1997, 23 per cent fewer nurses were in training than in 1991.[65]

The 1997–2002 Fianna Fáil/Progressive Democrat government was a study in contrasts. Cowen began with a commitment to tight budgetary discipline, further reducing nurse training numbers in his first year, when the number of nurses employed in the health service also fell.[66] Although current health spending increased by nearly 7 per cent in real terms in 1998, the health boards complained of inadequate budgets. As the national finances improved, Cowen and his successor, Micheál Martin, oversaw very significant real increases in health spending and recruitment. Martin's 2001 health strategy then advocated massive sustained investment in health over a ten-year period.

Cowen presented an uncompromising face for his first year, when legislation to make health boards more accountable for delivering services within budget, which had been announced by Howlin[67] and introduced by Noonan,[68] came into full effect. By December 1998, as health boards attempted to live within budget, an estimated 800 beds were closed to patients.[69] Cowen received his party's backing for his insistence that "it's important these local issues are dealt with locally".[70] Rory O'Hanlon, now party chairman, expressed "the united view" of the parliamentary party "that it doesn't seem to make any difference how much money goes into the area".[71]

This scepticism about the efficacy of health spending reflected a widely shared failure to appreciate the depth of the cutbacks and the low base from which investment must build. As public concern about the health service grew, the government became persuaded of this case. In 1999, Cowen more than doubled the real increase in spending to nearly 14 per cent. Increases stayed in double digits for the rest of the government's term. Over the five years to 2002, current health spending increased in real terms by an annual average of over 12 per cent and spending on hospitals by over 10 per cent. By 2002, current health spending was 78 per cent above its 1997 level in real terms and spending on hospitals was 67 per cent up. Capital investment had doubled in real terms.

When, in 1998, Cowen admitted that there was a shortage of nurses, it had become apparent that student nurses' lessened availability on wards, combined with the reduction in training places and the competing attractions of the booming private sector, had dramatically reversed the traditional over-supply – particularly in Dublin, where the cost of living had soared.[72] By 2000, the government had increased the number of funded training places for nurses by over 50 per cent but, with health sector expansion, shortages persisted in 2002, despite overseas recruitment.[73]

In 1998, a report on the waiting list initiative recommended further study of hospital capacity as "a matter of urgency". Some hospitals were "either at or near full physical capacity" and Ireland's bed occupancy rates were the highest in the EU. Short-term solutions would not end waiting lists.[74] In 2001 the new ERHA concluded that the east needed an increase of one-third in its acute beds over the next ten years,[75] injecting a much-needed note of urgency into the official response to the health care crisis, which provoked the Department into a belated study of national bed needs. Not until the publication of the 2001 strategy and the looming 2002 general election would the government commit itself to increasing bed capacity.

Evidence of the overloaded hospital system was there to see. In January 1999, Liz McManus, the Democratic Left spokesperson on Health, warned that the Dublin hospitals were in crisis. "Every hospital in the Dublin area was full last night," she said, and the Minister had "virtually disappeared from view".[76] Little had changed when Cowen left Health a year later. In January 2000, a winter 'flu' epidemic swamped hospitals all over the state.[77] In January 2003, after the government had secured re-election with promises of thousands of new beds – which it then appeared unwilling to fund – hospitals again turned away patients. A "cold spell" always brought an increase in admissions, Micheál Martin explained.[78]

Looking younger than his 39 years, the fluent and likeable Martin had been an inspired appointment to replace the surly Cowen in the urgent task of convincing the electorate that the government could solve this crisis. A former teacher and Lord Mayor of Cork, he had been judged a success in his first ministerial appointment of Education. In the mid-1980s, when still a young local councillor, Martin had described himself as a social democrat, "left of centre in economic terms", and his motivation in politics as "a genuine desire to effect change in Irish society".[79]

Within days of Martin's appointment in January 2000, Liz McManus tabled a comprehensive Dáil motion drawing attention to the "crisis" in the hospitals. A former architect, novelist and Rainbow Minister of State, McManus had first been elected to the Dáil in 1992, an achievement which had eluded her husband, the general practitioner and former Workers' Party health spokesperson, John McManus. This political couple had been consistent advocates of equal access to state-funded care. In 1977, John McManus advocated a free GP and hospital service, an end to private beds in public hospitals and the payment of doctors by salary.[80] In 1994, Liz McManus supported the extension of free GP care to all by 2000 and "a shift toward equal access for private and public patients" to hospital care.[81] In 1998, she argued for access to hospital care based on need and funded "through either a universal insurance system, with those on low incomes being subsidised by the state, or else funded simply through direct taxation".[82]

Now speaking for the merged Labour and Democratic Left, she asked the Dáil to note "that the current two-tier system of medical care discriminates against those who are unable to pay for private cover" and to condemn "the fact that public patients with life-threatening conditions are left on waiting lists for long periods because they are unable to pay for private care". She called on the government to increase resources and staff levels, improve bed numbers and commit itself to "the introduction of a universal health insurance system which will ensure that access to health care is determined by medical need rather than ability to pay".[83]

Battle had been joined. The long silence of the 1990s on the two-tier system was finally over. For the next two years, until the general election of May 2002, the debate on the future of the health service would increasingly engage the interest of the electorate and draw in many new voices in demands for fundamental reform.

The 1990s was a period of stasis in health care reform. The acceptance of the 1991 formula of designation of public and private beds, with its illusory offering of equity, had silenced debate within and beyond the political system. Politicians and administrators complacently promoted the fiction that it was possible simultaneously to promote private health care as a source of funding for the public hospital system and to deliver equitable access. Only when the intoxicating economic recovery and growing health care spending failed to deliver adequate improvement in the system did an appreciation gradually grow that the reform options so summarily rejected in 1991 needed to be revisited. In health care, as in the broader economy, it became apparent that all the boats had not risen with the tide. And as the tide ebbed, inequities in income and in access to health care emerged once again from beneath the waterline.

7

THE POLITICS OF BLOOD

"The whole health care system is on trial."
– *Raymond Bradley, solicitor for the Irish Haemophilia Society.*

The scandal of the infection of large groups of patients – haemophiliacs, pregnant women and others – by contaminated blood products, while not unique to Ireland, became in Ireland a saga of immense complexity. Over a thousand people were infected, many suffered severe illness and many died, or may yet die, prematurely. Two tribunals of inquiry investigated the circumstances of their infection. The investigations extended as far back as 1975. Four Ministers for Health gave evidence to the tribunals. Further inquiries are anticipated. Many reputations suffered but no prosecutions followed.

By the 1990s, public disquiet about the health service was not confined to its underfunding or its inequity. The blood scandals provoked deep concern about the quality of care and encouraged further patients with unhappy experience of the health service to seek explanations and redress. The tribunals' investigations illustrated that cutbacks, negligence and lack of accountability had real – and tragic – human consequences. It became apparent that underfunding had contributed to the patients' infection and to inadequacies in the health service's subsequent response. Motivated by financial concerns, politicians resisted the victims' demands for justice and accountability.

This decade of stasis in health care reform was also a decade of reckoning for the health service. The tribunals' inquiries put the Department of Health under intense scrutiny from the mid-1990s, which while revealing the need for greater investment in and oversight of the services under investigation, necessarily distracted from the wider issues of reform. Having been obliged to administer the cutbacks of the late 1980s, the Department remained under pressure, further evidenced when the Ombudsman concluded, in a report on nursing home care, that there had been "maladministration" by the Department and the health boards in the 1990s.

The infection of pregnant women with hepatitis C

Brendan Howlin's political antagonists like to point out that he got out of Health just in time. On Thursday February 17th 1994, a deputation from the Blood Transfusion Service Board (BTSB) came to see the Minister. Howlin and his senior officials had just returned from assistant-secretary Gerry McCartney's funeral. It was to be, in the words of an official, "one of those shocking days".

The representatives of the BTSB explained that evidence had emerged that there was a possible link between their product Anti-D immunoglobulin and hepatitis C. On Monday February 21st 1994, the BTSB asked women who had received Anti-D to come for screening in case they had contracted hepatitis C from an infected donor.[1] By October, 55,000 women had been tested and over 1,000 had antibodies to hepatitis C. Howlin had decided on immediate publicity once he was informed of this emerging scandal. He also appointed an expert group chaired by Miriam Hederman O'Brien to investigate the events leading to the women's infection.

Because the coalition government collapsed in November 1994, the expert group reported to Michael Noonan of Fine Gael in January 1995. To Noonan fell the task of responding to what he himself described as "the greatest scandal" in public health since the foundation of the state.[2] Women infected with the virus had formed a lobby group called Positive Action. As evidence of how they had become infected began to emerge, they sought compensation for victims and demanded a full public inquiry. The Minister offered them a private no-fault tribunal that would provide speedy payments but would require a waiving of their rights to legal action against the state. "I always took the view that rather than analysing the past, we needed to look after the health care needs of the victims," he said later.[3]

However, for many of the victims compensation was not the central issue. They wanted explanations and they wanted accountability for what had happened to them. When a severely ill Donegal woman, Brigid McCole, courageously took a High Court action against the state, the

National Drugs Advisory Board (NDAB) and the BTSB, the state fought her every step of the way. Just days before her death from liver failure on October 2nd 1996, the BTSB finally admitted liability and negligence and apologised to her.[4] While offering to pay her compensation, the BTSB denied liability for aggravated damages and informed her that should she seek to pursue these and fail in her bid, the BTSB would seek an order for costs against her.[5] The day before she died, Brigid McCole agreed to settle. This protracted legal hounding of a dying woman by the state agency that had infected her would cause huge public outrage.

Noonan had received legal advice from the Attorney General, Dermot Gleeson, that, while the state was not liable in the case, the BTSB was. Noonan's successor, Brian Cowen, later challenged him as to why this advice had not been communicated to the BTSB so that "the State could have avoided much anguish for Mrs McCole and others".[6]

Noonan countered that the BTSB, although a state agency, was not under his control. He pointed out that, in an examination undertaken at Cowen's request of how the state and the BTSB's defence had been conducted, senior counsel, Fidelma Macken, had reached the view that "it would not have been permissible for the BTSB to have in fact abdicated its decision on how the case would be run to the Minister because 'this would likely jeopardise its indemnity entitlement under its insurance'".[7] However, Macken had added that if the state had acknowledged it would pay compensation on behalf of the BTSB, the issue of insurance would have been redundant and "the Minister could say that, as the paymaster, the Minister should have a say in when and how liability is admitted". This did not arise because the state was itself claiming indemnity from the BTSB.[8]

Speaking to the Dáil the day after Brigid McCole's death, Noonan had resisted demands for a judicial inquiry. He was apparently motivated by concern about the potential cost:

> I sat in this House when people shouted for a judicial inquiry to get to the bottom of the beef scandal. After £35 million of legal fees, did we get to the bottom of that matter? I suggest we are much further down the road in respect of this issue.[9]

Within a week, however, the Minister capitulated and announced the establishment of a judicial inquiry chaired by the High Court judge Tom Finlay. Noonan was struggling but he had yet to make his truly disastrous gaffe. In a statement to the Dáil on the McCole case on October 16th 1996, two weeks after Brigid McCole's death, he questioned her lawyers' handling of her case, as if the case had not been motivated by her own desire for justice and accountability. The Minister asked:

> Could her solicitors not, in selecting a test case from the hundreds of hepatitis C cases on their books, have selected a plaintiff in a better condition to sustain the stress of a High Court case? Was it in the interest of their client to attempt to run her case not only in the High Court, but also in the media and the Dáil simultaneously?[10]

A group of women from Positive Action were watching from the public gallery of the Dáil and walked out. In a nearby hotel, they drafted a statement demanding an apology or resignation. The Minister later "unreservedly" apologised. Noonan had started his statement in the Dáil by describing Brigid McCole's experiences as a "major personal tragedy" and her infection and that of others a "public health disaster" and a "scandal". These were not the statements which would be remembered. The Minister was roundly condemned and political commentators immediately foresaw that this issue would continue to haunt him. "The hepatitis C issue has seriously undermined the political career of Michael Noonan and created a wave of anger against the Coalition Government," wrote Denis Coghlan, chief political correspondent of *The Irish Times*.[11]

Noonan found a courageous defender in his government colleague Liz McManus of Democratic Left. Then Minister of State for Urban Renewal, McManus acknowledged that Noonan had been

> grossly insensitive to the feelings of hepatitis C victims. He is not the first man in this House to wound the feelings of women and, in the nature of human discourse between women and men, it is unlikely that he will be the last. He did wrong in what he said and he did right in apologising so swiftly and unreservedly.

However, she added, he should be judged by his actions:

> He has inherited a complex and as yet not fully told saga of damage and neglect. It extends back over 20 years and over the stewardship of many Ministers for Health. None of these Ministers can be held responsible for the tragedy. In meeting the needs of those so terribly affected the Minister has shown himself not just to be a good Minister but also a good man.[12]

Noonan was elected leader of Fine Gael in February 2001. The party considered him a better bet than John Bruton to lead it to victory in the next election. In January and February 2002, RTÉ television broadcast a dramatised account of the fight for justice of the women infected with hepatitis C. In the series *No Tears*, Noonan emerged as the "TV villain".[13] Even Mary Quinlan, who had followed Brigid McCole in suing the state, took issue with the portrayal of the former Minister as "a stage villain". The series, she said, portrayed Noonan as responsible for making all the decisions regarding the state's legal strategy in the McCole case. "I think he got bad legal advice."[14]

Fianna Fáil chose to run a presidential-style campaign in the May 2002 general election. Huge posters of the popular Bertie Ahern covered the country. Fine Gael did not manage its campaign particularly well but, had its politics been more convincing or its platform more engaging, with this dramatisation of Michael Noonan's handling of the hepatitis C scandal fresh in the minds of the voters, the Fine Gael leader was unlikely to emerge as the popular choice for Taoiseach. As the scale of Fine Gael's electoral collapse emerged, Noonan resigned from the leadership. Reflecting a month later on the election outcome, he would not accept that *No Tears* had been a factor. "It had an effect on my personal ratings but not on the election. Our canvassing reports and qualitative research did not pick it up."

This view was not generally shared. A political rival, who was personally well-disposed to Noonan, expressed the more common held view: "he was unelectable. *No Tears* really destroyed him. It was a killer blow. It made him a monster, which he is not."

Ironically, Fine Gael had polled well in the preceding election of June 1997, gaining in seats and votes, although the hepatitis C controversy was then an ongoing political issue. The Finlay Tribunal had conducted public hearings between December 1996 and February 1997 and had heard evidence not only from victims and from employees of the BTSB and NDAB but also from no less than 18 present and former officials of the Department of Health, from Brendan Howlin and from Michael Noonan. The Tribunal had reported on March 6th 1997 and had effectively supported Howlin and Noonan's handling of this crisis. In general, Finlay considered their actions "adequate and appropriate". Howlin and his department, he judged, should have acted more rapidly to ensure there was independent counselling available for the victims. They should have more closely supervised the BTSB's recall of the infected product once the scandal broke. And they should have agreed to the recommendation from a group of liver specialists about the criteria for treatment of infected women.[15] Noonan and the Department should have been quicker to introduce the legislation providing for health care for the victims.[16] With the exception of these criticisms, the Tribunal supported the two Ministers' actions.[17]

While the reverberations of this health scandal had significant political consequences, of much greater significance was the inescapable fact that over a thousand people had been infected with a debilitating, depressing and potentially fatal disease by an agency of the state. The Tribunal uncovered a history of negligence, although it did not use that term, which stretched back through decades of the administration of the health service. It found that the BTSB had breached its own standards for donors, "failed properly to react" to reports of infection in women who had received transfusions, failed to prevent infection by recalling blood products even when it knew that there was concern about contamination, had acted unethically in using a patient's plasma without her consent[18] and had been motivated in "wrongful acts" in part because of "a reluctance to admit the possibility of having been wrong".[19] When the existence of infection had been brought to its attention there had been "a total refusal to face the consequences"[20] apparently motivated by "a sort of vague and irresponsible hope that the problem might go away".[21]

The Tribunal named the officers of the BTSB whom it regarded as responsible. It also found that the National Drugs Advisory Board had failed in its obligations to inspect the BTSB. Ultimately, the Tribunal's scrutiny travelled up the chain of command and into the past to the era of Brendan Corish and found that

> in the period 1975 to 1994 successive Ministers for Health and the Department of Health failed adequately and appropriately to supervise the NDAB in the exercise of its functions concerning the licensing of the manufacture of products by the BTSB and the authorisation of products by the BTSB, in that they failed to provide the NDAB the appropriate resources for carrying out those functions.[22]

By pinpointing inadequate funding as key to this failure, the Tribunal by implication found that not only Ministers but also entire governments must share some responsibility for the scandal. Had sufficient funding been allocated for appropriate oversight of the BTSB, reactions of recipients of Anti-D in 1976 and 1977 to the contaminated product might have been revealed and further investigated, the Tribunal suggested.[23] The Department of Health had also been at fault for its slowness in giving permission for the introduction of screening for hepatitis C in blood donors when a reliable test became available in

1991, a responsibility which the Tribunal assigned to officials rather than the then Minister, Rory O'Hanlon.[24]

Shortly before the 1997 election, Brigid McCole's daughter Brid said that Michael Noonan should resign because of the state's legal strategy in her mother's case.[25] *The Irish Times* commented in a leader a few days later:

> To a certain extent, Mr Noonan has become the political victim of a situation which he inherited, a situation which was the responsibility of his predecessors in office. To a greater extent he has become the victim of a political parsimony which would try to protect the taxpayers' interests.

The Minister had responded with too little, too late but "it is doubtful that any other Minister for Health, from whichever political party, would have responded in any different manner."[26]

The infection of haemophiliacs with HIV and hepatitis C

The validity of the *Irish Times'* assessment was supported by the experience of haemophiliacs who had been infected with HIV, and who met even greater resistance than the women infected with hepatitis C to their efforts to seek redress from the state. The general election of 1989 had been provoked by the unwillingness of Charles Haughey's government to increase financial assistance to the infected haemophiliacs. Rory O'Hanlon had offered a mere £50,000 to the Irish Haemophilia Society (IHS) for counselling.[27] When Fianna Fáil was re-elected in a coalition with the Progressive Democrats, this new Haughey government eventually responded to the IHS's demand for £14.5 million compensation by paying £8 million on a no-fault basis in 1991. By then 18 of the 103 haemophiliacs whose infection had been certified in 1989 were reported to have died and a further 33 had developed full-blown AIDS.[28]

The Haughey government's approach to compensating the infected haemophiliacs had been a great deal more grudging but, in principle, was conducted on very similar lines to the Rainbow government's approach five years later to compensating the women who had received Anti-D. Although compensation was eventually wrung from the state, it had to be on a no-fault basis. In their case, the government was influenced by its mistaken belief that overseas pharmaceutical companies had produced all the infected products that the BTSB distributed, although the BTSB had been aware from 1986 that its own product might have contributed to infection. That the state nonetheless shared some responsibility, if not legal liability, for their infection was then an alien proposition.

With many of its members severely ill and dying, the IHS reluctantly accepted the 1991 compensation package. After the establishment of the Finlay Tribunal in 1996, the society unsuccessfully sought a broadening of the Tribunal's terms of reference to include the infection of haemophiliacs. Although it was granted limited representation at the Tribunal, the society eventually withdrew and sought an inquiry that would be specific to haemophiliacs. In January 1997, the Rainbow government agreed to establish a new tribunal. Following the change of government that year, it took a further two years before the Fianna Fáil/PD government appointed a Circuit Court judge, Alison Lindsay, to chair the Tribunal, which only opened in September 1999.

Whereas people with haemophilia and their families had first been most concerned about their infection with HIV, the potential consequences of infection with hepatitis C were now better understood and of growing concern. Of the estimated 400 people with haemophilia in Ireland in 1999, at least 217 had been infected with hepatitis C since the mid-1970s. During the 1980s, 104 people had been infected with HIV. In all, the Tribunal eventually estimated at least 252 people had been infected with either disease or both.[29] These two diseases had caused all but two of the 68 deaths among haemophiliacs over the 15 years before the establishment of the Tribunal. Most people had died from AIDS-related illnesses.[30]

The Tribunal heard harrowing evidence: how boys and men with this inherited disorder had been infected by blood transfusions, how many had suffered greatly and died from the consequent infections. This was the anticipated evidence. The unanticipated evidence was the disclosures of how the sufferers and their families had been treated: of the absence of counselling, the insensitivity of some hospital personnel, the refusal to allow relatives to see or touch the body of their loved one, which would be immediately sealed in a body bag, the unaccountable delays in informing parents of their sons' infection. One woman described hearing that her three sons had been infected with hepatitis C – four years after they had tested positive.[31]

It had been anticipated that once more the BTSB and its paymaster, the state, would be in the dock. It had not been anticipated that the entire health care system, the treatment of the most vulnerable patients by their carers, would be subject to such intense public scrutiny. "The whole health care system is on trial. It's about the way doctors deal with patients, about the way doctors ensure that patients understand the consequences of any diagnosis, about what support or counselling is put in place," argued Raymond Bradley, solicitor for the IHS.[32]

The Tribunal uncovered that whereas the majority of haemophiliacs had been infected by imported blood products distributed by the BTSB, in addition products made by the BTSB itself had been responsible for some infections. Although the BTSB had been alerted as early as 1986 that its own product might have caused infections,[33] it was "reluctant to acknowledge" this and the government remained unaware of it throughout its negotiations with the IHS in 1991. Consequently, as both Rory O'Hanlon and a former official of the Department of Health acknowledged, the government's decision to oppose compensation in the late 1980s and its 1991 negotiations had been informed by inaccurate and incomplete information about the extent of the state's responsibility for the infections.[34] Rory O'Hanlon told the Tribunal that had he known that Irish-made blood products had been responsible for infections, the government's approach to the Labour Party's 1989 motion calling for the establishment of a trust fund for haemophiliacs would have been different and the government might not have collapsed. He had discovered that he had given incorrect information to the Dáil and would now seek leave to correct the Dáil record.[35]

The Tribunal also established that whereas the Department of Health believed that from January 1st 1985 the BTSB was only distributing heat-treated products, which would therefore be HIV free,[36] in fact the BTSB continued to distribute non-heat-treated products until late that year and only withdrew old stock in mid-1986, a delay which caused the infection of a number of patients.[37] Barry Desmond told the Tribunal he was "appalled" that he had been given incorrect information, which led him to assure the Dáil in November 1985 that the BTSB had been making heat-treated blood products for haemophiliacs when in fact it was continuing to supply an untreated product. He said he had only learnt at the tribunal that he had given incorrect information to the Dáil.[38]

The Tribunal concluded that the Ministers could not be blamed for believing the information supplied to them by their civil servants.[39] How the Department had been misled remained an open question. The IHS continued to believe after the publication of the Tribunal's report that there had been "a deliberate cover up and some wilful misleading of the Department".[40]

Although accepting that the Department of Health might reasonably expect to rely on the BTSB's expertise, the Tribunal did not absolve the Department. While it recognised that the Department had been active in attempting to ensure the safety of blood products and had recommended the use of heat-treated products only, the Tribunal said that it should have pursued the BTSB to ensure that it was complying with this recommendation. In addition, the Department's failure to address structural weakness and staffing problems in the BTSB had made it very difficult for the blood service to respond to the risk of AIDS. The Department had been slow to respond to requests for counselling facilities and remiss in failing to ensure that patients were aware of the risks attached to the products with which they were being treated.[41]

Desmond and O'Hanlon were the two Ministers who had been at the helm of the health service during the worst cutbacks in health spending. If evidence were needed that the cutbacks had had real human consequences, the Tribunal supplied it. In the hospitals, there were insufficient haematologists to treat patients and insufficient social workers to counsel them. The BTSB was understaffed, badly structured, essentially relied on the sale of blood to break even, lacked funds for capital projects and, in the early 1980s was in financial crisis. When AIDS emerged as a threat in 1982 and 1983, the BTSB was ill-equipped to respond.[42] While the Tribunal did not accept that the BTSB's decisions about which products it supplied were compromised by commercial considerations,[43] the publication of its report did not allay all such suspicions, especially because a BTSB employee had been a founder shareholder in an importer of commercial blood products that were believed to have caused infection.[44]

Although the Lindsay report was widely criticised for failing to apportion blame as the Finlay report had done, its findings confirmed the earlier Tribunal's picture of negligence in the BTSB: its slowness in restricting its supply to heat-treated blood products; its slowness in checking whether earlier donations from an infected blood donor were infected;[45] the inadequacy of the measures it adopted to seek a source of blood which was free from hepatitis C.[46] After the report's publication, the state blood service apologised to haemophiliacs for the first time for their infection.[47]

While sympathetic to medical staff, who had been harshly criticised by many victims and their families, the Tribunal faulted the National Haemophilia Treatment Centre at St James's Hospital in Dublin for an "unacceptably long" delay in preparing a policy response to the risk of AIDS;[48] for not pursuing the BTSB more about the availability of heat-treated products;[49] for not acting faster in switching to such products;[50]

for not providing blood products safe from hepatitis C sufficiently early;[51] and for not keeping doctors in other hospitals informed of developments.[52] The delay in telling patients about their infection had been "unacceptable".[53] The Tribunal also judged that the centre's director, Professor Ian Temperley, had made a major contribution to services for haemophiliacs and at times carried "an almost impossible workload".[54]

When the Lindsay Tribunal reported in September 2002, 79 haemophiliacs had died from illnesses relating to their infection from blood products. It was already apparent that the story would not end there. The Tribunal's chairwoman had decided that she would not investigate the role of pharmaceutical companies whose products were responsible for more than 90 per cent of the infections. While the Minister for Health, Micheál Martin, made a commitment to holding an inquiry into the drug firms, the Minister for Justice was sceptical about its prospects for success.[55]

In March 2002, Micheál Martin was served with a writ from an infected haemophiliac.[56] The IHS planned to serve him with weekly writs to force the government to deliver on a commitment made in 1999 to overturn the 1991 compensation settlement, which the government had acknowledged as being unfair. The society's timing was good. The general election was imminent and, after the recent screening of *No Tears*, Fianna Fáil and the Progressive Democrats did not want the public to understand that Noonan's failings in 1996 had been eclipsed by their earlier treatment of the haemophiliacs. With only a few weeks to go to the election, legislation was rushed through the Dáil to extend access to the hepatitis C compensation Tribunal to haemophiliacs and their families. Compensation and reparation for 1,453 victims of hepatitis C infection had already totalled €370 million between 1996 and 2001[57] and, with victims also taking recourse to the courts, the eventual cost to the state was unquantifiable.[58]

In June 2002, the Minister was forced to announce still another inquiry into the affairs of the BTSB, now renamed as the Irish Blood Transfusion Service (IBTS). A blood donor who had tested positive for hepatitis C in 1991 but had not been informed of this until 1993 had initiated a suit for damages arising from that delay against the BTSB and the state. Up to 27 women and men were believed to have shared that donor's experience.[59]

Medicine in the dock

The hearings of the Lindsay Tribunal put the practice of medicine in the dock in an unprecedented way. The anger and distress of the victims of contaminated blood products and their surviving relatives at how they had been treated following their infection seemed to rival their distress about the infection itself. In a culture where doctors had been revered and largely unchallenged figures, the victims' and their families' demands for accountability were evidence of a significant cultural change. Other patients and their families followed in seeking redress for unhappy experiences of the health service. In 2001, 65 legal actions were taken by women who alleged that a consultant obstetrician had performed unnecessary hysterectomies after they had given birth by Caesarean section. The High Court upheld one woman's case in 2002.[60] A patients' advocacy group sought another judicial inquiry and compensation tribunal.[61]

"A Department under pressure"

As well as revealing shortcomings in the Department of Health, the investigation of the blood scandals placed enormous pressure on the Department in the later 1990s and partly explains this period of stasis, when the political parties' failure to seek a mandate for reform was matched by the Department's failure to generate new ideas. The tribunals' inquiries sapped the energies and divided the loyalties of this small department, which, in a climate of financial constraint and health union militancy, was attempting to meet growing demands for health and social services and to address hitherto neglected needs, such as the protection of children at risk and the care of the intellectually disabled. The Department also came under the critical eye of the Ombudsman, whose investigation of state subventions to nursing home care for the elderly disclosed how cutbacks and their aftermath not only contributed to the failure of the health service to respond adequately to the blood scandals but also had created enormous difficulties in other areas administered by the Department.

By the time the Lindsay Tribunal ceased hearing evidence, it had been sitting for two years and had heard 148 witnesses. It had delved back 20 years into the history of the state's health service and its administration. This had followed the shorter hearings of the Finlay Tribunal. The Department of Health had become engulfed in keeping abreast of the proceedings. Officials had disagreed in their evidence. Personal relations had become soured. The internal disarray was publicly aired in 1998 in a High Court action taken by an official who claimed she had been denied promised promotion because her evidence to the Finlay Tribunal about the Department's slowness in authorising screening for blood donors conflicted with the secretary general's account. The court did not accept that the failure to promote her had been motivated by malice.[62] The case had been pending for two years and senior officials were aligned on opposing sides. This did not make for a happy or productive atmosphere in the Department. "Affidavits were flying, lawyers were being briefed. It damaged the image of the Department," an official recalled. "The biggest casualty" was the Department's development of strategy. Although the Howlin strategy's action plan expired in 1997, its successor was not launched until 2001. "There was little or no work done on it until 2000."

In 2001 the Ombudsman found that "maladministration had occurred on a significant scale" when he pursued complaints from the public about the operation in the 1990s of a scheme of state support for elderly people requiring nursing home care.[63] He concluded that, despite the existence of a statutory right to long-stay care, in the 1990s health boards insisted on taking into account the income and means of an elderly person's children in determining the level of state support for their care. The Department was aware of this, he said, but although there were internal concerns about a possible legal challenge, it made regulations in September 1993 that had the practical effect of including children in the means test.

> Clearly, financial pressures played a large part in the decision eventually made. Nevertheless, the conclusion is unavoidable that the Department made a regulation in the knowledge that it was almost certainly invalid or, at least, highly unlikely to survive a legal challenge.[64]

The Department vigorously contested the Ombudsman's interpretation of events, rejecting in particular "the suggestion that it knowingly engaged in illegalities". It disputed the existence of a statutory right to long-stay care, arguing that eligibility for a service was not synonymous with entitlement and did not confer a legally enforceable right.[65] The Department insisted that there was a distinction between the intent of its regulations and how the health boards implemented them. It had made difficult decisions in the context of limited resources "at all times in good faith" and based on its understanding of the "legal parameters".[66] While recording the Department's objections, the Ombudsman nonetheless reached the "inescapable conclusion that the Department presided over a set of practices for a period of more than five years in the knowledge that these practices were legally indefensible". He added:

> With regard to mitigating circumstances, it has to be accepted that, as a result of the cutbacks of the 1980s and the rationalisation of the hospital

system, the Department could no longer deliver on the entitlements provided for in earlier legislation. In addition, serious funding constraints continued to apply ... What was done represented, in the eyes of the Department, a pragmatic response to a difficult situation; one, in which, in effect, the Department (along with the health boards) was expected to achieve a particular objective without being given the means to do so. The Department always had the option to declare that what was expected, viz. the creation of a nursing home subvention scheme, was simply not achievable.[67]

The Ombudsman found no evidence that the alternative of amending the legislation had been seriously discussed or that such an "unpalatable" option was put to any Minister. Department officials apparently took the view that implementing the scheme in a limited way would improve care without alarming the Department of Finance about the cost of a more comprehensive scheme. The Department began discussing how to regulate the subvention scheme from shortly after the Nursing Homes Act was passed in July 1990, when Rory O'Hanlon was Minister. The regulations came into force when Howlin was Minister and remained in force through Noonan's period and for over half of Cowen's ministry. Family assessment was finally discontinued in January 1999. In the dialogue between the Department of Finance and the Department of Health the "controllers" were talking to the "controlled" and their primary concern was financial damage limitation. "What seems to have been lacking from the dialogue is an acceptance that, increasingly, human rights, including economic and social rights, have to be addressed," the Ombudsman commented.[68]

Even when funding for health began to increase significantly from 1999, the Department remained beleaguered. In a review of customer service in the health care sector, presented to a committee of the Oireachtas in June 2001, the Ombudsman observed that Health "exhibits all the signs of a Department under pressure".[69] As the former secretary of a government department, Kevin Murphy was qualified to recognise such signs. Like many government departments, Health was by then suffering from severe under-staffing due to cutbacks in civil service recruitment in the earlier 1990s and its inability to recruit and retain staff in competition with the rewards on offer in the booming private sector. Later that year it was reported that 20 per cent of the Department's approved positions remained unfilled.[70]

The Department's slowness in the 1990s to confront the political establishment with the aftermath of the 1980s cuts and to calibrate the inability of the health service to meet the needs of Ireland's rising population reflected a deeper demoralisation, which appears to have taken until 2000 to lift. A seasoned health administrator observed: "in the Department of Education, after the 1980s cuts, they gradually rebuilt the pupil/teacher ratio over the next 10 years but in Health there was no rebuilding of acute capacity".

Irish society has yet to come to terms with the full implications of the blood scandals for the administration and funding of the health service, for the relationship between politicians and the people whom they represent, and the relationship between doctors and their most vulnerable patients. What greater failure of the health service could there be but that a state agency should have been the means of infecting large numbers of people with potentially fatal diseases and should have failed to act, even when this became apparent?

The victims' campaigns for accountability forced governments to a reluctant acceptance that the state shared responsibility, if not legal liability, for the actions of the BTSB. Underfunding had played a role in the inadequacy of the BTSB's response to the blood crises. The state had not done all it could to provide a safe supply of blood.

The human, political, medical and compensation cost of these infections has had some practical consequences. Patients with inherited blood disorders are now treated with genetically engineered products, so that Irish treatment "compares very favourably" with treatment in other states, according to the Lindsay report.[71] Such treatment is, however, "enormously expensive", as the Department of Health testified to an Oireachtas Committee, in one of its periodic attempts to explain health inflation.[72]

In the atmosphere of a tribunal of inquiry, the disclosure that concerns of cost have affected treatment sounds indefensible. Yet cost dictates quality of care throughout the health service. While health spending cannot expand infinitely, the need for better quality care, higher standards and greater accountability is inarguable. Until these are delivered, the next scandal will remain just around the corner.

8

Ethics, Ownership and the Catholic Church

"If the Catholic Church in Dublin wants a voluntary Catholic hospital, the Catholic people will have to want that and work it, because we won't be there."
– *Helena O'Donoghue of the Sisters of Mercy, owners of Dublin's Mater Hospital.*

At the end of the 20th century, the state continued to accord considerable influence to the Catholic Church in the running of voluntary but state-funded hospitals, although declining numbers forced religious orders to review their health care role. During the 1990s, the Church sought: to prevent liberal legislation in areas affecting sexuality, despite concerns about the threat of AIDS and the consequences of unplanned pregnancies; to prevent abortion in any circumstances; and to influence legislation on bioethics. The Medical Council became contested ground as conservatives and liberals fought to influence the code of professional ethics. While campaigning Church organisations remained advocates of equity in health care, they lost influence when the liberal tide within the Church receded.

Conflict was inevitable between an ageing hierarchy, selected by a conservative pope, and an increasingly youthful and heterodox society. Whereas, in the 1980s, the Catholic Church view was shared by a majority of the electorate in the referendums on abortion (1983) and divorce (1986), in the 1990s and afterwards, these victories were overturned, with the Church's stance defeated in subsequent referendums on abortion (1992 and 2002) and divorce (1995). By 2002, only 48 per cent of Irish Catholics attended Mass each week, compared to 91 per cent in 1973[1] – although in 1999 over 90 per cent of the population retained a religious affiliation, compared to as few as 60 per cent in some European countries.[2] The

124

number of religious fell from a peak of 30,000 in the mid-1960s[3] to 13,393 in 1999, of whom nearly half were retired and two-thirds over 60. There were 59 religious under the age of 29 working in Ireland in 1999.[4]

Despite the writing on the wall about lay alienation and falling vocations, the Catholic Church fought to retain its power. In religious-owned but state-funded voluntary hospitals, the orders sought means to ensure that the laity who replaced them would continue to restrict medical treatments to those considered permissible in Catholic ethics – efforts mirrored in the schools where they sought to ensure continued Catholic control after their departure.[5] Despite a backlash against clericalism provoked by the Church's mishandling of clerical paedophilia – manifest in majority support for the resignation of Cardinal Desmond Connell, Archbishop of Dublin, in 2002[6] – Ireland had yet to develop a political groundswell in support of systems of health care and education which respected the values and rights of non-observant Catholics, citizens of other denominations and those of no denomination. Even as Connell pondered his future, he remained president of the holding company which controlled Dublin's Mater Hospital, chairman of the board of Holles Street maternity hospital and chairman of the committee of management of Our Lady's Hospital for Sick Children in Crumlin, where a courageous challenger of his response to paedophilia had been abused by a Catholic chaplain when a 13-year-old patient in 1960.[7]

Fifty years before, in McQuaid's era, the Church was confident in its place as the provider of most of Irish education, much of its health care and many of its social services. Thousands of religious worked for little material gain, ploughing their salaries back into their orders or employing institutions. But behind the accepted face of a caring, albeit authoritarian institution, it was one of the unspoken realities of Irish life that the Catholic Church could also be cruel and violent. In the 1990s, victims of institutional violence and abuse by religious discovered their voice. As books, films and television programmes told their secret history, Ireland responded with guilt, grief and anger. Yet the state's failure to respond adequately to the social needs which it had formerly consigned to the Church, evidenced in inappropriately staffed childcare institutions and growing numbers of homeless, intimated that future generations might put the state in the dock in the Church's place.

AIDS, condoms, sterilisation and bioethics

It took three legislative attempts in the early 1990s before the sale of condoms ceased to be restricted. The retreat to conservatism within the

Church was evident in its reaction to proposals to liberalise Desmond's contraceptive legislation, advanced in 1991 by the Fianna Fáil/Progressive Democrat government of Charles Haughey. The hierarchy's spokesman, Joseph Duffy of Clogher, said that it was the duty of Catholic legislators to take the bishops' teaching into account when framing contraceptive legislation, a marked contrast to the view of the Catholic primate, Tomás Ó Fiaich, in 1977 that churchmen should not bring pressure to bear on legislators.[8] The hierarchy now contained a number of conservative papal appointees, notably Ó Fiaich's successor Cahal Daly in Armagh and Connell in Dublin.

Public health experts and campaigners wanted the Department of Health to advocate the use of condoms to prevent the transmission of AIDS but, under existing legislation, homosexual activity was criminalised and the sale of condoms was limited to over-18-year-olds in chemists and health care institutions. The Minister, Rory O'Hanlon, was perceived as a conservative Catholic.[9] Eventually, after the Irish Family Planning Association was fined for selling condoms in a record store, the Taoiseach, Charles Haughey, promised to amend the law.[10] In cabinet, he found that only two ministers supported reducing the age for purchase of condoms from 18 to 16[11] and both government parties were divided on the issue. The 74-year-old Catholic Cardinal Cahal Daly warned that to change the law would have "profound implications for the moral quality of life" in Ireland.[12]

O'Hanlon's 1991 Bill, which would have required health boards to regulate the sale of condoms, was not enacted and was eventually superceded by legislation introduced by John O'Connell which dropped this provision but retained a ban on vending machines and restricted the sale of condoms to over-16-year-olds.[13] Catholic reaction had now become relatively muted, perhaps reflecting recognition of the degree of popular support for legislative change. The hierarchy issued a statement only after the passage of the Act, which said that sexual intercourse outside marriage was sinful but "there are many things which are sinful and which the law cannot reasonably be expected to prohibit". Labour's Brendan Howlin brought this saga to an end with further legislation in 1993 that no longer defined condoms as contraceptives, permitted their sale from vending machines and their purchase at any age.[14] The Bill was passed without opposition in the Dáil the day after a spokesperson for the hierarchy had restated its response to O'Connell's Act.[15]

The Fianna Fáil Minister for Justice, Máire Geoghegan-Quinn introduced legislation to decriminalise homosexuality in 1992. The Labour Minister for Education, Niamh Breathnach, circumvented

Catholic opposition to introduce a Relationships and Sexuality Education (RSE) programme in schools in 1997 but did not make it compulsory. In 2000, nearly 60 per cent of post-primary schools had still not implemented the programme.[16] A Mid-Western Health Board survey of secondary schools in 2001 discovered that, within the previous three years, 31 of 41 schools had pregnant pupils.[17] Teenage mothers considered sex education inadequate, a study published in 2002 revealed.[18]

Due to the dominance of the Catholic voluntary hospitals in Dublin, in the 1980s and early 1990s it remained more difficult to obtain female sterilisations in Dublin than in the regions where the major hospitals were publicly owned.[19] Dublin's Mater and St Vincent's hospitals, respectively owned by the Sisters of Mercy and the Sisters of Charity, continued to ban sterilisations in 2002.[20] The Mater's ethical policy still incorporated the ethical code issued by Archbishop Ryan in 1978.[21] At Vincent's, the Sisters of Charity's code for their health care institutions prohibited sterilisation "to prevent or eliminate fertility"; the promotion of "artificial contraceptive practices"; in-vitro fertilisation; and any other procedure which put embryos at risk.[22]

Holles Street maternity hospital had eventually managed to escape such strictures. Following pressure from patients and from doctors, who were averse to referring patients elsewhere for sterilisation, its ethics committee lost the power to prevent sterilisations from 1992, although individual cases still required the approval of the Master until the later 1990s. In 2002, Holles Street was actively planning to offer in-vitro fertilisation, then only available in two other hospitals.[23] Although Desmond Connell was Holles Street's titular chairman, its governing committee included many doctors and representatives of the Minister for Health and Dublin Corporation, who reflected contemporary opinion rather than Church teaching.

In 2002, Donal O'Shea, the chief executive of the ERHA, said that in the preceding two years, "the issue of ethics has never arisen". If a hospital were unwilling to provide a legal procedure which patients required, he suggested that this would have to be made explicit and the ERHA, as a commissioning authority, would be obliged to ensure its availability in another hospital.[24] It would seem that Dublin patients and their GPs were so accustomed to limited availability of services that they had never thought to complain to the authority.

The Catholic stance on ethical issues provoked a matching defence of its "ethos" from the board of Dublin's Protestant Adelaide Hospital, when it was merged with two other hospitals, one of which had a strongly Catholic ethos, and relocated to the new Tallaght hospital in the 1990s. By 1989, the Adelaide was the last voluntary teaching hospital in the state under Protestant management.[25] The refusal of Catholic nurses in some hospitals to cooperate with the performance of sterilisations had been a major barrier to access to the procedure in the 1980s.[26] The Adelaide wished to provide all legal medical services.[27] Its protracted battle to retain a Protestant ethos was only eventually resolved in 1996, when the new hospital's charter was approved by the Oireachtas. The hospital's board would have a majority of members appointed by the Adelaide Hospital Society or by its president, the Church of Ireland Archbishop of Dublin. While the hospital would have a "multi-denominational and pluralist character", admission to its Adelaide School of Nursing positively discriminated in favour of Protestant and other non-Catholic applicants. The hospital's charter affirmed that it would provide lawful medical and surgical procedures.[28]

In the 1990s, the political establishment no longer feared to challenge the Church. Howlin's 1994 strategy stated that a "comprehensive family planning service" in each health board area would include "ready access" to all legal methods of contraception, including sterilisation.[29] However, a study in 1995 found that contraceptive services were generally limited.[30] In one health board area, they were "non-existent or unsatisfactory" for nearly half of medical card holders.[31] Michael Noonan announced that year that sterilisation and most other forms of contraception would be free to medical card holders and published a list of hospitals offering tubal ligations, which Desmond had feared to do in the 1980s.[32] Although protests by militant lay Catholics and doctors provoked the North-Eastern Health Board to close a vasectomy clinic at Letterkenny General Hospital in 1997, after Noonan pointed out that the board had a statutory obligation to provide a wide range of family planning services it reversed its decision.[33]

Access to contraceptive services remained unsatisfactory. In 2002, it was reported that medical card holders in one small town must pay privately for a prescription for oral contraception because the sole GMS doctor's religious beliefs prevented him from prescribing contraceptives.[34] A 2001 study of health needs in the west-Dublin suburb of Tallaght recorded that 56 per cent of the women's most recent pregnancies had been unplanned.[35]

By 2002, the Catholic Church was not the most significant obstacle to developing a comprehensive contraceptive service. The deficiencies in the service reflected more general deficiencies in primary care. The tardiness of the approach of the Fianna Fáil/Progressive Democrat government contrasted with the approach of Labour and Fine Gael ministers in the early and mid-1990s. In contrast to the 1950s, when Fianna Fáil was less supine than Fine Gael in the face of Church moral strictures, Fianna Fáil had become the most conservative of the political parties on issues of reproductive morality. Although the party had supported Howlin's liberalisation of contraceptive legislation in 1993, when dependent for Dáil support on independent deputies with fundamentalist views in the later 1990s Fianna Fáil's chameleon qualities made preventing abortion a higher priority than preventing unwanted pregnancy.

By 2000, many other bioethical issues were arising which could lead to conflict between the Catholic Church and the state. Religious belief could dictate differing approaches to such issues as the right to die, amniocentesis, IVF, the use of foetal tissue in medical treatment and reproductive cloning. Micheál Martin established a Commission on Assisted Human Reproduction. In a submission to the Commission, the Adelaide Hospital Society supported greater availability of IVF and research on human embryos of up to 14 days, which it was "widely accepted internationally" might be of "considerable medical value" in areas like stem cell research.[36] While the ethics of embryo research were exercising governments internationally and, were by no means solely of concern to Catholics, if the eventual Irish state stance in this area were to deviate significantly from other states', this would give some indication of the Catholic Church's power over Irish medical practice in the 21st century.

Abortion

A catalytic event in the slow process of liberalising Ireland's confessional legislation was the so-called X case of 1992. X was a 14-year-old schoolgirl, who was pregnant as a result of rape by a family friend. The High Court prevented her from leaving Ireland to secure an abortion in England, under the terms of the 1983 amendment to the Constitution which accorded an equal right to life to the foetus and the mother. However, the Supreme Court permitted her to go abroad for the abortion because it had been argued that she was suicidal.

The spectacle of the girl's ordeal educated voters on the social realities behind abortion. The climate of opinion had changed since 1983. When, in 1992 and again in 2002, Fianna Fáil/Progressive Democrat governments asked voters to overturn the Supreme Court's judgment and amend the Constitution to remove the threat of suicide as grounds for abortion, the electorate declined to do so. In other referendums in 1992, voters supported amendments to the Constitution to protect the right to travel, which had been initially denied to X, and to permit freedom of information on services lawfully available in other states. This second amendment was required to counter an escalation of censorship, occasioned when militant lay Catholic groups invoked the 1983 abortion amendment in legal action against any group or publication offering abortion information.

In 1992, the Catholic Church opposed the protection of the rights to travel and information. The amendment that proposed to remove the threat of suicide as a ground for abortion was more problematical for the Church because it would also have permitted abortion when there was a physical risk to a pregnant woman's life, "not being a risk of self-destruction".[37] While the Irish Bishops' Conference took a neutral stance on this amendment, Connell and a number of other bishops declared their opposition to it[38] and found themselves making common cause with liberals, who regarded it as too restrictive. Following the defeat of this amendment, Ireland had a potentially liberal abortion regime, since the Supreme Court judgment permitting abortion to a suicidal woman stood, but, as no doctors performed abortions in Ireland, women still travelled to England for their abortions.

Although the 1992 Fianna Fáil/Labour government promised in its programme for government to legislate to regulate the existing position,[39] and John O'Connell had produced the heads of a draft Bill to provide for abortion where there was a threat of suicide, Howlin did not advance it, having concluded that "the Bill would not be supported by a majority of Fianna Fáil backbenchers".[40] In this legal vacuum, anti-abortion activists resurrected the old alliance of bishops and doctors. The Medical Council, the profession's self-regulatory body, published new ethical guidelines in 1994 which stated that where the life or health of either the mother or the "unborn" were endangered, "it is imperative ethically that doctors shall endeavour to preserve life and health".[41] While not explicitly prohibiting abortion, the guidelines made clear that a doctor ran the risk of being struck off the medical register if he were to perform one.

In the Rainbow Coalition, Noonan's success in 1995 in establishing a legislative framework, within which Irish women could discuss a crisis pregnancy with their doctors and receive information on abortion services in the UK, was an early high point in his subsequently embattled tenure as Minister for Health.[42] This government also succeeded in securing a slim majority for the removal of the constitutional prohibition on divorce, in what was widely regarded as a watershed in Church-state relations.

In 1995, 8.5 per cent of all conceptions among Irish women and 25 per cent among unmarried women were terminated.[43] An opinion poll in 1997 revealed that 77 per cent of voters believed abortion should be permitted in limited circumstances, while only 18 per cent believed it should not be permitted in any circumstances.[44] This did not dissuade the Medical Council from stating in its 1998 ethical guide that "the deliberate and intentional destruction of the unborn child is professional misconduct".[45] The Fianna Fáil/Progressive Democrat government published a non-committal green paper on abortion and failed to achieve a consensus on how to proceed in an all-party Oireachtas Committee.

While the government was deliberating, the balance of opinion on the Medical Council had changed. In June 2001, the Council passed a motion supporting the option of termination of pregnancy when there was a threat to the life of the mother or when the foetus was no longer viable. This changed stance appeared to open the door to the government to legislate for the Supreme Court judgment in the X case and regulate for the provision of abortion in Ireland. It provoked a backlash from anti-abortion activists in the medical profession and, eventually, in September, new ethical guidelines were adopted which, while recognising that termination could occur in the case of a threat to the mother's life, additionally stated that the Council subscribed to the views of the Institute of Obstetricians and Gynaecologists, who had taken a minimalist stance on when doctors might acceptably endanger a foetus in order to treat a woman and did not include the threat of suicide as grounds for a termination.[46] These ambiguous guidelines did not refer to termination in the case of an unviable foetus. Opinions differed as to how much discretion a doctor might have in interpreting them.[47]

In 2002, the government once again asked the people to row back the Supreme Court judgment, which had permitted the threat of suicide as grounds for abortion, and to make abortion a criminal offence carrying a 12-year sentence. The Taoiseach Bertie Ahern's motivation was regarded as a combination of personal conviction and political expediency: his government depended on the support of independents, with strong anti-abortion stances, and he did not wish the issue to emerge during the imminent general election.[48]

The terms of his proposed constitutional referendum posed a dilemma for many doctors, since while the government sought to remove the threat of suicide as a ground for abortion, it also sought to support traditional medical treatments that might result in harm to a foetus. Doctors who wished to have the latter protection might not agree with the former objective. The profession was divided down the middle during the debate: psychiatrists disagreed with one another on whether the risk of suicide should be grounds for abortion;[49] obstetricians and gynaecologists disagreed on whether it was necessary to amend the Constitution to protect obstetric practice;[50] some doctors formed a pro-choice organisation.[51] A Dublin mother of two, Deirdre de Barra, concentrated minds on the barbarity of current medical practice by describing how, in order to avoid carrying an unviable foetus to term, she must travel overseas for an abortion.[52]

Church of Ireland bishops described the proposed amendment as "disastrous";[53] the Methodists recommended a "No" vote;[54] the Presbyterians commented that the Constitution was not the place to deal with this issue;[55] the Catholic bishops actively campaigned for a "Yes" vote, despite their concern that the amendment would not protect the foetus prior to implantation. They said it was vitally important that embryos were "never treated other than as human persons".[56]

Three days before the vote, the X-case rapist, who had served a reduced sentence because he was considered unlikely to reoffend, was again jailed for the sexual abuse of a young girl.[57] The amendment was defeated in a low poll by a very slim margin. By either voting against or staying away, more than three out of four Catholics had ignored their bishops' call for a "Yes" vote.[58] Abortion hardly emerged as an issue in the general election two months later. Although the Supreme Court judgment in the X case still stood as the law of the land, and the Medical Council's ethical guidelines remained open to interpretation, the government's programme did not mention abortion. Could a doctor now legally perform an abortion in Ireland, if he considered his patient suicidal? If he could do so legally, would the Medical Council decide he had acted unethically? Could he terminate a pregnancy in the case of an unviable foetus? These issues remained unresolved.

The Catholic Church as an owner of hospitals

By 2002, the falling numbers of religious had provoked varying responses from the owners of Catholic hospitals: sale to new private owners – in 2000, the Sisters of Mercy sold the Mater private hospital to a management group to be run for-profit; sale to the state – in 1997 the Medical Missionaries of Mary sold Our Lady of Lourdes Hospital in Drogheda to the North-Eastern Health Board (NEHB); or continued religious ownership but with a new structure to protect the Catholic ethos under eventual lay control – as in the case of the Mater public hospital. Even private sales of private hospitals such as Aut Even hospital in Kilkenny, under negotiation by the Sisters of St John of God in 2002, were made contingent on a continued Catholic ethos.

The state continued to invest massively in voluntary hospitals. Ongoing projects in 2002 included a state investment of an estimated €340 million in the Mater Hospital, which would incorporate a children's hospital – the biggest health care investment in the National Development Plan;[59] and an estimated €200 million in St Vincent's – the biggest investment in the hospital's history.[60] The state remained content to invest heavily in health care institutions that limited the treatments on offer according to Catholic ethics and were owned and controlled by unanswerable religious institutions. Although the closure and sale of religious-owned but heavily state- and community-supported schools were contentious because communities lost their schools, religious control and disposal of hospitals remained an accepted part of Irish life. "Quite extraordinarily in Ireland, the state uses the voluntary sector in the city of Dublin as a vehicle to provide the health services that it's obligated to do. That's unusual in any other city, in any other state," observed Helena O'Donoghue, the provincial leader of the Sisters of Mercy – the order who controlled the future of the Mater Hospital.[61]

When the Medical Missionaries of Mary sold their Drogheda hospital to the NEHB, the eventual price was below its market valuation following an agreed evaluation of the state's capital investment, according to Donal O'Shea, chief executive of the NEHB at the time. In this instance, the hospital became a health board hospital, in which sterilisations were eventually performed.[62] However, despite the considerable state funding for the voluntary hospitals, at the beginning of 2003 there was no agreed formula for the state to secure its investment in the event of a subsequent sale. The Department of Health had established a group to "examine" the issue and had opened discussions with the Mater about agreeing a formula.[63] The state was hardly negotiating from a position of strength, given that its investment was already committed.

In 2002, only five Mercy sisters remained in the Mater public hospital and the order anticipated that soon there would be none. Most Mercy sisters were over 70 and the few younger religious had lost interest in running large institutions for the state. Having opened their private hospital to complement the public hospital by "attracting the best medical expertise", they had come to see it as a draw on their resources and to realise that serving the better-off was putting their "own ethos at risk", Helena O'Donoghue admitted in 2002.[64] They sold the private hospital to a management group but made the sale contingent on the continuation of Catholic ethics, to be overseen by the Catholic

Archbishop of Dublin whose nominee would sit on the hospital's board. For their public hospitals, the new children's hospital and the Mater public hospital, they developed a company structure to retain Catholic control even when their direct involvement would end. While the overarching holding company would be a charity controlled by the order, it now involved representatives of the Archbishop and lay Catholic groups, such as the Catholic Nurses' Guild.[65]

"Looking ahead five, ten or fifteen years, if the Catholic Church in Dublin wants a voluntary Catholic hospital, the Catholic people will have to want that and work it, because we won't be there," O'Donoghue foresaw.

Some Catholic lay people were willing to take up where the religious left off. Already, Jimmy Sheehan was imposing Catholic ethics in the Blackrock Clinic and intended to do so in other private hospitals. In St Vincent's, the Sisters of Charity also introduced a company structure in 2000 that, while still under their ownership and control, involved more lay people. Their arrangements differed from the Mater's in that they did not involve the Archbishop and they retained ownership of their private hospital, never as high-tech as the Mater private. The consequence was that, whereas some consultants in the Mater were now shareholders in a private, for-profit hospital, this option had been denied to consultants in St Vincent's, to the disappointment of some. While the Sisters of Mercy had ceased to have direct involvement in the promotion of private medicine, they had, by their sale of the private hospital, permitted the potential emergence of an aggressively commercial health care institution, which the Sisters of Charity had so far been unwilling to countenance.

The voluntary hospitals, which continued to dominate the delivery of health care in the east of the state and were virtually wholly funded by it, not only eluded state control in the kind of treatments which they might offer but, in 2002, were also still permitted to operate their own selection procedures for medical staff. The archdiocese had coordinated the voluntary hospitals' opposition to efforts by the Department of Health under Desmond to develop a common selection procedure for all public hospital consultants.[66] Although the government committed itself in 2001 to extending the role of the Ombudsman to voluntary hospitals,[67] this had not taken place by the end of 2002.[68]

The progressive voice of the Catholic Church

Although, in the early 1990s, the Church focused on unemployment as an issue of greater concern[69] and, in the mid-1990s, was distracted by the scandals of clerical sexual abuse, Church groups nonetheless maintained an interest in health care reform, which became more vocal towards the end of the decade and into the new century. The Irish Commission for Justice and Peace, a commission of the Irish Catholic Bishops' Conference, lobbied for constitutional provisions for social and economic rights, including a right to health.[70] The Commission was represented at the hearings of the UN Committee on Economic, Social and Cultural Rights in 2002, which recommended that the state should revisit the 2001 Health Strategy to include a human rights framework.[71] The most media-savvy group was the Conference of Major Religious Superiors (later renamed CORI or the Conference of Religious in Ireland) which, while initially established to defend Church interests in social provision,[72] later provided a platform for religious to campaign on issues like health cutbacks, the two-tier system, the "exorbitant" salary demands of hospital consultants[73] and to participate in social partnership. As the numbers of religious sharply declined, the positive witness of individuals – like the priest Peter McVerry and the nun Stanislaus Kennedy who worked with the homeless – confronted an increasingly self-interested society.

Ireland's deafness to the Church's exhortations extended to its campaigning voice, which was undermined by internal contradictions. In 2002, CORI simultaneously defended the generosity of the state's agreement to indemnify religious orders for claims from victims of institutional abuse and argued for social justice. The religious orders' insistence on applying Catholic sexual morality in their hospitals contrasted with their tardiness in recognising that proprietorship of private hospitals or two-tier access to care might be at odds with a broader view of ethics. Ultimately, despite the genuine commitment to social justice of many religious, as long as the Church remained an élitist and undemocratic institution, it would be in a weak position to lecture the state about civil rights.[74]

As Helena O'Donoghue of the Sisters of Mercy foresaw in 2002, health care would soon have to get by without the religious orders – "we won't be there". She envisaged a future in which "the Catholic people" must provide their own Catholic health care. But, in 2002, who were the Catholic people? The 48 per cent of Catholics who still attended weekly Mass? Or the nominal Catholics, who had voted for the legalisation of divorce, refused to ban abortion when there was a risk of suicide and elected governments that legislated for wide availability of contraception, including sterilisation, nonetheless denied to patients in state-funded, religious-run hospitals?

When the Catholic bishops fought their rearguard action against "socialised medicine" in the 1940s and 1950s, at least as great a concern as socialism was that the state would take control of sex education and permit contraception.[75] While socialism receded as a concern and the Church became a supporter of the state's role in health care, this in no way diminished its desire to control sexuality, as evidenced by its interventions in the debates on contraceptive legislation and the continued ban on sterilisation in Catholic hospitals. The referendums on abortion saw the emergence of an aggressive lay Catholic movement, whose views on sexual morality were far to the right of the majority of the electorate. If the religious orders were to transfer control of the major Dublin voluntary hospitals to the laity, would this movement dictate which medical procedures were ethically permissible? And, given the massive state investment in these institutions, would the state countenance this? How would the state recover its investment if a major voluntary hospital were closed? While, in 2002, the religious orders had thought hard about the future of voluntary health care, there was no evidence that the state had done so.

PART THREE
A FAILED SYSTEM

9

TWO-TIER HOSPITAL CARE

"There are significant inequalities in the system at present."
– *2001 Government Health Strategy.*

Having evolved without a unifying vision and with capricious funding, Ireland's health care system fails in the most essential way – it fails to deliver adequate patient care. Too many people cannot receive care when they need it, either because they cannot afford to access primary care or because they must wait so long for treatment in hospital. Too much care is delivered by junior doctors, many outside formal training programmes and in sub-standard hospitals. Too much care is delivered in hospital instead of at community level, because primary care is underdeveloped.

Irish society today faces two major challenges: to fund the health care system adequately; and, within that system, whatever its level of funding, to deliver care equitably, giving priority to those in greater need. Before exploring the arguments for greater funding, it is necessary to understand the deeper-seated failures of the contemporary health care system: how it discriminates between patients to an extraordinary degree; how it puts local politics before patient safety; and how, at the very first point of contact, the family doctor, it excludes many citizens from care.

At the heart of the health care system, in Irish hospitals, there is a discrimination between patients that other European states would not tolerate. In public hospitals, there are two forms of apartheid: two-tier access and two-tier care. Waiting lists for public patient care are only the most obvious manifestation of this pervasive system of discrimination, which has deep roots in how hospitals are organised, how doctors are employed, trained and paid, and how health care is funded. The reality of two-tier access is not in dispute. It exists, it is institutionalised and it has been getting worse.

This is a system in which patients are treated according to income rather than need. Private patient care is delivered promptly and, generally, by consultants in person. Public patient care comes tardily and is frequently delivered by doctors in training. Public patients may wait so long for care that they are effectively denied it. Death may intervene. When they are treated, their care may be of inferior quality to private patients'. Only in the accident and emergency departments of public hospitals is there a levelling, so that the insured and uninsured alike find themselves confronted by the chaotic, inadequate face of Irish public health care.

That many patients yet emerge from hospital cured and happy is testimony to the efforts of the many medical, nursing and other staff, who work long hours with competence and dedication in difficult circumstances in under-resourced hospitals. How very much more they might achieve were they not asked to work in such an invidious system. Some of the most vocal critics of two-tier care are among those who must deliver it.

Experiences of two-tier care

"GPs experience both shame and frustration in trying to work the system for our patients. Shame because the system increasingly favours those who can pay rather than those who need it. Frustration because of difficulties with patient access to hospital and consultant work practices, especially in the bigger urban centres."

– Tom O'Dowd, general practitioner and TCD professor of general practice.[1]

Case study one: suing for care

In June 2001, 39-year-old Janette Byrne sued the Irish state, the Eastern Regional Health Authority and the Mater Hospital to gain access to the chemotherapy treatment that she had been told would save her life. She had undergone an eight-hour operation to remove a tumour nearly five months earlier, after she was diagnosed with non-Hodgkins Lymphoma. Since then, she had received some chemotherapy but, again and again, her scheduled treatment had been cancelled, due to the unavailability of beds in the Mater Public Hospital in Dublin.

She was a public patient, a medical card holder. She argued that the state had failed to ensure her right to health care and was failing to vindicate her right to life, as protected by the Constitution. She stated that she was "terrified" because of the delays in getting treatment. "I felt that, while I was at home waiting for a bed, the tumour was growing again. I had been advised my cancer was treatable but time was of the essence."

The case was settled after she was offered an immediate course of treatment in the Mater Private Hospital, treatment which would have been readily available had she been a private patient. The High Court judge advised her to accept the offer because pursuing the case would take time. Had it proceeded, the case would have tested the obligation of the state to vindicate the right to life of its citizens.[2]

Case study two: buying access

In August 2000, a Dublin woman in her late seventies, living alone, developed gangrene in both feet. A consultant told her that she would have to wait six weeks for a bed in the local hospital. Her GP suggested she should take a taxi to the outpatients department and wait there for admission. Members of the St Vincent de Paul, a Catholic charity, called each evening to her home to put her to bed and again each morning to get her up. Once the St Vincent de Paul offered to pay for her bed, the local hospital made a private bed available that same afternoon.[3]

Case study three: dying on the waiting list

In November 1990, Peter Sheridan, a farmer with a young family from Tourmakeady, County Mayo, died from a massive heart attack after six months on a waiting list for a heart bypass operation. He had suffered an earlier cardiac arrest. His GP remains convinced that, had he been a private patient, he would have had his bypass prior to the attack. "He died because he didn't have the money," Noel Rice concluded. In 2002, more than ten years after Peter Sheridan's death, Rice, a former chairman of the Western Health Board, found his public patients suffering equal discrimination. The two-tier system remained "hugely wrong". "It makes me so angry," Mary Sheridan, the dead man's widow, told RTÉ television. "If I could have afforded insurance, probably he would have had the bypass straight away, probably in a week or three weeks or so."[4]

Two-tier access

Getting to see the consultant

The apartheid in hospital care runs very deep. From the moment patients visit their family GP, their status is defined by their ability to pay for care, either through private insurance or out of their pockets. General practitioners refer patients onwards to specialists' outpatient clinics. The hospital consultants or specialists will then decide whether the patient requires hospital treatment. Private patients may see consultants at their outpatient clinics or may be given an appointment at their private rooms. When there is a significant wait to see a consultant at his outpatient clinic, a private patient will inevitably be referred to the consultant's private rooms. Public patients have no option but to attend the public clinic. While some specialists, in great demand, may have waiting lists of some months before they will see private patients, public patients may wait years before they get their foot even on this first rung of the ladder.[5] Even though patients may spend years waiting to see a specialist after their GP's referral, they are not counted on waiting lists. Not until after a specialist has seen them and prescribed surgery and they have then waited *a further three months* will such patients appear on official Irish waiting lists.

Case study four: waiting to wait

In June 2001, it was reported that a 12-year-old Tipperary boy, whose mother was dependent on social welfare, had waited over five years for an initial consultant appointment to assess his breathing difficulties. His mother had been told he was 150th on the consultant's waiting list.[6] He would not be counted on any official waiting list. Such a routine investigation would be scheduled within weeks for a private patient. The mother accepted an offer of the proceeds of a charity auction to pay for private treatment.[7]

Case study five: waiting ... and waiting ... to wait

During the 2002 general election campaign, rheumatologists disclosed that, in the Galway area, patients with disabling arthritis were waiting up to four years for an initial outpatient appointment. By the time some patients managed to reach a rheumatologist, their joint damage might be so disabling that they would require surgery. They would then find themselves waiting for an initial appointment with an orthopaedic surgeon. Neither wait would qualify them for inclusion on an official waiting list. Private patients in the Galway area wait no more than a few months to see a rheumatologist, according to local GPs.

Getting a date for surgery
  "I monitored the attendance and quality of our outpatients services and

challenged the inequity. I was accused of being opposed to private practice."
> *– a nurse's story recounted to a workshop at the Irish Nurses' Organisation 2001 annual conference.*[8]

After a patient is seen in outpatients, the apartheid becomes explicit. Private patients are generally given a date for surgery: public patients, except those in immediate need of treatment, are given a place on the list. Commenting on a detailed study of waiting lists by the Harvard Association of Ireland, UCD professor Ray Kinsella observed:

> At the heart of management at this point is the simple issue: does the patient have private health insurance? If he/she does, then the patient is usually given a date to come in for surgery often at a convenient time and/or, in some cases, at the location of his/her choice. If not, they may – depending on their categorisation – get locked into the public waiting list system.[9]

That private patients might opt to use their insurance to expedite their date of surgery, ahead of public patients, raised "major issues of equity and of equality of access", he commented.

As Fine Gael's Richard Bruton foresaw when the Fianna Fáil/Progressive Democrat government declined to introduce a common waiting list for public and private patients, and instead opted for designating a ratio of public to private beds within the public hospital system, two-tier access to care would become institutionalised. The 1991 legislation was "enshrining in our system a permanent separation, a fast lane for those who can afford and a slow lane for those who cannot".

The waiting list system is neither transparent nor consistent. Waiting lists have been, in effect, "owned" by individual consultants. The November 2001 government health strategy promised the innovation – radical in Ireland, overdue in any logical system – that lists should be managed at specialty, rather than at individual consultant, level. "This will aid referral of patients to consultants with shorter lists."[10] A new National Hospitals Agency would develop guidelines to prioritise patients and the lists would be published on an intranet site for GPs, the strategy proposed. Under the existing system, neither the patient nor their GP might know that they had been unfortunate enough to be referred to the consultant with the longer list. Unfortunately, the introduction of a new system appeared to be a receding possibility in late 2002. Removing waiting lists from the ownership of individual consultants depended on negotiations on a new consultants' contract. In the meantime, it was variously reported that consultants' sense of ownership of "their" patients on "their" lists was constituting an obstacle to government plans to treat public patients in the private sector, since some consultants were objecting to patients on their lists being referred for treatment to other consultants, and that plans for a unified computer system for the state's hospitals had been abandoned because of health cutbacks.[11]

In autumn 2002, the reluctance of some consultants to cooperate with a new Treatment Purchase Fund, set up to secure treatment for the patients who had waited longest, was causing concern that the Fund would not be able to take up all the capacity for treatment that it had purchased in English private hospitals. "It's very wrong," commented one health administrator, who was observing this process. "There are all sorts of reasons being found not to refer patients."[12] The most sympathetic interpretation of consultants' motivations for so denying their patients care was that they were doing so from a misplaced wish to bring home to government their objection to feeding the private system when underfunding was thwarting their own efforts to treat within the public system.

Finbarr Fitzpatrick, secretary-general of the IHCA, who insisted that consultants were willing to cooperate with the Fund, nonetheless sympathised with this stance. He described talking to consultants in a regional hospital who predicted that their public elective work would be cancelled on budgetary grounds and that they would then be encouraged by the health board "to take their public patients down the road" to a neighbouring private hospital and "be paid for them, if they wanted, from the Treatment Purchase Fund. It is revolting that you scale down your public facilities and you send the patients to a private hospital, which is a mile down the road."[13]

Other consultants were reluctant to cooperate with the Fund because they were not impressed by the skills of their private hospital colleagues. Some public consultants even considered it morally wrong to benefit from the Fund and resolved to devote any private earnings from the Fund to research.[14] A less benign motivation was the desire to protect opportunities for private practice. Under the Howlin Waiting List Initiative, consultants could have expected to treat "their" public waiting list patients privately. They had in effect been offered an economic incentive to keep lists in existence. The organisers of the Fund were determined to avoid this. Their principles of operation stated that no consultant should "predominantly treat patients from his or her own public list" when providing private care commissioned by the

Treatment Purchase Fund.[15] In specialties with few consultants, this might be unavoidable but many consultants would indeed see some of their public patients depart to the care of another. Not only would they lose potential for private practice, but also they would lose their most potent argument for extra resources and staff – a long waiting list.

At the end of 2002, fewer than 20 of 400 places reserved for treatment of Irish patients in England had been filled, a shortfall which the Fund's director, Maureen Lynott, put down to consultants' "resistance". "This new initiative has not yet been accepted by consultants."[16] Whatever the motivation, there could be no justification for consultants to stand between their patients and care. So serious was this problem of non-cooperation that Micheál Martin held a number of press conferences in late 2002 to publicise the work of the Fund and encourage patients and their general practitioners to seek treatment. Since the Fund's hotline had received hundreds of calls from eligible patients, most of whom had not been referred by their consultants, the Fund's organisers decided in early 2003 to wait no longer for consultants' referrals and to ask GPs to refer their patients directly for treatment overseas, in effect to reclaim ownership of their care from consultants' lists.

For the patient waiting, the arbitrariness of the traditional waiting process, the sense that their treatment is dependent on the decision of an individual consultant about their relative need, has often engendered a sense of helplessness, which the Fund was hoping to dissipate. Kinsella reported:

> Once a person on the public list is referred for surgery, they are not generally routinely contacted again until they are called for surgery. However, some people/families will continually contact the Admissions Office who, while they cannot change a person's priority status, can refer them back to OPD [the outpatients' department] where they may be given a higher priority rating but keep their initial date of referral for surgery, thus increasing their chances of being called at an earlier date. In effect, he/she who shouts the loudest may gain faster access, while a less vocal person may be disadvantaged; there is, at the same time, a very real risk of a person deteriorating while they are on the List.[17]

Prior to the creation of the Treatment Purchase Fund, with its emphasis on treating people who had waited over a year, many such patients might never have received treatment. Their low-priority rating would ensure that they would perpetually stay at the bottom of the list. As one hospital manager observed, some consultants placed patients on their list without any expectation of treating them. By seeing, diagnosing and ranking these public patients, they might hope to win from the patients' GPs further referrals of private patients. In the meantime, their presence on the list would help in arguing for better facilities.[18]

On the waiting list

Significant numbers of patients wait for care in Ireland. In September 2002, over 29,000 patients were waiting for public inpatient or day treatment in Ireland. Government spokesmen frequently attempted to diminish the significance of these numbers by contrasting them with the hundreds of thousands treated each year. It was an invalid comparison, a classical confusion of apples and oranges. Economists consider it nonsensical to compare a stock (those waiting) with a flow (those passing through beds). Compare like with like – those actually in acute hospital beds with those waiting for them – and quite another picture emerges. For every public inpatient being treated at any given moment, there were more than two waiting, one of whom had been waiting for over a year.

Official waiting list data give very little information on waiting times. The list published each quarter by the Department of Health provides information for certain targeted specialties on the number of adults who have been waiting for over a year (after their three months' wait to be considered "waiting") and the number of children who have been waiting for over six months. No one inquires just how much longer than that these patients may have been waiting. For the first time, in September 2002, waiting lists for day treatment were published, although day treatment constituted nearly 70 per cent of non-emergency hospital activity.[19] No waiting times were available for over one-third of day patients and one-third of the remainder had long waiting times.[20]

Irish waiting lists compare poorly with those in other states. The UK's NHS, despite its well-publicised difficulties, does remarkably better. In September 2002, in England, only 6 patients in total had waited longer than 18 months for either inpatient or day treatment. Only 3 patients in every 10,000 people had waited for over a year. This compared to 21 adult patients in every 10,000 people who had waited for over a year in the Republic.[21] In France there are, quite simply, no waiting lists. All surgery is planned under a booking system in which the patient is given a date for surgery immediately it is prescribed, although this may involve a few months wait. In Canada, where waiting times have been a political issue, what is defined as "waiting" would not warrant inclusion on an Irish "waiting" list.

Failure of the waiting list initiatives

Targeted waiting list initiatives have had limited impact. After the impressive reduction in the lists achieved by Brendan Howlin, when he introduced the first such initiative in 1993, the number of patients waiting exceeded the 1994 level in each subsequent year.[22] Not only have these initiatives failed to solve the problem of waiting lists, the proportion of patients waiting for longer periods has remained high. In 1996, when the Department of Health first started to count the numbers of adults waiting for over a year and children waiting for over six months in targeted specialties, they constituted 42 per cent and 65 per cent respectively of these waiting lists. In September 2002, 42 per cent of adults and 66 per cent of children on these targeted inpatient lists remained waiting for over 12 and 6 months respectively.[23] A study of patients on waiting lists in the west-Dublin suburb of Tallaght in 2001 found that 62 per cent had waited over 6 months and 33 per cent over a year.[24]

Waiting lists are a function of many shortcomings in the health care system – too few beds, too few staff, an underdeveloped primary care system and inadequate convalescent and geriatric facilities. But Irish waiting lists are not only much worse than in other countries, they are also distinguished by the fact that they are experienced by one class of patient. While public patients wait uncounted years for care, the wait for private patients, insofar as it exists, is very much shorter.

A telephone survey of 2,620 people, conducted by the ESRI in 1999, found that of those on waiting lists for inpatient surgery, not one insured person had waited for more than a year, whereas 22 per cent of the uninsured had done so.[25] A further survey of 1,250 people in 2000 found that, whereas 56 per cent of the insured had experienced no wait for day treatment, not one uninsured person had been admitted for day surgery without a wait.[26] Confirmation that private patients' faster access is not just a consequence of the availability of private hospitals but reflects their privileged access to public hospitals was provided in a 2002 Eastern Regional Health Authority survey, which disclosed that the average waiting time for private patients in public hospitals was 3.4 months, whereas the average waiting time for public patients was 6.7 months.[27]

Why people take out private health insurance

The Irish people are in no doubt about the reality of the two-tier system. Surveyed in July and August 2000, almost 90 per cent of them believed that hospital care could be obtained more quickly in the private system than in the public system.[28] The proportion of the population with private health insurance rose from under 22 per cent in 1977 to 46 per cent by 2001.[29] The insured are generally better educated and paid than the uninsured. Nearly 70 per cent of third-level graduates have insurance compared to 40 per cent of early school leavers; 75 per cent of professionals and managers have insurance compared to 21 per cent of unskilled manual workers.[30] Eloquent testimony of lack of faith in the public system is provided by the fact that over one in ten of the poorest 10 per cent of the population had taken out health insurance in 1994.[31] The cost of insurance is the chief deterrent to purchasing it: in 2000, 67 per cent of the uninsured had not purchased it because it was too expensive; only 31 per cent were without insurance because they were satisfied with the public health system.[32]

People take out private insurance to avoid large bills and to be sure that they will be treated quickly and well. Surveys reveal that these motivations are of growing significance. Other reasons which are of lesser and diminishing importance are: being assured of a consultant's care, being able to choose a consultant, arranging the timing of treatment and having a private room.

Table 9.1 Reasons for having private insurance

Reasons for having private insurance	%
Avoid large bills	88
Ensure quick treatment	85
Ensure good hospital treatment	73
Ensure consultant care	59
Arrange time of treatment	57
Choose consultant	43
Private bed	25
Private room	22

Source: Dorothy Watson and James Williams, *Perceptions of the Quality of Health Care in the Public and Private Sectors in Ireland*, ESRI, 2001. Based on a survey in July and August 2000.

Acknowledgement by all of "glaring inequalities of access"

"I feel guilty that I haven't spoken out. Our hospital is in crisis. We are constantly cancelling our day services. It is the public patients who are cancelled, not the private patients. The consultants take the decision, on medical grounds they say. But we see the notes, we can't see any difference."

– a nurse's story at the INO's 2001 annual conference.

Equity in access to health care, which had been a silent issue for so much of the 1990s, resurfaced with a vengeance in the new millennium. The government acknowledged the existing inequities in its 2001 health strategy. "It is clear that there are significant inequalities in the system at present, which must be addressed, such as unacceptably long waiting times for public patients for some elective procedures."[33]

The National Economic and Social Forum referred to "glaring inequalities of access between public and private patients" in a report published in July 2002, its first study of the health system since its establishment in 1993 to advise government on social inclusion and equality issues.[34]

While the NESF grappled with these issues at public meetings during 2001, the health administrators, who wrote the 2001 strategy document, were meeting in private to address the same concerns. The report of an informal working group established by the Department of Health commented:

> There is broad consensus that the current inequity of access for public patients is unacceptable ... The issue of equity of access to treatment is most marked in regard to non-emergency and elective care for public patients, where the waiting lists and waiting times in certain specialties has proven exceptionally difficult to reduce even with targeted measures, and for which private patients do not experience material waiting times.[35]

This group first met in May 2001 as part of the preparatory work for the new strategy, with a mandate to "consider specific immediate issues relating to the public/private mix".[36] It is an interesting statement about Departmental perceptions of inequity that the group limited its discussions of the public/private mix to the acute hospital sector and did not consider the mix in primary care. Of its 24 members, 16 were officials of the Department, including the secretary-general, Michael Kelly, and four were employees of health boards. Chaired by Maureen Lynott, a management consultant who had formerly worked at a senior level in both the VHI and BUPA (Ireland) and was subsequently appointed director of the National Treatment Purchase Fund, the group produced a report that could fairly be taken to represent the considered views of the Department, and remained within its four walls until released under the Freedom of Information Act.[37]

Not only did public patients wait longer but also their position relative to private patients had deteriorated, the working group found. Analysis by a sub-group revealed that planned admissions of private patients for inpatient care in public hospitals rose by 2.4 per cent between 1999 and 2000, while admissions of public patients fell marginally, by 0.4 per cent. Emergency admissions of private patients rose by 0.8 per cent while emergency admissions of public patients fell by 2.2 per cent.[38] The favouring of private patients was most marked in the growth of day surgery, where there was a 12.5 per cent increase in private day patients between 1999 and 2000, compared with an increase of only 0.5 per cent in the number of public day patients.[39] Private patients were clearly gaining significantly preferred access to this most rapidly growing area of hospital activity. Day patients were 33 per cent of all patients discharged from hospital in 1999, compared to 13 per cent in 1990.[40]

Two-tier care

Inferior treatment for public patients

Public patients not only find it harder to access hospital care. When they reach hospital, they may also experience inferior treatment. This was acknowledged by doctors themselves as early as 1975, when an Irish Medical Association working party report said that public patients were

> less likely to have an operation performed by a consultant surgeon. They are less likely to receive their day-to-day medical attention from resident staff … Patients attending out-patients' departments are treated less well, first because of long waiting and poor physical conditions, and secondly because they are often seen by residents who, in our opinion, may not be competent to deal with their problems.[41]

This reality had not changed when the Tierney Report in 1993 stated:

> Medical services in hospitals are provided, to a large extent by NCHDs [non-consultant hospital doctors] who by definition are not fully trained. The bulk of emergency work is carried out by NCHDs under the supervision of consultants but this can often be of a nominal type.[42]

It remained unaltered in 2001 when the Medical Manpower Forum reported that there was "inappropriate staffing" of hospitals and "limited availability of senior clinical decision-making".

> Frontline services are mainly provided by non-consultant hospital doctors many of whom are in the early stages of their training or not in formal training posts. Long waiting times, additional tests, referrals to other junior doctors and a reluctance to seek senior opinion at times have serious implications for both diagnosis and treatment of the patient.

Participants in the forum included the medical organisations and consultants' representatives.[43]

Case study six: when a consultant wasn't consulted – death of a public patient

In September 1998, a man died in the operating theatre of an Irish hospital – in itself not unusual. The hospital staff had done their very best to save him. What was unusual was the series of events preceding his death, which had taken place in another hospital, whence he was transferred. It was sufficiently unusual that the dead man's family asked the Ombudsman to investigate. Following a detailed investigation, the Ombudsman concluded that the dead man's care in the initial hospital had been inadequate. Although the Ombudsman is precluded from commenting on the exercise of clinical judgement, he nonetheless recommended that the health board, hospital and medical staff should bring "greater clarity to the working relationships between junior and senior medical staff".[44]

There is a danger zone, a *terra incognita*, in many Irish hospitals. This is where patients are left to the care of junior doctors, under the nominal but absent supervision of their superiors. The most dangerous time of all is the weekend. This man's condition deteriorated on a Saturday. By Sunday evening he was dead. Over Saturday evening and night he had been under the care of an orthopaedic senior house officer (SHO) assigned to the hospital on a six-month training rotation. This junior doctor had been on call continuously from 9 am on Saturday and would remain on call until 9 am on Monday, when he was due to commence a normal 9 to 5 shift. The patient had been admitted the preceding Wednesday, following a referral by his general practitioner for assessment of lower back pain. He had seen an orthopaedic consultant. The consultant was off-duty for the weekend and expected to see the patient again on Monday. As the patient's condition deteriorated over the weekend, the consultant was never contacted. In the hierarchy between him and his struggling junior was another, more senior non-consultant doctor, the orthopaedic registrar. Not until Sunday morning did the SHO tell the registrar that he had concerns about the patient. The registrar was knowledgeable enough to realise that the surgical team should immediately be involved in the patient's assessment. The surgical SHO later examined the patient and telephoned the locum consultant surgeon on duty from the ward. The consultant surgeon recommended the patient's immediate transfer by ambulance to a neighbouring hospital, which had a vascular unit. It had become apparent that the back pain was in fact a manifestation of a vascular problem, later identified as an aortic aneurysm, or swelling of the aorta. The eventual rupture of this aneurysm caused the patient's death.[45]

Over that long Saturday and into Sunday morning members of the man's family had kept vigil at his bedside. They testified that he was suffering severe pain from which medication gave him no relief, his right leg was becoming cold and he had trouble moving it; his lower back and front torso were discoloured. The orthopaedic consultant later accepted that, if the family's observations were correct, then "something catastrophic must have been going on". If the doctor on duty had made those observations, he would have expected him to contact a more senior doctor immediately.[46] The SHO, whom the family found "dismissive" when they raised their concerns during the night, and whom the consultant suggested might have been significantly deprived of sleep, later said he had not observed the discoloration and would have expected the nursing staff to have brought it to his attention. During the Ombudsman's investigation, the SHO initially could not recollect if the patient's leg was cold or had a poor reaction to stimulus and later asserted that this was not the case.[47] Nursing records supported the family's observations that the patient was in severe pain. The Ombudsman observed that the paucity of available records made it difficult to establish what precisely had happened.[48]

After reviewing the case, the Ombudsman recommended the adoption of "an administrative protocol outlining the circumstances in which a junior member of a medical team should consult with his or her consultant when a patient's condition gives cause for concern, and the corresponding obligation on consultants to be accessible for such consultation". The health board accepted these recommendations. Not only was the patient's care inadequate, but also the Ombudsman found that his medical notes "left a lot to be desired". He criticised the handling of the family's subsequent complaints and recommended that senior health board and hospital management should apologise in person to the family.[49]

The distressed family complained to the Ombudsman neither vindictively nor as a prelude to litigation, he observed. They sought answers, apologies and an assurance that the experience of their dead husband and father would not be repeated. "It should not have been necessary for the family to come to the Ombudsman to get that," he commented.[50] The Ombudsman noted that, in the UK, where a complaint refers to clinical judgement and is not resolved locally, the complainant may ask for the establishment of an independent review panel.

How health professionals view two-tier care

"You know when the SHO hasn't a clue. A patient was in cardiac arrest – the doctor hadn't a notion what was going on. At one stage I gave the drugs because she hadn't a clue. No one is supervising them. No one is training them."

"I see public patients ringing everyone they can think of to try to get to speak to a consultant. I see the consultant saying to the private patient in the bed 'give me your husband's mobile phone number and I'll phone him about your progress'."
– nurses' accounts from a workshop at the 2001 INO annual conference.

"At its worst the present public-private divide constitutes a kind of caste system. The public caste perceives its care as largesse, the private caste perceives its care as service."
– Sean Conroy, a doctor and programme manager with the Western Health Board.[51]

"The patient is VHI positive."
– overheard remark recounted by the former chief executive of Tallaght Hospital, David McCutcheon.[52]

Consultants have traditionally delivered private patient care personally. Public patient care is under their supervision – "consultant-led" not "consultant-provided". In the 21st century, the manner in which consultants work and are employed perpetuates the discrimination between paying and charity cases operated by their early 20th century predecessors. Care of the poor was a form of charity in voluntary hospitals where it offered useful training for young doctors. Even after 1981, when the first consultants' common contract provided all doctors with a salary for their public work, this attitude of *noblesse oblige* persisted. "You made your money in private practice but you looked after the underprivileged," as cardiac surgeon and Blackrock Clinic co-founder Maurice Neligan expressed it.

The delegation of care

Under their contract, consultants have been permitted private practice limited only by its location. Still, in 2003, consultants might opt for essentially two different forms of contract: category one, which only permitted them private practice in the hospital of their appointment; and category two, which permitted them to engage in private practice off-site. There were also some consultants with full-time academic appointments. In January 2003, 91 per cent of hospital consultants were engaged in both public and private practice. Of 1,731 public hospital consultant posts, 57 per cent were category one and 34 per cent were category two.[53] Many consultants in Dublin, in particular, treat patients in private hospitals that are distant from the hospital where they have their public contract, inevitably making them less accessible to public patients.

It is an unwritten understanding of consultants' terms of employment that they attend personally to their private patients' care, while they may opt to delegate as much as they wish of their public patients' care. They receive their public salary for a 39-hour week (of which 6 hours are set aside for "episodic activities" such as planning and meetings)[54] yet their contract does not insist that for the remaining 33 salaried hours, they dedicate themselves to public patients. On the contrary, under the terms of the contract, they may delegate the treatment of public patients for whom they are responsible to more junior doctors, while they earn fees for the treatment of private patients.

The 1997 version of the consultants' common contract, still unamended at the beginning of 2003, stated: "The consultant may discharge this responsibility [for investigation and treatment] directly in a personal relationship with his patient, or, in the exercise of his clinical judgement, he may delegate aspects of the patient's care to other appropriate staff."[55]

In 2001, the Department of Health remained far from happy with the terms of the contract. The report of the working group on the public/private mix commented:

> The contract does not stipulate that the 39 hour contract is solely for public patients, and while it specifies such extent will be subject to national review, this has not been operative, nor is the stipulation that off-site private practice is subject to the consultant satisfying the employing authority that he is fulfilling his contractual commitment within public hospitals.[56]

A Departmental sub-group report deplored the practical consequence of this lax arrangement:

> Within this 33-hour commitment, they may practice privately (varying between on-site and off-site depending on category) subject to meeting commitments to the public hospital and to the ratio of public/private beds in the hospital. This provision must be changed so that the needs of public patients are fully met and that consultants are no longer effectively paid twice for "private" hours worked within the 33-hour commitment. In addition the 33-hour public commitment should be scheduled so that each consultant is available on-site every day (five days) at each public hospital to which he/she has a commitment in order to facilitate patient discharges.[57]

The hospital system has been predicated on the assumption that public patients will not receive the same degree of consultant attention as private patients. There are, quite simply, not enough consultants to offer individual attention to every patient. Nor are they required to do so. When public patients are unable to track down their consultant, it is not (with occasional exceptions) that he is on the golf course. Their consultant is after all only expected to work 33 hours a week in the public hospital for his sizeable public salary. He is permitted to delegate their care to others. He regards his public salary as a baseline on which he builds his income from private practice. Cormac MacNamara, former president of the IMO, has observed:

> The overwhelming majority of consultants operate in a paradigm where they have huge, unrealistic workloads in the public sector, which they can only address by delegating. And they have income expectations, which can only be met by undertaking supplementary workloads in the private sector.

A medical politician, MacNamara was careful to add:

> I have no personal experience of anyone not performing to contract. I hear the stories of the handful of consultants who don't give value to the public sector, who are forever in their private rooms. They are an embarrassment to the 99 per cent who do work more than their 33 contracted hours for the public sector.[58]

Hospital managers did not share MacNamara's sanguinity. Deloitte and Touche management consultants, who examined value-for-money in the health system, found among health board and hospital managers "widespread concern that the private health care system is reducing the resources available for public health care". While there was "no evidence to support any widespread abuse of public sector responsibilities by consultants", there was no monitoring or evaluation of the impact of private practice on public patients' care or any hard evidence on the amount of activity in private hospitals carried out by individual consultants.[59] "There are some consultants who don't touch a public patient," an experienced public hospital manager observed in 2002. A study in 2002 disclosed that almost a quarter of patients said they rarely or never saw their consultant.[60]

The same consultants, by and large, staff the public and private systems, which are, in many respects, one system. In 2002, 790 consultants, aided by about 70 juniors, provided care in private hospitals. The public hospital system formally employed 592 of those 790 consultants. Public hospital care was provided by 1,731 consultants aided by 3,932 juniors.[61] It is in the large cities, like Dublin and Cork, that opportunities for private practice are greatest and the competing demands on consultants' time most intense.

> Consultants in these larger centres have particular contracts and working practices that entail servicing the consultation needs of a rapidly escalating population of very sick public patients in public hospitals, while at the same time running a busy private practice at both inpatient and outpatient level. This is an enormously crushing burden to fulfil, particularly since private medicine is exclusively a consultant-delivered service, sometimes off-site from the public hospital campus. Delivering intensive private health care in such a personalised individual way, without the support of junior doctors ... is not sustainable in the long-term.[62]

So Muiris FitzGerald, dean of medicine at UCD and a consultant physician at St Vincent's Hospital in Dublin, has described the work practices of his peers.

A study in one general practice of the diagnostic care of patients with coronary heart disease provided evidence of the differing care received by public and private patients. The study of 30 private and 40 public patients found that 77 per cent of private patients and 25 per cent of public patients had had angiograms; all but one of the private patients had had an exercise electrocardiogram; 15 of the public patients were not offered this test.[63]

Even when patients are admitted through accident and emergency departments, where immediate medical need should be the determinant of a patient's treatment, their insurance status may decide the nature of the care they receive, as an A & E nurse recounted:

> A young man came in, about 30. I saw the name of who was on call. I thought he's dead, anyway, before he starts. Then I saw he was in the VHI. Thank God, I thought. So I said to the patient "you are requesting the cardiologist, aren't you? Mind you, I am not saying this, but you are requesting the cardiologist, because it's the diabetes doctor who is on call." If that had been a public patient, I could have done nothing for him.[64]

The reasons for two-tier care and two-tier access

Two-tier care in modern Irish hospitals may be a carry-over from 19th century social attitudes but, in its modern manifestation, it is institutionalised: in how doctors work, the manner in which they are paid and the nature of the medical hierarchy in hospitals; in how hospitals are organised and allocate beds; and in how the state subsidises private care.

Winner-takes-all medicine

Irish hospital medicine is characterised by a winner-takes-all system. At the top of the hierarchy is the hospital consultant, who has the potential to earn a very large income indeed. There are too few consultants. On this, the profession, the Department of Health and every published report agrees.[65] Where differences in opinion emerge is on the issue of how extra consultants should work: whether more consultants should mean cheaper consultants, more answerable to hospital management and with reduced or no opportunities for private practice.

Retaining this small élite corps of high-earning consultants at the top of the medical pyramid has had serious consequences for medical care and for the careers and lives of their colleagues who have not climbed to the top. Ireland produces its own doctors from among its best and brightest but, traditionally, it has not retained them. Up to the late 1990s, Irish graduates would typically leave the hospital system after three to four years and go abroad for further training or take up other career choices. Young doctors refused to stay because much so-called training was unsupervised work, running the system for their absent consultant superiors for long hours and poor pay, with dubious promotion prospects at the end. In England, they could walk into well-organised training programmes, with guaranteed consultant jobs at their conclusion. Only a few specialties in Ireland ran comparable training programmes, centred on larger hospitals, in which Irish doctors in training continued to contribute to the Irish system. "There are", the Medical Manpower Forum observed in 2001 "relatively few fully trained doctors in Ireland in their thirties". The vast majority of consultants were 40 or over. Irish doctors in their 30s were "working abroad with little prospect of returning to a consultant post in Ireland".[66]

The consequence of this exodus has been that the state, despite heavily subsidising the medical education of its young people, staffs its hospitals to a great extent with youngsters and immigrants, many of whom are not in formal training posts. In 2002, the public hospital sector employed 1,731 consultants and 3,932 non-consultant hospital doctors, of whom 2,145 were interns or house officers, generally within their first three years of training after leaving medical school, in training rotations that would move them from hospital to hospital every three to six months.[67] These young, recently qualified doctors treated patients "with, at times, insufficient supervision and guidance at ongoing senior level", as Muiris FitzGerald, dean of medicine at UCD, has attested.[68]

At the intermediate level in the hierarchy, between house officers and consultants, are the registrars, ostensibly in another training grade, except most registrars remain outside formal training programmes. In 2002, approximately one-third of registrars were "specialist" or "senior" registrars engaged in four- to five-year training programmes, changing jobs each year. The remaining two-thirds of the registrars were not in recognised training posts. Of the 593 specialist registrars, the majority, 77 per cent were Irish. Of the 1,193 generic registrars, the majority, 72 per cent were not Irish. In 2002, while non-nationals comprised 53 per cent of all NCHDs, they were close to or over 90 per cent of registrars in five health board areas.[69] They were in the dead-end posts that Irish doctors would not fill. Smaller hospitals in particular have been "virtually totally reliant on non-EU nationals, mainly from the Indo-Pakistan subcontinent", according to FitzGerald.[70] Some of these registrars might remain decades in small Irish county hospitals, having never been offered the opportunity of accredited training and of progressing to a consultant post.

Since the late 1990s, a growing number of young Irish doctors have remained in Ireland to train as specialist registrars. Two developments have convinced them to stay. Since the negotiation of a new NCHD contract in 2000, basic pay and, in particular, overtime rates for NCHDs so increased that junior doctors could earn more in Ireland than in many other states. But, more importantly, driven by further improved training in the UK, most specialties in Ireland felt belatedly obliged to offer structured training. When these specialist registrars emerged from their structured training programmes, and, in 2002, the first cohorts were just beginning to come through in significant numbers, they were now qualified to work as specialists in any EU state. They constituted a time bomb in the Irish medical manpower system. For as they emerged fully trained, the only permanent post on offer to them in Ireland was that of consultant and, unless the number of consultant posts increased dramatically and consultants' method of working consequently changed, there would be nowhere for most of them to go in the Irish system. They also feared that their emigrant classmates would win the contest for whatever consultant posts become available in Ireland. If the medical hierarchy remained unreformed, a minority would become the winners who take all and many fully trained doctors would face a choice between emigration and remaining in training grades.

Muiris FitzGerald has compared the medical hierarchical system to an army consisting of 1,700 "Five Star Generals" (the consultants) assisted by 3,900 "soldiers, most of whom are privates or NCOs [interns and house officers] – these 'lesser ranks' rotating from barracks to barracks every three to six months".

> Walk into any Accident and Emergency Department and you will find that an average of eight out of ten doctors staffing this area will be house officers, typically two to three years qualified, and who will work in this Department for usually no more than 3–6 months. Walk into a public outpatient clinic in the first week of July each year, in most hospitals in Ireland, and you will find that, apart from the consultant, there has been a complete turnover of staff with rarely a single doctor remaining, who was at the same clinic in the last week of June. A similar scene is re-enacted on the wards of most acute hospitals on the changeover date of July 1st – apart from the consultant, all the other doctors have moved on. This makes for huge problems in continuity of care, team work and maintenance of expertise for specialist patient groups.[71]

It is in Accident and Emergency departments that private patients receive a rare insight into how public patients may be treated. At this coalface, all the problems of the hospital system converge. Not only may patients spend the night on trolleys awaiting admission because there are too few beds to accommodate them, but they may be subject to the inexperienced ministrations of junior doctors.[72] Seriously ill patients, who have been referred by experienced GPs, might be seen eight times out of ten by very junior doctors on a brief training rotation, who will cautiously conduct tests and consult each other and, "an unacceptably long number of hours later", decide to admit the patient.[73] Less-ill patients may be admitted unnecessarily because of the absence of trained senior doctors to see them.[74] Patients may wait many hours to be seen. The government's health strategy proposed a "substantial programme of improvements in accident and emergency departments" including the appointment of more A & E consultants and designation of a member of staff to liaise with patients awaiting diagnosis and treatment.[75]

Case study seven: a "death by misadventure"

On a Saturday evening in September 2000, 76-year-old Josephine Hanbury was brought by ambulance to St James's Hospital's Accident and Emergency department in Dublin. She was suffering severe abdominal pains. Half an hour after she arrived she was vomiting blood. Over a number of hours, she was alternately seen by various members of the surgical and medical teams in the A & E. She did not see a consultant surgeon. At 3.30 on Sunday morning, she was sent home. At 9 that evening, she returned and was admitted to the A & E observation ward. When, finally, a consultant surgeon saw her on Monday morning, he immediately sent her to intensive care. She subsequently underwent surgery for a perforated duodenal ulcer and died on Wednesday. A post-mortem found that she had died of acute peritonitis or inflammation/infection of the abdominal cavity, caused by the perforated ulcer. A coroner's inquest issued a verdict of death by misadventure. At the inquest, the consultant surgeon, who had been on call that weekend, said that the initial decision to send Mrs Hanbury home in the early hours of Sunday morning had been an error of judgement. It was difficult if not impossible to say whether she would have survived had she been admitted 24 hours earlier. The coroner noted that, following this death, the hospital had introduced a policy that no patient in a similar situation should be discharged without review by a senior surgeon.[76]

"The right type of consultant"

Improving the quality of care for all public patients requires the retention of Irish graduates in a structured and supervised medical training system and a graduated system of promotion. Gerard Bury, a general practitioner and UCD professor of general practice who, as president of the Medical Council, has campaigned for more demanding standards in Irish hospital care, sees "no reason why the state should be denuded of graduates. The haemorrhage could be arrested by making it attractive to stay here and providing appropriate training."[77]

Making it attractive to stay would require changing the way in which the medical hierarchy is organised. Muiris FitzGerald has been an outspoken advocate of change in the winner-takes-all system. At a public lecture in 1997, speaking at the invitation of the IMO, he suggested that the profession should "radically review the current inflexible hierarchical system"; consider changing the title "consultant" to "specialist"; appoint fully trained doctors at an earlier age; provide a system of career progression based on achievement; shift the emphasis from solo practice to team participation; and "predetermine the level of permissible private practice to ensure a full contribution by specialists/consultants to the public hospital".[78]

His consultant colleagues have not always welcomed his message. Peter Kelly, a consultant pathologist at the Mater Hospital and IHCA negotiator, responded to a later report of FitzGerald's views:

> Prof FitzGerald, oh Prof FitzGerald, what can I say? The "many consultants who disagree with the IHCA" [about changing the nature of consultants' work practices] have remained resolutely silent while he persists as a lone voice in expressing his views. This invisible and shy army is truly without number. His manpower model would have some currency in a large metropolitan hospital in New York or Boston but has little functionality in a small hospital in Ireland.[79]

FitzGerald's offence was to challenge the consultant-as-god model. Gods do not work in teams, have careers whose progress depends on achievement or agree on their private earnings in advance. FitzGerald retained his aplomb. A year later, he told a public meeting of the National Economic and Social Forum that, if 1,000 extra consultants were to be appointed, it must be the "right mix of the right type of consultants". To shift the equity balance, there must be "an incentive for consultants to choose a contract with limited or no private practice".[80]

The consultant as god

> "Who controls access to the hospitals? The medical profession. The politicians won't take them on although they know what's going on. It is a conspiracy against the patient to keep power vested in the medical profession."
>
> "The consultants treat managers with utter contempt. Our management are not educationally equipped to cope with consultants and control them."
>
> – *nurses' accounts at the 2001 INO annual conference.*

> "The doctor has the status of a mini-God. There are no votes in saying I am going to disturb 1,000 consultants. If a politician appears in argument with a doctor on the evening news, the doctor always wins."
>
> – *a health system manager.*[81]

Consultants' terms of employment are extraordinarily anomalous in the Irish public sector. They are salaried and yet they are private practitioners, with all the attitudes of the self-employed. Their independence – arrogance in some – presents enormous challenges for hospital managers. If Irish hospitals are badly run, it is chiefly because the outcome of years of stormy negotiations between consultants and the Department of Health has been a contract which does not make clear who is in charge. The 1997 contract, still current in 2003, stipulates that the proportion of a consultant's on-site practice accounted for by private patients should reflect the proportion of designated private beds in the hospital and that this should be subject to an ill-defined review which, in the words of the 2001 Department of Health working group, "has not been operative". Although the contract additionally states that "it is important to ensure the co-existence of public and private practice does not undermine the principle of equitable access", "there is no mechanism in place to monitor this in practice",[82] according to the working group, which concluded that "changes to the current Common Contract are critical to improvement in the current equity situation".[83]

When Deloitte and Touche examined value-for-money in the health system, they discovered that consultants were "not subject to effective management from a non-clinical perspective". They were absent "from any formal reporting structures". Under the terms of their contract, the quality of their work might be assessed by peer review, but "it is evident that not all consultants participate in this type of audit" and "there is no great desire to introduce the system at consultant level".

"A consultant must decide on what the balance in his practice will be between emergency and elective clinical work and between teaching, research or other work. The employing authority has little control over what that balance should be." The consultants' profile of work "may not necessarily match the overall needs and priorities of the employing authority".[84]

The management consultants further observed that "senior clinical decision-making is not available within our system at all key times". This became an industrial relations issue in early 2002, when nurses took limited industrial action in protest at overcrowding and excessive workloads in A & E departments. The Irish Nurses Organisation sought the appointment in every hospital with an A & E department of a nurse as bed manager who, when overcrowding was occurring, would have the power and the full support of the hospital's chief executive to cancel elective work and "to insist that additional ward rounds are undertaken by consultants" or their senior staff, to ensure the earlier discharge of patients. The INO said that existing bed managers were required "to effectively mediate between in-house consultants and others about how future planned elective work can be maintained, notwithstanding the problems in A&E departments".[85]

This uppity attempt by nurses to fill the management deficit in hospitals provoked a predictably choleric response from the IHCA, which, in a letter to the Health Service Employers Agency, argued that to accept it would be to breach the consultants' contract, since consultants carried "full clinical responsibility for patients under their care". That this meant consultants must take the final decision about which patients were ready for discharge, and that no one else should make that judgement, was a reasonable stance. But the IHCA went much further: "We cannot accept that any consultant be obliged to undertake ward rounds at any time other than a time of their own choosing." How, then, was anyone – nurse, accountant, or medical colleague – to manage an Irish hospital?

The IHCA identified "unwarranted and unacceptable insinuations" in the INO's plan:

> The clear implication of the INO's demands is that consultants are not fulfilling their obligations. That is a charge that we cannot and will not accept ... There is no evidence to suggest that the causes of delayed discharge are the fault of consultants ... Anecdotal evidence exists that many consultants will identify conditions under which individual patients can be discharged, even when the consultant is absent from hospitals.[86]

A month after the IHCA's assertions, they were undermined by the publication of the Comhairle na nOspidéal report on A & E services. This consultant-dominated body found that amid the factors contributing to delays in finding beds for emergency patients was "the need of consultants [due to shortage of beds] to delay discharging their patients in order to ensure bed availability for their incoming patients". Delays in discharging patients also occurred "over weekends and other times when senior clinical decision-makers are not available".[87] The Department of Health working group had already privately reached the conclusion that "consultants and hospital management should address measures needed, if they work off-site, to ensure problems of delayed discharge due to the absence of the consultant, are remedied".[88]

Since consultants do not respect lay managers, the thrust of policy has been to encourage consultants themselves to manage – to develop "Clinicians in Management" (CIM). Although the 1997 contract made provision for CIM, the concept remained "too dependent on local enthusiasm and initiatives"[89] and "in its infancy",[90] reviews in 2000 and 2001 concluded. Clinicians who do take on management roles frequently find themselves regarded as having "gone over" to the other side and meet from their colleagues the same resistance to their efforts to manage as any lay manager.

How consultants are paid

"If a publican paid her barman by the hour for covering the bar and by the drink for covering the lounge, it would be hard to get served in the bar."
– *Sean Conroy, a doctor and programme manager with the Western Health Board.*[91]

At the heart of the discrimination in access and care in Irish public hospitals is the manner in which hospital consultants are paid: by salary for their public patients and by fee-for-service for their private patients.

There is abundant evidence that doctors, like everyone else, respond to the incentive structure they face. Depending on how doctors are paid, they behave differently. From what health economists know about the effects on care of how physicians are paid, I believe that a change in methods of remuneration could go a long way towards solving the problem of the two-tier system of care for Irish hospital patients.

So argued Dale Tussing, the US economist, who, having exercised considerable influence on debate on Irish health care in the 1980s, returned to the fray when the reform debate reignited in 2000.

Problems arise when a physician is paid according to different principles for different classes of patients. Irish consultant specialists are paid what amounts to a salary to treat public patients and by fee-for-service for private patients. Such hybrid systems are full of mischief and will tend to produce a bias in care between the two groups ...

If a doctor is paid by fee-for-service (FFS) for one group of patients, and by capitation or salary for another group, he or she is being given economic signals to increase treatment of the first group and another set of signals to reduce treatment of the second group. Ireland appears to have created such hybrid systems in two circumstances. Firstly, Irish GPs are paid by capitation for medical card holders, and by FFS for private patients ... Similarly, Irish consultant specialists are paid by what amounts to salary to treat public patients, and by FFS for private patients. A health economist would predict that the consequence of this unhappy combination would be that consultants would, consciously or unconsciously, favour private patients in the allocation of their time and resources. The extent of this bias doesn't really depend on the levels of salary and fees. Even where a doctor is paid a truly handsome salary, the incremental revenue for treating one more public patient is nothing ... Of course, one could try to combat these strong incentives through a system of careful monitoring of consultants' use of time. Trying to overcome economic incentives with regulation is often unsuccessful.[92]

Despite the differences in how public and private patients are treated, doctors hate to admit that their financial relationship with their patients affects the nature of the care they offer. For some doctors, the level of their remuneration may be a matter of indifference. There are as likely to be altruists among doctors as among any other group of people. Most people, however, are influenced by how, and how much, they are paid. The Review Group on the Waiting List Initiative, which included 5 consultants in its 12 members, observed in 1998 that international experience indicated that among the reasons why it was very difficult to eliminate waiting lists entirely was that "some hospitals or consultants may find it attractive to maintain a public waiting list because a proportion of those waiting may opt to be treated privately".[93]

This theme was taken up by the Joint Oireachtas Committee on Health and Children, which, in a comparison of waiting lists internationally, quoted a Canadian study suggesting that "greater access to private care appears to be generally associated with longer public sector queues – particularly where physicians operate in both sectors". In Ireland, the committee commented, "there is in effect an inherent incentive within the system for consultants to create waiting lists for treatment".

Private hospitals piggyback on cash-strapped state-funded institutions as they rely hugely on consultants from the public sector. Financial incentives available to consultants in the private sphere, coupled with the lack of monitoring of work carried out under public contract, leaves open the *potential* for disproportionate time to be spent with the lucrative private market, further shifting the balance against the public patients.[94]

Peter Kelly, the consultant pathologist who chaired the IHCA negotiating committee that agreed the 1997 version of the consultants' contract, challenged that Tussing's analysis of the effect of incentives on doctors' behaviour progressed simplistically from a premise to a solution but his premise was unproven. There was no evidence to show that consultants who carried out private work in public hospitals were neglecting their public patients, he responded. Private practice rights had existed for decades, yet no action had ever been taken against a consultant for breach of contract.[95]

The consultants' contract in fact permits discrimination: the delegation of public patient care to juniors; the earning of private fees while on a public salary. A consultant may act as a rational economic agent in response to the incentives on offer to him, may treat as many private patients as can be accommodated in the beds allowed to him by the hospital, may oversee his public practice at arm's length and may do so without ever being in breach of his contract.

Hospital managers are aware of consultants who do not fulfil their public requirements. "There are some consultants, who don't touch a public patient. We know them. We can name them in the different hospitals," an experienced hospital manager observed in 2002. He added, "However, if you were to look at the percentage who behave in this way, it is minimal, when you consider the potential."[96]

Even when a consultant's work does not meet the contractual requirement that his private practice on-site should reflect the proportion of designated private beds in the hospital – when he treats more private patients than he should – this is highly unlikely to lead to disciplinary action, because, in the words of the 2001 Department of Health working group, the contractually ill-defined system of reviewing this requirement "has not been operative". Consultant trade unionists like Kelly attribute this to failures of management. And in support of his view, a senior health system administrator observed in 2002 that some hospitals were much more effective than others in their monitoring of consultants' public and private commitments. While in St James's in Dublin, a leading hospital in developing a clinical role in management,[97] "management would sit down with clinical directorates and engage with consultants on the level of clinical activity", other hospital managers failed to do so.[98]

The success of monitoring appears to depend on the culture and governance of the hospital, reinforcing Tussing's view of the difficulties inherent in "trying to overcome economic incentives with regulation". One manager in a large public hospital explained "I know which consultants are pulling their weight or not but the time and effort it takes to go after one consultant could bring a whole institution down." He favoured focusing on the performance of specialty groups rather than individuals and relying on peer pressure to bring individuals into line.[99]

Managers are attempting to police the 1997 consultants' contract, which emerged as a much woollier version of its 1991 predecessor, because consultants and managers failed to work the practice plans in the 1991 version and, in an atmosphere of militant threats, consultants resisted attempts by the Health Service Employers' Agency to insist on greater accountability, during the 1997 negotiations.

How much do hospital consultants earn – and does it matter?

Consultants' earnings vary hugely. Few full-time consultants earned less than the Taoiseach's €133,000 in 2002. The highest earners made many multiples of this. What differentiates high and low earners is their specialty and the size of their private practice.

Hospital consultants have a number of sources of income: their state salaries; payments from health insurers for treating private patients; outpatient fees paid by private patients, which are not fully reimbursed by insurers; and out-of-pocket payments from patients without insurance who opt for private treatment. In 2002, consultants' state salaries ranged from €115,000 to €142,000. The few remaining consultants on the public-only contract, which was no longer offered from 1997, earned €149,000. Consultants with fewer opportunities for private practice received higher salaries. One-third of consultants opted for lower salaries, which they received for a 33-hour week in a public hospital with the potential for unlimited off-site private earnings. On-call and emergency allowances could add a maximum of €28,500, only fully achievable by working extraordinary hours. The Department of Health estimated that consultants' average state earnings were €151,694 in 2002.[100]

Consultants' earnings from private practice remain a closely guarded secret but may be estimated from insurers' payments to them, an aggregate €192.5 million in 2002.[101] When academic consultants and those in specialties with few opportunities for private practice, such as paediatrics, geriatrics and psychiatry, are excluded, the average income from insurers for the remaining two-thirds of consultants was €130,000 in 2002, effectively doubling their basic salary and suggesting an overall average income for consultants in both public and private practice of some €280,000, even before patients' unreimbursed payments are taken into account. Consultants in rural areas have much fewer opportunities for private practice, so their earnings would be lower than this average while their city counterparts would have correspondingly larger incomes.[102] Consultants in private practice also incur costs – such as rental of rooms and payment of staff. Opportunities for sizeable additional outpatient earnings arise disproportionately for some consultants, such as surgeons, and hardly at all for others, such as anaesthetists. Some consultants could also earn significant sums for legal work in the lucrative personal injury industry. It was reported from legal sources in 2002 that a small pool of consultants might earn some thousands of euro per day for expert evidence.[103] It can be stated with confidence that a significant minority of consultants earn in excess of €500,000 per annum, while the very top earners would exceed €1 million a year.[104]

Even the verifiable incomes of Irish consultants are high compared to their peers' in other countries. In Finland in 2002, the average hospital specialist earned €45,000, the Hanly task force on medical staffing reported in 2003.[105] In the UK, consultants' public salaries ranged from €80,808 to €138,873 (stg£52,640 to £90,465), with a small minority earning up to €205,071 (stg£133,588) through a system of merit awards.[106] The majority of consultants worked on NHS contracts, which limited their private earnings to 10 per cent of their salaries.[107] When Scottish consultants voted for a new contract in 2002, an Irish medical graduate who had worked for eight years as a consultant in Edinburgh and was earning €108,992 (stg£71,000) welcomed the opportunity to increase her income to €128,948 (stg£84,000) by working more reimbursed on-call hours for the NHS.[108] In Denmark in 2002, the salary of a consultant was €87,996 (653,612 Dk), while a "managing consultant" earned €99,626 (740,000 Dk).[109] In New Zealand in 2002, the top of the public hospital salary scale was €79,712 (NZ$159,578).[110] In 2001, doctors with significant private practice could earn in excess of €125,000 (NZ$250,000).[111] In 2002 in France, where pay rates vary widely, salaried public hospital doctors earned a maximum of €83,000 and had very limited opportunities for private practice.[112] Doctors in university hospitals earned some 50 per cent more. In Canada in 2001, surgical specialists earned an average €213,872 ($303,377) and medical specialists an average €162,401 ($230,366).[113] To rival Irish consultant earnings, it is necessary to look to the United States, where in 2001 cardio-vascular surgeons earned a median income of €515,000 (US$459,000) and oncologists and anaesthetists approximately €314,000 (US$280,000).[114]

Far more significant than how much Irish consultants earn is how they earn. Consultants' public earnings constitute a fraction – some 3 per cent[115] – of the overall public health budget. Their private earnings from insurers, although of huge value to some consultants and of lesser importance to others, are insignificant in the context of national health spending – equivalent to 2 per cent of the public health budget. It is not how much consultants are paid but how they are paid, their pursuit and defence of fees for private practice, which props up the two-tier hospital system. Were they paid higher salaries – or fees – for a full-time public commitment in a system that ended discrimination between classes of patients, the majority might conceivably earn comparable incomes but they would no longer be serving two masters – the public and private systems.

However, were the Irish hospital system to employ many more consultants to ensure public patients' treatment by fully qualified doctors, their number would have to increase to 3,500, the Hanly task force on medical staffing estimated.[116] If this body of consultants expected the state to reimburse them for a full-time commitment to the public system with earnings rivalling those of consultants with significant private practice under the present system, the pay bill – €280,000 p.a. for 3,500 consultants – would total nearly €1 billion, or one-eighth of the 2002 public health budget. Were these consultants to be paid at the rate of their Irish colleague in Edinburgh, the bill to the state would be more than halved. Therefore, it does matter how much consultants earn – more consultants must mean cheaper consultants.

More readily available beds for private patients

The system of designation of public and private beds introduced in 1991 has not worked to ensure access to care for public patients. Private patients have four routes into hospital: they may be treated in private hospitals, which supply some 2,300–2,500 beds[117] exclusively dedicated to elective surgery, since they have no emergency departments; they may be treated in some of the inpatient beds designated for consultants' private patients in public hospitals – 2,350 in 2002; they may be admitted as emergency cases in public hospitals and treated wherever a bed could be found; and they may be treated as day cases. Public patients have more limited options: admission as emergency cases to whatever bed is available in public hospitals; treatment as day cases; and admission to inpatient beds in public hospitals, of which 8,650 were theoretically designated for their use in 2002. However, since 70 per cent of all public hospital admissions are emergencies,[118] elective surgery is frequently displaced. In addition, because public hospitals treat the more complex cases and a disproportionate number of the elderly, disabled and chronically sick, who can not afford health insurance, all of whom have greater lengths of stay and may become marooned in hospital awaiting convalescent or nursing home care, there are immense competing demands for the beds that represent public patients' only route to elective surgery. Under the waiting list initiatives, a public patient may be funded for care in a private hospital but, to qualify for this, he will have to have survived a significant wait.

As if it were not enough that the hospital system should be so weighted in favour of treating private patients, they have further benefited from the failure to implement and police the system of bed designation introduced in 1991. The Department of Health's working group reported that the 80/20, public/private bed designation "has not held to that level of mix in some key areas affecting equity of access". The 2001 National Health Strategy observed that in the case of elective admissions, the very area where waiting lists arise, the ratio was "less than satisfactory".[119] In 1999 and 2000, private patients accounted for over 23 per cent of all admissions to public hospitals; accounted for over 29 per cent of planned inpatient admissions; and increased from 21.8 per cent of day patients in 1999 to 23.8 per cent in 2000.[120] In 2001, private patients accounted for 30.9 per cent of patients discharged after elective inpatient treatment and 25.5 per cent of patients discharged after day treatment in public hospitals. In the Eastern Regional Health Authority's area, private patients comprised 28.7 per cent of elective inpatient discharges in 2001; in the mid-west nearly 45 per cent; in the south 34 per cent; and in most other health board areas close to or over 30 per cent.[121] Private patients, on average, have shorter stays in hospital than public patients, reflecting their relative youth and good health,[122] which contributes to this level of throughput but does not explain why it so exceeds the 20 per cent private bed designation.

It is hardly surprising that private patients have been gaining preferential access to day treatment, as 33 per cent of all designated day beds were private in 2002,[123] up from 27 per cent in 1991, having apparently evaded the 80/20 split from the start.[124] In Limerick Regional Hospital, 50 per cent of day beds were private. In Cork Regional

Hospital, 40 per cent of day beds were private.[125] Furthermore, because of the changing nature of day treatments, these official figures failed to reflect the full bias in day patient activity in favour of private patients, a bias which was worsening by the day, with a 12.5 per cent increase in private day patients between 1999 and 2000, compared to an increase of only 0.5 per cent in public day patients.[126]

While day beds are a small proportion of the total bed complement of the state's acute hospitals, day activity has come to dominate elective treatment and many treatments do not require beds at all. Whereas in 1980, only 8,000 day case treatments were recorded, a mere 2 per cent of non-outpatient hospital care, by 2000 there were 320,000 day cases, representing 38 per cent of all hospital activity, 50 per cent of all surgical admissions[127] and 68 per cent of all elective activity.[128] This shift has made the 1991 system of bed designation virtually redundant. As much as a quarter of day case treatment can take place in a "side room", for which there is a specific "side room charge". The patient may be accommodated on a chair, a trolley or in a recliner. The explosion of day activity has led to an explosion of day places, which the old monitoring system fails to capture, a realisation that apparently only dawned on the Department during the course of the detailed preparatory work on the 2001 health strategy. It then emerged that the mismatch between the growing throughput of private patients and the formal designation of private beds could not be adequately explained by private patients' shorter length of stay or the blocking of public beds by older or sicker patients, for whom convalescent places could not be found. In 2002, the Department had yet to devise a means of measuring these new day places, never mind formulate a policy response to their subversion of the monitoring system.

It might be argued that, since the privately insured have now grown to almost half the population, hospitals might be expected to treat growing numbers of private patients and that private patients' medical need might legitimately require their prior allocation of this share of public hospitals' resources. The evidence suggests, however, that it is not greater medical need which secures private patients their growing access to public hospitals. In the Eastern region, where private patients comprised over 28 per cent of public hospitals' elective inpatient discharges, public patients waited twice as long as private patients on average to gain admittance to public hospitals. What this evidence confirms is that hospitals accord the privately insured faster access than public patients, independently of their need, and that the bed designation system, which purports to protect public patients' access, has failed to do so.

In this discussion, an important distinction needs to be borne in mind. Private patients – those who can afford health insurance – have been shown in surveys to be as a group younger, healthier and higher earners than public patients. Poor health makes one less rather than more likely to have insurance. Although, by 2001, 46 per cent of the Irish population had taken out private health insurance, this was a self-selecting group. Among over-65 year-olds, for instance, only 31 per cent of the population had subscribed to private insurance, presumably reflecting the drop in income experienced by people when they retire.[129] Private patients therefore require hospital treatment less often than public patients. When admitted to hospital, their stay is generally shorter. On the other hand, medical card patients, the poorest 30 per cent of the population, are as a group older and sicker than the rest of the population. In public hospitals in 1996 and 1997, they accounted for over half of all bed days[130] and stayed in hospital on average 25 per cent longer than non-medical-card patients.[131] Yet, in 2000, private patients accounted for 27 per cent of bed days in public hospitals, further evidence of slippage in the 80/20 ratio.[132]

It is against this backdrop that the bed designations need to be seen. Private patients – this generally younger, healthier, wealthier group – have unimpeded access to the beds in private hospitals. There is no competition for these beds from emergency admissions. Scheduled surgery goes ahead as planned. Hence, private hospitals have gained a spurious reputation for greater efficiency. In addition to their exclusive access to this population of beds, private patients are admitted for elective surgery to the designated private beds in public hospitals in advance of public patients in greater need. No matter what the length of the public waiting list, no matter how much sicker the people on that list may be, private patients may take up beds in public hospitals. And, even if privately designated beds are not available, they may receive their treatment as day patients on any resting place which escapes definition as a bed.

Even were the 80/20 system of bed designation observed, there would be discrimination against public patients. This system is state-sponsored discrimination, which exists independently of the terms of the consultants' contract. In the words of the Department of Health working group, "the system involved separate waiting lists for public and private beds".[133] However, for private patients to have acquired a one-third designation of all day treatment beds in public hospitals in 2002, running counter to stated government policy, and to have gained further, as yet unenumerated access to day procedures in side rooms,

172

exacerbated this discrimination and was little short of scandalous. Who was to blame: consultants or hospital management? If some consultants were responding to their economic incentive to treat more private patients, why were hospital managers permitting an upward drift in the number of privately designated beds in their hospitals and growth in private day procedures outside designated beds? Bed designations, at least, are under the control of hospital managers.

In the 1980s and early 1990s, hospital managers encouraged growth in private beds to increase private income for their hospitals. Private beds rose from 10 to approximately 20 per cent of the total between 1972 and 1987[134] and, even after the introduction of bed designation, designated private inpatient beds rose from 19 per cent in 1991 to 20 per cent in 1993, while designated private day beds increased from 27 per cent to 31 per cent.[135] The Department of Health effectively colluded in this. As one long-serving administrator put it: "There was a period in the late 1980s and early 1990s,when the Department was happy enough if hospitals were getting a higher percentage of their income from the VHI."[136] The VHI eventually sought to limit additional private bed designations and, in 1996, introduced a system of prior approval for new private beds.[137] If the agreed ceiling of private beds were exceeded, the VHI would not fund the private maintenance in hospital of these further patients, even though it covered their private consultants' fees. Since permitting increased numbers of designated private beds would no longer provide additional income to the hospital, it might appear that hospital managers' incentive to permit growth in private beds had disappeared. This was not entirely the case. As one manager of a major hospital described in 2002, he would still on occasion take the pragmatic decision to allocate further beds to private patients, "even though the VHI won't give me credit for it, even though I will get nothing". He unapologetically explained that he did so because, by offering increased potential for private practice, he could retain consultants working on site and available to public patients, who would otherwise develop their private practice in a private hospital. "I'd prefer to have them here, doing a few extra private cases, than going to Timbuctoo, Blackrock or somewhere else."[138]

It emerges, therefore, that whatever the theory of bed designation, in practice the nature of the consultants' contract puts pressure on public hospitals to facilitate private practice to an even greater degree than the legislation intends, because public hospitals are effectively competing with private hospitals to keep their most senior medical staff working on-site.

The Department's working group report observed that there was a "major lack of clarity" about the bed designation system. Private patients admitted through accident and emergency might be accommodated in public beds, while opting to be treated privately. They would pay the consultant's fees but not the bed charges.[139]

Inequitable from the start, unclear in its application, the bed designation system has been overtaken by developments in medicine. It is neither working to ensure equitable access nor was there ever any prospect that it would do so.

State subsidy for preferential access

Two-tier access to care is not only institutionalised in Irish hospitals but it is also subsidised by the state. In 2002, private health insurance premiums continued to receive tax relief, at an estimated cost to the Exchequer of €94 million.[140] Charges for private hospital beds, even after an increase in August 2002, still contributed less than half the actual cost of providing care.[141] This was despite the commitment in the 1999 White Paper on private health insurance that economic pricing of private beds in public hospitals would be phased in over five to seven years.

The consequence of these state subsidies is that preferential access to care comes cheaply for private patients. In announcing an 18 per cent increase in premium rates from September 2002, the VHI pointed out that the average private health premium was 3 times higher in the UK than in Ireland and up to 12 times higher in the US.[142] In 1999, out of a total national health spend of €5 billion, private health insurance contributed approximately €444 million or a mere 9 per cent.[143]

Defenders of the two-tier system occasionally argue that people who pay for private health insurance are paying twice for health care that they have funded by their taxes. However, the reality is that their taxes pay for public care, which is equally available to all and which they are not denied the right to claim. What private patients achieve by a relatively marginal extra payment is the right to jump public queues and gain superior care, which is denied to many other members of the community who also pay or, in the case of the retired or unemployed, have paid taxes. This leaves aside the more basic argument of whether a civilised or even a self-interested society should base its citizens' access to necessary health care on their ability to pay tax. The preferential access accorded to the insured is analogous to a public educational system which would permit parents of children seeking entrance to over-subscribed national schools to bribe their way in. As one former official with the Department of Health observed: "There is huge dishonesty about how we organise the health services. We are giving one set of taxpayers more rapid access to better treatment for the payment of very little extra money."[144]

While the contribution of private health insurance to the running of the health service is marginal, for individual hospital consultants this private income is significant and a considerable incentive to develop their private practice. For public hospitals, this marginal income from fee-paying patients is an incentive to keep supplying private beds. Insurers too have an incentive to have their members treated in public hospitals, where private treatment is subsidised by the state and therefore cheaper than treatment in private hospitals. The Departmental working group report on the public/private mix commented that treatment in public hospitals was "at an average cost of half that of care in private hospitals" and the hospital's charge was "on average half the cost of care". Consequently, more insured patients are treated in public hospitals than in private hospitals, even though 50 per cent of private beds are in the private sector. While some insured patients are admitted to public hospitals for procedures that could not be performed in the private sector, this is not generally the case. The working group observed that the high volume private cases in public hospitals are procedures that are available in private hospitals and dominate the public waiting list.[145]

Two-tier access and care are realities in Irish hospitals. They explain the scramble to buy health insurance, even among those who can least afford it. They reflect deliberate government policy, expressed in the system of bed designation, and the traditional work practices and self-interest of hospital consultants, expressed in their common contract. Since 2000, there has been a reigniting of debate about the inequities of this system. The failure of contemporary Irish health care is not only reflected in two-tier hospitals, however, but also in the delivery of care in a network of sub-standard hospitals and through an underdeveloped primary care system – further challenges for the reformers.

10

THE POTENT POLITICS OF HOSPITAL LOCATION

"We considered the arguments in favour of placing a General Hospital there [Monaghan] but we are satisfied that the location of the town in relation to the area which it would serve is unsuitable for this purpose."
– FitzGerald Report, 1968.[1]

There are few more potent issues in Irish politics than the local hospital. Although experts argue for the concentration of resources in regional centres of excellence, communities fight to retain local services and politicians dare not deny them. The intense battles over the organisation of hospital services, which so incite local fears and loyalties, too often obscure the more urgent debate about the quality of care which patients receive. There is abundant evidence that too many hospitals offer less than acceptable care. If this were not more than sufficient reason for reform, the continued funding of poor care in inadequate hospitals is bad value for money for patients and for society as a whole. In the absence of political will to confront these issues, pressure to rationalise local hospital networks has come from other quarters: from insurance companies fearing the cost of litigation, from the efforts of medical professionals to improve standards and from the inability of hospitals to find staff. Patients' voices generally seem to make themselves heard only after a tragedy forces them to seek recourse in the courts.

Repeated political failure to remedy inadequate care in sub-standard hospitals has focused attention on decision-making within the health care system. It has become increasingly clear that to reform Irish health care will require reform of the system of health administration – and, critically, of its relationship with the political process.

The patchy pattern of Irish hospital care

In 2002, the Department of Health published a review of bed capacity which concluded that Ireland needed 3,000 additional acute hospital beds – a 25 per cent increase. When re-elected, the government committed itself to providing the beds.[2] The Department of Health then began the much more challenging – and political – second phase of its analysis: determining where the beds should go and assessing whether existing beds were of the right type, in the right places and being used to deliver the right kind of care.[3] Ever since the FitzGerald Report of 1968, the question of hospital location had bedevilled Irish politics. The argument for rationalising small rural hospitals to concentrate resources on providing better care in centres of greater expertise – although broadly accepted by health managers and many, but not all, professionals – remained political dynamite. The Irish electorate had yet to accept the connection between inadequate health services and the duplication of resources in small, out-of-date hospitals. Yet there was plentiful evidence that medical care was not uniform throughout the state.

Death rates at the same age from coronary heart disease (CHD) varied significantly around the country, it was reported in 1999. The Department of Health's chief medical officer, Jim Kiely, concluded in his 1999 annual report that there was regional inequity in access to services which was "clearly unacceptable". The 1999 report of the cardio-vascular health strategy group also found evidence of "inconsistent implementation of internationally recognised best practice" in treatment of patients.[4]

Death rates from the same conditions varied in hospitals around the state, the Medical Manpower Forum reported in 2001. Its report recorded that analysis of mortality from common diseases and procedures like chronic bronchitis, myocardial infarction, mastectomy, fracture of the hip, appendectomy and diabetes found "considerable variation with regard to the mortality from these conditions in Irish hospitals".[5] No research had been undertaken to explain these differing death rates.

It was reported in 2002 that, while patients arriving at accident and emergency departments might have the good fortune to arrive at a hospital where their care would be supervised by a fully trained specialist in emergency medicine, they would be equally if not more likely to find themselves under the care of a doctor from outside the EU, who had come to Ireland to train but had been put on the frontline providing emergency care without any formal postgraduate training.[6] A 2002 report from Comhairle na nOspidéal, the body that advised the Minister for Health on the organisation of hospitals, suggested that appointing more consultant and senior medical staff to emergency departments could improve the quality of care and reduce "the number of errors attributable to junior staff inexperience" – not altogether reassuring for those dependent on current care. The number of complaints might go down too, it added.[7] Above all, patients should be brought to the hospital most capable of providing appropriate care, which meant that each region must have a specialised "trauma receiving" hospital.

"It is almost certain that people are dying from road traffic accidents, who should be saved, and the proportion is probably quite high," was the considered view of University College Dublin's professor of surgery, Niall O'Higgins, in 2002. "We in the College of Surgeons have repeatedly urged local politicians and administrators that, when some one is badly injured, they should be brought to the nearest appropriate hospital and not necessarily to the nearest hospital." Bringing severely ill patients to unsuitable hospitals had not only resulted in avoidable deaths but also long-term disability "with its economic, human and personal costs":

> There is absolutely no doubt about this. We see it all the time – people coming into our hospital [St Vincent's in Dublin] who have been brought to another place where the standard of care is less and where they have not been treated well.[8]

Incredibly, up to 2002, Ireland still lacked a comprehensive system of hospital accreditation. Although professional bodies might inspect hospitals to see if training for doctors was adequate, in the absence of their interest no one was ensuring that patient care met approved standards.[9] In 2002, a new Health Services Accreditation Body was established but, while it might advise on standards, it did not have the statutory power to impose them.

The debate about hospital location

The debate about hospital location, which was opened by the FitzGerald Report in 1968, had mutated into a debate about "centres of excellence" 30 years later. Whereas in the 1980s, hospital closures took place against a background of cutbacks, from the mid-1990s, health boards sought to achieve hospital "reconfiguration". Hospitals would be urged to come together to share services rather than duplicating them in small units. Thus a "regional centre of excellence" in a specialty could be developed.

"We are really talking about centres of competence," a senior medical administrator acerbically explained.[10]

> We are trading convenience for safety. From the initial bad political decision to keep small hospitals open comes a cascade of consequences. Patients avoid them and go to the bigger centres. The sort of people you want to work in the system won't go to them and the Medical Council does not regard them as suitable for training.

In 1968, the FitzGerald Report had recommended the rationalisation of the hospital network into 4 regional and 12 general hospitals, with other hospitals becoming community health centres.[11] The 1993 Tierney Report, a cooperative document from the Department of Health and Comhairle na nOspidéal, took up where FitzGerald left off and concluded that equitable hospital services could only be achieved throughout the country by "having viable hospitals with a critical mass of work to be done and sufficient staff and facilities of the highest calibre available to do it". A population of about 100,000 was required to make this possible, the report argued, yet many areas with such a population currently had two acute general hospitals.

> We do not envisage the closure of any such hospital. Instead we envisage pairs or groups of hospitals in a viable catchment area co-operating to provide a more comprehensive range of services than it is feasible to provide in small, autonomous and often rival units.[12]

This approach was adopted as government policy in the 1994 strategy, *Shaping A Healthier Future*.[13]

Thus, the logic went, two hospitals, each with a small maternity unit, should centralise the unit in one of the two while the other might take on another area of care. But making this case would remain an uphill battle. Communities might even argue that small maternity units should remain open because of the "county jersey" argument – "how can we have a local GAA team when no one is born in the county?" The depopulated county of Leitrim eventually provided a precedent. After the maternity unit in Manorhamilton closed, Leitrim babies took their county status from their home address not their place of birth. Communities would, however, remain vigilant about any evidence that their hospital was being downgraded to the kind of community health centre which FitzGerald had recommended. If geriatric care and dermatology were staffed up and acute care shifted to another hospital, then the odds were a hospital action committee would soon be formed.

By 2002, the Medical Council's statutory control over the training and registration of doctors had become a potent force for change. The Council could insist that doctors who had qualified outside the EU, and were therefore temporarily registered, must work in accredited training posts. The simple, overdue but devastating requirement that such hospital doctors should be adequately trained was forcing reforms in the rural hospital network which no politician had dared contemplate. The president of this body of self-regulating medical professionals was Gerard Bury, a practising family doctor and professor of general practice at UCD. He had been re-elected three times, had held the position from 1996 and would retain it until 2004. Bury had clear views of the rationale for moving from the general care offered by small local hospitals to a more specialised service in the region. He cited "excellent evidence in the medical literature" that:

> A surgeon who works almost exclusively on breast or bowel cancer has much better results than a general surgeon. Three or four working together have far better results than someone working in isolation. There needs to be a catchment area of some 200,000 to 300,000 people for doctors working in an acute hospital to maintain their expertise. There is probably a threshold below which people served by an institution get less than acceptable care.[14]

The Council had no power to reform or advise on hospital networks but it was required to satisfy itself as to the suitability of medical education and training. With the reduction of working hours for junior doctors from 1989, the Irish hospital system had come to depend on ever-increasing numbers of doctors from outside the EU – one-third of all junior doctor posts by 1992.[15] Nominally they came to Ireland to train. In reality they "were propping up the hospital system", in Bury's words, assigned to small hospitals where their posts were not accredited for training, which meant they could not sit postgraduate professional examinations. A survey in 1995 of house officers and registrars had identified that 56 per cent of them had never received a job description, 57 per cent were not in training schemes, 50 per cent considered their training "less than good" and 68 per cent did not know whether a particular person had been designated as responsible for their training.[16]

The implications for their professional formation were not good but, more importantly, the implications for the patients in their care were alarming.

Doctors who had qualified in Ireland or other EU states, and had better professional options, would not generally fill posts which were not accredited for training. Hospital services in five of the eight health boards (midlands, mid-west, north-east, north-west and south-east) were, by the end of the 1990s, virtually totally reliant on non-EU nationals, mainly from India or Pakistan, who had entered Ireland without any examination to establish their competence. Bury recalled:

> It was clearly inappropriate and it was not acceptable for patient care. The Irish public had no assurance of the competence of these doctors. We remained the only system in the Western world that didn't have some form of competence assurance for overseas doctors.[17]

From 1998, doctors who had qualified outside the EU were required by the Council to sit a medical examination and pass a language test. For the Irish public, the reassurance was not total. Driven by concerns for staffing – since the introduction of the exam caused an immediate hospital staffing crisis – rather than for the quality of patient care, the Dáil passed amending legislation in 2002 which excused non-EU doctors who had entered the state before 1998 from the requirement to take the exam.[18] Two years previously the length of time that non-EU doctors already present in the state could remain for "training" had been extended from five to seven years.[19] In addition, Irish or other doctors who had qualified within the EU, and were therefore fully registered, but who, unusually, might not harbour ambitions to go beyond their basic medical training, might still fill posts which were unaccredited for training, because the Medical Council had no power to insist that fully registered doctors should work in accredited posts.

The Council's battle to ensure that doctors working in Ireland should be adequately qualified, and should then be further trained when in the state, had deep-seated consequences for smaller rural hospitals. The quid pro quo for the doctors who passed the exam was that they should be placed in training programmes and "not just dead-end, unaccredited posts", as Bury put it. The Medical Council set out to achieve this by inspecting hospitals, which were then required within six months to set up training programmes agreed with the relevant postgraduate institution. If the hospital could not provide such training, then the posts would not be accredited and non-EU doctors could no longer fill them.

From 1998, the Medical Council set out on its tour of inspection and by 2002 a minority of posts remained to be reviewed. This tour of inspection had radical ongoing consequences for the status quo in smaller Irish hospitals.

In the 2002 general election, two independent deputies were elected solely on the issue of their local hospital. In Clare, James Breen, a farmer and disaffected member of Fianna Fáil, had campaigned for Ennis General Hospital to be upgraded. In Monaghan, Paudge Connolly, a psychiatric nurse, said that he had been asked to stand by consultants and GPs in the town who wanted to keep facilities in Monaghan Hospital.[20] Already in the preceding election, Monaghan had returned a Sinn Féin TD, Caoimhghín Ó Caoláin, who had campaigned on the issue of Monaghan Hospital. Ó Caoláin was also returned to the Dáil in 2002. The location of health services was a hot issue all over the state. On a visit to Waterford, the Taoiseach, Bertie Ahern, was jeered and pelted with daffodils, more typically sold to raise funds for cancer care, by protesters demanding a radiotherapy unit for cancer patients in the South-East.[21]

It remains illuminating to read how the 1968 FitzGerald Report viewed the hospitals that so exercised local feelings in 2002. Of Ennis, the report said that, since it was only 23 miles from Limerick, "we could not contemplate its development as an independent hospital centre". Ennis should become a community health centre and the general hospital needs of the area should be met from the general hospital in Limerick. With only 86 beds and fewer than 5,000 admissions in 1999, Ennis nonetheless still ran an accident and emergency department.[22]

As to Monaghan, the FitzGerald Report instead favoured Cavan as the location for a general hospital because of its central location in the north midlands area. Monaghan's location was "unsuitable". Monaghan still had 107 beds and just over 5,000 admissions in 2001. Its accident and emergency department saw an average of nine new patients a day.[23] However, Monaghan appeared to be fighting a losing battle, which explained the local groundswell that carried Paudge Connolly into the Dáil.

Monaghan General Hospital – survivor of the old politics, casualty of the new

On December 11th 2002, in the 25th week of her pregnancy, Denise Livingstone gave birth to her daughter, Bronagh, in an ambulance on the side of the road between Monaghan and Cavan. Her baby died in Cavan

General Hospital three hours later. Denise Livingstone had first sought help at Monaghan General Hospital but, although nursing staff there believed her delivery to be imminent,[24] she had been sent onwards to Cavan in an ambulance, accompanied by neither nurse nor doctor. Although the chance of survival of such a premature baby was under 10 per cent even in the best of circumstances, and of survival without significant disability even less,[25] and, although the baby's death was attributed to her immature lungs,[26] her roadside birth caused widespread outrage.

In the variegated annals of Irish hospital politics, Monaghan had been notorious long before the birth and death of this baby girl. Ironically, the hospital which had not admitted Denise Livingstone had for long been regarded as the hospital that wouldn't close. In the 1970s and 1980s, local resistance defeated the attempts of two Labour Party Ministers, both serving in Fine Gael-led governments, to follow the recommendation of the FitzGerald Report and direct Monaghan patients to Cavan and other hospitals in the region.

When Brendan Corish published a hospital development plan in 1975, which proposed to reduce the number of general hospitals from 54 to a maximum of 33, he told the Dáil "Monaghan County Hospital is not so sited or constructed as to be capable of expansion into the kind of general hospital envisaged by the guidelines." He announced that he would develop a general hospital in Cavan, while Monaghan would become a community hospital.[27] In the 1977 general election, Fianna Fáil's health spokesman, Charles Haughey, made considerable political capital of the proposed downgrading of hospitals like Monaghan. Once Haughey became Minister for Health, it was the government's stated policy "to preserve the role of the county hospital in providing the necessary level of services to the local community".[28] "All the promises were kept. All the hospitals Fine Gael tried to close have been kept open," Haughey told the Dáil.[29] Monaghan had been reprieved.

Development of the new Cavan hospital, recommended by FitzGerald and planned by Corish, did not begin until 1984 when Barry Desmond was Minister. The new hospital was intended to subsume the functions of the existing sub-standard hospitals in Cavan and Monaghan. Desmond initially intended to close down Monaghan altogether but met such intense local opposition that he instead proposed merely to move the maternity and paediatric units to Cavan. "I was getting advice from Comhairle that they were totally opposed to single-handed units like Monaghan with no peer assessment, no peer relationships," Desmond later recalled.[30]

Local people took Desmond to court. When they failed in the High Court, they went to the Supreme Court. There, the former Minister for Health, now Chief Justice, Tom O'Higgins, and his two colleagues unanimously upheld their case. The court ruled that the Minister did not have the power under the 1970 Health Act to discontinue services in a hospital, although he might close the hospital, provided he held a local inquiry first. The court decided that, although the Act gave the Minister power "in relation to the arrangements for providing services" in a hospital, this meant he could provide for the doing of something but not for its cessation.[31]

The Minister responded to this curious judgment by announcing his intention to amend the 1970 Act. This never happened. "I wouldn't have got it through government because the Fine Gael deputies in the area would have been so violently opposed," Desmond explained.[32] For Desmond's successors, and indeed anyone else who hoped to see a Minister implement rational hospital reform, the legislation would remain "a minefield", in the words of one health board official. Monaghan then proceeded to live a charmed life, for the next Minister was Fianna Fáil's Rory O'Hanlon, who represented the county. Monaghan survived the cutbacks of his era, which were driven by the need to save funds, not by any rational planning to allocate local resources in the optimal way.

By 2002, a new politics had emerged. Policy-makers were now privately relying on a pincer movement to change the role of the poorly resourced and staffed hospitals which their political masters feared to touch: medical professional bodies would no longer certify them as suitable for training; insurance companies would not provide cover for staff working in them; and, once junior doctors' working hours were reduced as required by the EU, it would no longer be possible to recruit a sufficient army of junior doctors to staff them.

Mick Molloy, a campaigning junior doctor and later president of the Irish Medical Organisation, predicted in 2000 that, when the EU insisted on reduced hours for junior doctors, the staffing crisis would become so extreme, "this will end up rationalising hospitals very quickly".[33] In 2001, junior doctors were working an average of 77 hours per week. This was required to drop to 58 hours by 2005 and 48 hours by 2010.[34]

Monaghan was visibly caught in this pincer in the years before Paudge Connolly's election and provided the pre-eminent example of how the politics and policy of hospital location were now being decided. Monaghan remained one of five acute hospitals in the North-Eastern region, which now had a population of approximately 345,000. Clearly the expert advice from 1968, to 1993, to the present day agreed that this represented too many acute hospitals for the population of the region. More importantly, it was not possible for each to offer the level of medical expertise and care across a full range of specialties, which would ensure the best outcomes for patients. However, Monaghan hospital employed nearly 300 people: health was not the only issue at stake.

In September 2000, outside experts, who were assessing local hospital facilities for the health board, were so concerned about the "inadequate and unsafe" environment in the 60-year-old operating theatre in Monaghan that they made an early report. "Remedial action must be taken immediately to ensure a safe environment for surgical procedures," they said.[35] A temporary, purpose-built, pre-fabricated operating theatre replaced the old theatre until a permanent theatre was provided in 2002.

In February 2001, Monaghan's obstetric unit was closed after the health board was informed by its insurers that they would withdraw cover because of safety concerns.[36] The Institute of Obstetrics and Gynaecology had advised that 1,000 deliveries were required annually for doctors to maintain skill levels and that units should have a minimum of three consultant obstetricians. Monaghan had only one consultant obstetrician and in 1999 recorded 344 births. An expert report commissioned by the North-Eastern Health Board (NEHB) had recently recommended closing the unit.[37] Although the elected members of the board had rejected this advice, the insurers had effectively taken the decision out of their hands. Following the unit's closure, local people mounted a sustained campaign to have it reopened, despite evidence that premature babies and babies who did not breathe immediately after birth had significantly poorer outcomes if born in Monaghan than if born in a major regional hospital, such as Drogheda, which could offer on-site specialist paediatric care.[38] Eventually, following yet another expert report, the health board decided that it would open a midwife-led birthing unit at Monaghan for low-risk births.[39] This had yet to happen when Denise Livingstone gave birth.

In July 2001, the Medical Council's tour of inspection arrived in Monaghan. All junior doctors at Monaghan came from outside the EU, so the Council began the process that would require all of them to be in proper training programmes. In December, the Council published criteria for staffing, equipment and supervision in A & E departments that must be met before it would accredit non-EU junior doctors to work in them. Monaghan did not meet the criteria and was requested by the

185

Council not to receive any ambulance emergency cases from January 2002.[40] Here the story of Monaghan differs, depending on the source. The Medical Council discovered that, despite its strictures, the hospital was still "on call" and, consequently, determined to inspect again in May.[41] The Health Board later maintained that major trauma had ceased going to Monaghan by the end of January but conceded that the hospital had continued to receive some ambulance cases.[42] Supporters of the hospital argued that, since Monaghan strictly speaking only operated a "treatment room", the Council's A & E requirements did not apply. Following the reinspection by an exercised Medical Council in May, negotiations ensued between health board and Council about very limited circumstances in which Monaghan might receive ambulance cases, either minor trauma or emergencies requiring immediate stabilisation before transfer. This visit of the Council provoked the closure of Monaghan's child and adolescent unit, so that young people would receive the specialised care of paediatricians in the other hospitals in the region.

In the meantime, in January 2002, Paudge Connolly had organised a rally, which attracted 1,500 protesters, when the Minister for Health, Micheál Martin, visited the hospital. Connolly was then a member of the health board. In May, he was elected a TD for the area.

The Medical Council was not the only body interesting itself in the inadequacy of Monaghan's accident and emergency department. In June 2002, health board members objected to the recommendation by Comhairle na nOspidéal in its report of February that year that, of the four consultants in emergency medicine proposed for the region, three should be based in Drogheda, one in Cavan and none in Monaghan. The logic was that Drogheda should be the major trauma-receiving hospital of the area with emergency consultants available around the clock. In the Monaghan accident and emergency unit, general hospital medical staff, rather than specialised emergency consultants, would be available to provide "resuscitation and limited stabilisation" for the severely ill, before they would be transferred to Drogheda. Nurses in Monaghan would treat minor illnesses and injury in a unit with strong links to local GPs and primary care centres.

Given that only nine patients a day visited Monaghan's accident and emergency department or "treatment room", as the health board described it, it was hard to see how anyone could argue for a specialist emergency consultant to be based there. Residents of Monaghan or travellers passing through the county would stand a better chance of surviving a major accident, as Niall O'Higgins had argued, if they were transferred to a top-class trauma unit in the region, with sufficient staff to provide around-the-clock care.[43] Nonetheless the members of the North-Eastern Health Board passed a motion seeking the appointment of an emergency consultant to Monaghan.

In July 2002, the pincer movement was complete. Monaghan went off call. On July 2nd, the hospital was closed to emergency surgery and elective surgery was severely curtailed. Patients arrived for surgery to discover that their operations had been cancelled.[44] The health board opaquely explained "the issues behind the decision to temporarily suspend admissions to Monaghan Hospital relate to patient safety, professional standards and the need to comply in full with the Medical Council requirements on trainee doctors".[45]

Not only had the hospital failed to meet the Medical Council's A & E criteria, but now the College of Anaesthetists would no longer reprieve Monaghan from needing to meet its requirements for training posts. Ever since the Medical Council's inspection in 2001, the health board had known it had a problem with anaesthesia in Monaghan. The hospital offered neither the complexity nor volume of procedures to constitute an adequate programme to train anaesthetists. The health board had approached the College of Anaesthetists to ask for assistance in October 2001 and Monaghan was granted a reprieve until December, which was later extended until the following June. In July, Monaghan's time had run out. The Medical Council would no longer permit non-EU junior doctors to fill the hospital's traditional two junior anaesthetic posts. Overnight the entire workload had fallen on two consultant anaesthetists.

In mid-July in an atmosphere of rumour about the hospital's future, a small group of staff and patients travelled to Dublin to stage a sit-in in the Department of Health. Upstairs in his office, the Minister, Micheál Martin, gave a radio interview in which he explained "when the bodies responsible for safety make ringing declarations and statements to the effect that particular practices should not continue, then it's beyond the remit of the Minister to intervene". Monaghan might be caught in the pincer but the Minister was determined that it would not be seen as his doing.[46] At the end of July, Monaghan had 297 staff and 17 patients.[47]

How would Monaghan escape this pincer? The health board and the College of Anaesthetists put their heads together and came up with a training programme that would permit junior anaesthetists based in Cavan to spend a maximum of six months in Monaghan.[48] The board also awaited yet another expert report in an effort to find a consensus on the way forward for the region. It was becoming apparent that, to meet

187

the professional bodies' new requirements for quality of care and training, Monaghan would restrict its surgery to planned, elective procedures, many of which would be day cases. While its treatment room would see some patients, emergencies would be directed elsewhere. Monaghan could not continue to offer its former range of services, which had been largely provided, when all was said and done, by junior doctors whose training had been neglected. If some staff had to be redeployed, the pressurised hospitals in other rapidly growing counties in the region would be glad of their services. In December, on average 62 of the hospital's beds were filled.[49]

On July 31st 2002, Paudge Connolly had been at the head of an estimated 3,000 people from Monaghan, 6 per cent of the county's population, who marched through the streets of Dublin to the headquarters of the Department of Health. During the autumn, the hospital's supporters staged fasting vigils outside the Dáil. The protesters understood the political agenda. They knew their hospital was being downgraded but no one was willing to say openly that this decision had been taken. Instead they were watching services leave the hospital in response to the decisions of insurance companies, professional training bodies or expert groups. This was how the politics of hospital location would now be played out. To expect the Minister or the health board to announce an orderly winding down of acute services in Monaghan, as part of an overall plan for the North-East, would have been to require a form of overt political leadership that had last run aground with the 1984 Supreme Court judgment. Instead, the Minister and the health board would permit the reorganisation of the hospital services to hang on the medical profession's efforts to police higher standards, motivated in part by their own ethic but also now more urgently driven by professionals' and insurance companies' fears of litigation.

Five months later, after Bronagh Livingstone's birth and death, Monaghan politics became national politics. Initial comment tended to confuse many issues: the reasons for the baby's death, the handling of her birth, the appropriateness of maintaining an obstetrical service in Monaghan. A review conducted by the health board defended the decision by staff at Monaghan to transfer Denise Livingstone prior to delivery[50] but an independent review panel, established by the Minister, disagreed. It found that staff at the hospital had not followed a health board protocol that advised that if a mother arrived in labour and delivery was inevitable prior to transfer to another hospital, they should assist with the delivery.[51] It emerged that while nurses had believed delivery to be imminent, the junior doctor who assessed Denise Livingstone – a house officer in surgery – did not realise she was in labour.[52] Such "communication deficits" might have been resolved by the involvement of a consultant, suggested the health board review,[53] but a consultant was never called – that not uncommon omission.

The independent review panel concluded that junior medical staff were unfamiliar with the health board protocol, which had been circulated but never discussed on-site nor tried out in "fire drills", and that the protocol was insufficiently specific on key issues, such as the need to evaluate the imminence of delivery and how to handle an imminent delivery. The review panel recommended that the protocol should make it mandatory for a nurse or doctor to accompany a mother in an ambulance, if she were being transferred, and that it should be made clear in what circumstances a "flying maternity squad" should come from another hospital.[54]

When a hospital loses services, as Monaghan had, in a piecemeal way dictated by the concerns of insurers and professional bodies, over the objections of the community and not as part of a thought-through plan, one of the consequences is administrative and staff confusion – and this emerged clearly from the investigation into the Livingstone case. Monaghan Hospital had no assigned on-site manager in December 2002. As part of the "Cavan/Monaghan hospital group", all its top managers were based in Cavan. Staff cannot but have been aware that the obstetrics service had stopped for insurance reasons and they had been made insufficiently aware of the protocol that dictated how they should respond if a delivery was inevitable. They were "caught in the middle" in a "highly charged environment" leading to "vulnerability to error", the independent review observed.[55] Had the ending of the obstetrical service been planned and endorsed by local political representatives, or indeed been dictated by the Department of Health, then as an obvious corollary, procedures should have been put in place and explained effectively to hospital staff and the wider community to ensure a shared understanding of how a Monaghan woman facing imminent delivery should be treated.

For supporters of the hospital, the moral of the Livingstone case was that services should be restored to their former level. This flew in the face of the expert advice. For health service planners and the medical specialist bodies, who believed that patients should no longer be treated in small hospitals with too few patients to sustain professional standards, but who faced an uphill battle to convince the people of this, the moral must be that services should not be withdrawn without the substitution of appropriate alternatives to handle local emergencies.

While some defenders of local hospitals are motivated by concerns which have little to do with health care – defence of their jobs, of the status of their town, of spin-off local employment – the protests by the people of Monaghan and other small towns should also be seen against the backdrop of an underfunded, underdeveloped health service with significant financial barriers to access. Local communities may still regard their smaller, relatively low-tech hospitals as preferable to a high-tech centre in the next county for which the promised funding might never materialise. The "regional centre of excellence" might, after all, end up like the prestigious Dublin hospitals: with outlandish waiting times to be seen in accident and emergency and long waiting lists for elective surgery. The Monaghan protesters' resolve to defend their local hospital was stiffened by the sight of patients on trolleys in Cavan Hospital, where nurses went on a work-to-rule in June 2002 to protest about the overcrowded conditions in the A & E department.[56] On paper, a nurse-led accident and emergency department in Monaghan, linked to local primary care centres, might seem fine but where were the primary care centres? Until a government funded and implemented the primary care strategy announced in 2001, they were still by and large an abstract concept, even though Monaghan Hospital was admirably suited to provide the location for such a centre. In the existing system and for the significant numbers of people who found family doctors' charges prohibitive, it remained reassuring to be able to take the instant decision to take their child to the local emergency room, which, until the announcement of increased charges in July 2002, was cheaper than attending their local doctor.

Addressing local fears would require a Minister and government committed to sustained funding of a coherent, comprehensive and accessible health service. In the meantime, it was understandable that communities should fight to retain the health service they could see and access, however inadequate it might be. So the election of men like Paudge Connolly to the Dáil in 2002, although dismissed by some commentators as an expression of backward-looking local politics, might also be seen as people voting for accessible health care in the only way they knew.

The politics of breast cancer care

Until the death of Bronagh Livingstone, Monaghan had been a sideshow compared to the many other battles being waged about hospital location in 2002. During the general election campaign, Niall O'Higgins, UCD's professor of surgery, was judged to have struck "the heaviest blow landed on the government so far on health".[57] This diminutive, greying 60-year-old professor, with a precise and academic manner, made an unlikely political brawler. For two years, O'Higgins had been waging his own personal campaign to convince politicians, local electorates and some of his medical brethren that patient care must come before local pride or convenience. O'Higgins' particular battleground was breast cancer treatment. He had been chairman of a sub-group of the National Cancer Forum which recommended in its 2000 report that treatment for breast cancer patients should be concentrated in a smaller number of centres where specialised teams could offer patients a much better chance of recovery. Breast cancer was the most common fatal cancer in women. Ireland had well above the EU average death rate from the disease.[58] International evidence suggested that women treated in centres with a high volume of patients had a 15 to 20 per cent better chance of survival after five years. Conversely, the mortality rate for women treated in hospitals with little throughput could be up to 60 per cent higher. Translated into local politics, this meant that care should be concentrated in 13 hospitals.[59] O'Higgins explained:

> Patients with breast cancer have a much better chance of long-term survival when they are cared for in large, specialist centres that treat, at a minimum, 100 new breast cancers a year ... Such centres need a population base of 250,000 to 300,000 people.[60]

While improved survival would seem a sufficient argument for following O'Higgins' advice, he further argued that diagnosis in high-tech centres could save women "enormous distress and unnecessary operations" by substituting more sophisticated needle biopsies for "open biopsies" – breast incisions under anaesthetic – which general surgeons were still performing all over the state.[61]

Notwithstanding the strength of the report's case, its publication was the signal for the resurrection of traditional local inter-hospital rivalries. Letterkenny disputed the claims of Sligo in the North-West; Castlebar fought the centralisation of services in Galway in the West; Portlaoise did battle with Tullamore over breast cancer care in the Midlands – its supporters had already taken to the courts and streets when the 20-mile distant Tullamore was chosen as the centre for general cancer care. Although the report had recommended that transport to regional centres should be part of this new care regime, local communities – and doctors – campaigned for continued local care, despite the evidence that quality of care might suffer. It was, perhaps, understandable that local doctors, who had struggled to provide care for patients in the constrained health services, should resent the concentration of new investment in the next county, but their campaigning disturbed some of their colleagues. O'Higgins commented:

> The argument about downgrading local hospitals doesn't stand up because they never had a proper service to begin with. It's just pure local politics, nothing to do with medical care. Medical people, who really should know better and do know better, because they have the literature available to them, are pretty happy sometimes to call for the best but then when it comes to their local situation, they suddenly become non-medical and political.[62]

His frustration with lack of local political leadership on and inadequate resources for the development of regional cancer care became evident in an interview he gave during the 2002 general election campaign. "Since this report was issued two years ago, progress has been slow and disappointingly slow. It's fair to say that none of the units has been established, although some of the areas are more advanced in their planning than others."[63]

O'Higgins was elected vice-president of the Royal College of Surgeons in Ireland in 2002 and would assume the presidency in 2004. After the general election, he met the reappointed Minister, Micheál Martin. "I said this won't go away. There is going to be a maintaining of pressure because, for the people pushing this, it's not just an emotional feeling. This is evidence based and it's a life or death issue."

The provinces protest but Dublin suffers

The resistance of local hospitals to the development of regional centres of excellence has not only had implications for treatment in the provinces but also has affected care in the major urban centres. Some of the campaigners to retain local hospitals may take a different view of their hospital's services when they are in need of medical treatment. Patients frequently vote with their feet and, if they can afford to do so, travel to Dublin for treatment. Thus, a study by the Eastern Regional Health Authority, published in June 2001, revealed that a very large number of patients were being referred to Dublin for services which were universally or widely available around the country.

"The referral to the Dublin hospital or consultant is generally made by the patient's GP and the local hospital, the local consultant and the health board is unaware that this referral is being made," commented Donal O'Shea, chief executive of the ERHA. It was therefore not possible to take this pattern into account in managing the local service.

> Equally the acceptance for treatment of these referrals by the Dublin hospital or consultant is generally being made without regard to the availability of the local service, or without regard to, or probably knowledge of, the comparative waiting list in the referring region as against the Eastern hospital.[64]

The ERHA found that patients from outside the region used over 40 per cent of all bed-days for planned, elective surgery in the Eastern region. This 40/60 split had been constant for many years, despite a significant increase in consultants and services outside the East. Although it was appropriate to refer patients for national specialties, such as neuro-surgery, which were available only in major teaching hospitals, the level of referral for services that were well developed in all the regions was "surprisingly high". Hip-replacement surgery was available in every region, yet 36 per cent of hip replacements in the East were for patients from other regions with their own local service.[65]

The consequence for Dublin of these referrals from all over the state was that Dublin hospitals had the greatest pressure on beds, resulting in long delays in admission to hospital through accident and emergency departments and long waiting lists for public patients. Dublin had also lost disproportionately more beds during the 1980s cutbacks.[66] The ERHA calculated in its 2001 review of bed capacity that, despite apparently greater numbers of acute beds per head of population in Dublin, when referrals from outside the region were taken into account the East had 2.45 beds available per 1,000 population compared to 3.11 per 1,000 residents outside the Eastern Region.[67] The EU average in 2000 was 4.1 beds per 1,000 people.[68] In 2001, 60 per cent of patients waiting for elective surgery were in the Eastern Region,[69] which had 35 per cent of the population.

The flow of patients from the provinces to Dublin, even when facilities were available locally, reflected traditional referral patterns by general practitioners. GPs would also privately admit that they played the system. By offering a Dublin consultant the business of their private patients (who considered care in Dublin to be of a higher quality), they used this leverage to ensure that he would also care for their public patients. So, although long waiting lists would seem a deterrent to public patients' travelling to Dublin for care, they found it worth their while to make the journey. When Dublin maternity hospitals publicly warned of pressure on their services, health administrators nonetheless found them resistant to suggestions that they should give priority to patients from Dublin.[70] To prioritise local public patients would cut off the flow of private patients from the rest of the state. The inflow of patients for elective surgery in the East contained a higher proportion of private patients than among patients from the East, ERHA analysis for the first half of 2002 revealed.[71]

The reform imperative

Many observers of the inability of existing institutions to organise rational hospital services have concluded that there must be institutional reform. Debate has centred on the issues of how decisions about hospital location should be taken and by whom. Should the health boards lose their decision-making powers? Should hospital services be organised centrally? Should the Minister for Health legislate to recover the powers that he lost with the 1984 Supreme Court judgment?

While, on the face of it, the 1970 Health Act had given Ministers power to direct health boards to provide hospital services and to open and close hospitals, the Supreme Court judgment had limited the Minister's ability to act – he might no longer direct that services should be discontinued in an existing hospital. The legislation could quite simply have been amended to restore to Ministers the powers they had been believed to hold prior to the judgment. However, in the hot political climate of hospital location, it apparently suited subsequent governments to leave the ball in the health boards' court, even though the boards often appeared constitutionally incapable of taking unpopular decisions. This reflected their structure: the county councils and corporations in the region appoint a majority of the members of the boards; the remaining members are elected by local health professionals or nominated by the Minister. The boards are democratic bodies but, since a majority of members are local councillors elected to represent very small areas, they think locally not regionally. Their re-election depends on satisfying voters in a discrete local area. It is in their interests to retain dispersed services in smaller hospitals rather than to urge the development of superior services in one regional hospital. In an appeal for better regional development of services to remove pressures from the East, Pat McLoughlin, director of planning and commissioning at the ERHA, suggested in 2001 that health board members might instead be elected by a regional constituency so that they would put the needs of the region before those of the locality.[72] The 1970 Act had, in fact, provided for three regional hospital boards based on Dublin, Cork and Galway. By the late 1970s they were already regarded as an unnecessary tier of administration[73] and they were finally abolished in 1996.[74]

When they were established, the health boards were partially funded from the local rates so at least the local electorate had some interest in value-for-money in health spending. However, within five years the rates had been phased out and, as Ruth Barrington pointed out in her history of the health service, "with no financial consequences falling locally, every community had an incentive to fight for the development of its hospital to the standard envisaged for a few by FitzGerald".[75] Formerly an assistant secretary in the Department of Health and latterly chief executive of the Health Research Board, Barrington subsequently concurred with Pat McLoughlin that the boards should be elected by a regional constituency and further argued that they should once again be at least part funded by some form of local taxation. She favoured a Scandinavian model. In Denmark and Sweden, "local representatives are both accountable for raising taxation and spending wisely. Local authorities may vary the level of taxation, within limits agreed nationally, to fund developments over and above the minimum level of service that must be available to all."[76] She advocated

> a gradual introduction of financial flows between health boards for services provided for their population, for example, in hospitals outside the region. This would give health boards an incentive either to buy more services or provide them within the region, a choice they do not have at the moment.

Barrington is a defender of local democracy against those – in politics and medicine – who would prefer to see decisions on local hospital services taken at a central level.

> Politics cannot be taken out of health, no matter how much some professionals, technocrats or management consultants would wish. Health boards provide a decentralised decision making structure and a means to resolve conflict over health services in the interest of the public good. Despite a perception to the contrary, health boards have taken extremely difficult decisions about the development of health services, decisions that would not have been accepted if taken by officials or by a national body.

Barrington would, however, balance democratic representation by giving local politicians responsibility for raising the funding required for services.

Although local doctors are often at the centre of opposition to changing the role of hospitals, prominent members of the profession have urged the removal of politics from decisions on hospital location. Muiris FitzGerald, UCD dean of medicine, has suggested that health policies needed to be "politics proofed" against parochialism[77]; while Brendan Drumm, UCD professor of paediatrics and chairman of Comhairle na nOspidéal from 1996 to 2001, proposed that health services should be coordinated at national level by expert groups, representing patients, health care professionals and politicians. Drumm argued that the Dublin voluntary hospitals had been as "culpable" as rural hospitals in obstructing the rationalisation of specialised services. He instanced

> the attempt to develop five centres of excellence for the provision of cancer care in Dublin, when all international experience would suggest that this city, while providing routine cancer care on all hospital sites, should develop a centre of expertise for the country as a whole on one hospital site.[78]

The balance of opinion has been moving against local democracy in health politics. When the growth of health spending was curtailed from late 2002, the health boards bore the brunt of dissatisfaction with the health service. Since most decisions on health were health board decisions, every failing of the system from overcrowded accident and emergency departments to the mishandling of Bronagh Livingstone's birth began to be viewed as a failure of health board management. Medical and political voices joined in criticising the number and function of the boards. Growth in the number of health administrators became an exaggerated issue and the question of how health boards managed was confused with the quite separate question of how elected political representatives on boards affected local hospital organisation. The debate acquired an added edge because the Minister for Finance, Charlie McCreevy, perceived that health spending had increased without delivering commensurate improvements in care or defusing public anger about the health service.

Three bodies considered reform: a commission established by the Department of Finance and chaired by UCD professor of management, Niamh Brennan, was primarily concerned with management and control of health spending; Prospectus management consultants were appointed by the Department of Health to assess functions and structures in the health service; and a task force on medical staffing, involving a wide range of medical professionals, administrators and others, chaired by health consultant David Hanly and also reporting to the Minister for Health, was given a mandate to determine how care might be delivered by hospital consultants rather than junior doctors. To achieve any of their interrelated objectives – efficacious health spending, optimal organisation or consultant-delivered care – it was apparent that the hospital network must be organised differently and that achieving that would require a different way of taking decisions.

All these bodies had essentially been invited to reinvent the wheel. The FitzGerald Report might now be outdated in its details but its principles for hospital organisation had never been overturned. The Commission on Health Funding had pointed out in 1989 that "the simple question 'who is in charge?' cannot easily be answered for the Irish health services"[79] and had recommended that a national Health Services Executive Authority should replace the health boards, which would become health councils with the power to delay but not veto decisions on local health services.

Deloitte and Touche's value-for-money audit of the health service, undertaken for the Department of Health in 2001, had observed that, since the FitzGerald Report, there had been "no political will" to make "hard political decisions" about hospital rationalisation[80] and recommended a review of the role and number of the health boards which would focus on "mechanisms to de-politicise the implementation of Health Strategy and service delivery. If this is not achievable there need to be mechanisms in place to make Boards accountable for the non-delivery of VFM [value for money] associated with local political decision-making."[81] The consultants suggested that boards should be smaller and tighter and the focus of local political input should be on "representing the local population and not on a decision-making basis".[82]

In their early drafts, the Hanly task force rewrote FitzGerald for the new millennium, while the Prospectus and Brennan reports revisited the Commission on Health Funding. Three central questions remained: would the government have the political will to remove control of the direction of the health service from local political interests? Who then would take responsibility for deciding the shape of the health service? And, if local politicians were to lose their veto, how would the administration of the health service remain democratically accountable?

The work of the Hanly task force immediately confronted the

government with the need to remove decisions on local hospital care from the policy and political vacuum that had engulfed Monaghan hospital. The task force took the view that it could not design a system of consultant-provided care, rescuing patients from the ministrations of junior doctors in training or, worse still, not in training, without also designing a more rational basis for hospital organisation. It recommended that "hospitals should be structured rationally, on the basis of an objectively established national plan" and that a national hospitals authority should take responsibility for the planning and management of all acute hospitals.[83]

Already, the 2001 Health Strategy had announced that there would be a new National Hospitals Agency, which would prepare a strategic plan for the expansion of capacity in acute hospitals, provide "expert, objective advice" to the Minister for Health on the location of beds and configuration of hospitals and would "consult" health boards. The intent of the Minister's reforms had been far from clear. Although Micheál Martin suggested that only a brave Minister would refuse the advice of his new agency, it remained advisory and he appeared to accept that ultimate decisions on hospital location would be his.[84] The strategy stated that the government took the view that changing the number of health boards would not necessarily improve services, yet appeared to envisage that health boards would cede control over location of hospital services to this new agency.[85]

In early 2003, the Hanly task force was prepared to go further and recommended an empowered hospitals agency with national executive responsibility for management of hospitals, in which care would now be delivered primarily by consultants. Hospitals should then be organised according to a defined hierarchy: at the top would be hospitals providing a unique national specialty like transplantation; next would be "supra regional" specialties like neurosurgery, which would be confined to a few centres; then, in each region, there should be a large regional hospital, normally serving a population of between 350,000 to 500,000, which would offer a full range of acute hospital services. The rest, the Monaghans and other county hospitals which served smaller populations, would then become "associated" hospitals. They would no longer treat major traumas or medical emergencies, which would go to the regional centre. They would host outpatient clinics and offer elective surgery, mainly on a day basis. They would be staffed by teams of doctors coming from the regional hospital. Only low-risk patients would stay in these hospitals overnight and, if they deteriorated unexpectedly, they might be transferred to the regional hospital. The picture was familiar – the new dispensation in Monaghan writ large. The task force emphasised the positive: that these hospitals could be "dynamic, busy institutions" providing efficient services, where local general practitioners could, if they wished, retain responsibility for their patients' care. In general, acute hospitals would develop and work in close partnership with primary care.

The Hanly task force report was also clear, however, about the motivation for these recommendations – that fundamental reorganisation was required to deliver high quality care. "The importance of treating seriously ill or injured patients in a centre that is fully equipped to meet their need cannot be overstated." In answer to the fears of local people about seriously ill patients being asked to travel further for care, the report argued that many life-saving measures in emergencies were not affected by the immediate proximity of a hospital. It instanced that two-thirds of deaths from heart attacks happened before the patient reached hospital, while three of the most effective immediate responses – use of a defibrillator, cardiac resuscitation and "clot busting" drugs – could be delivered by emergency ambulance personnel. Similarly, after a serious accident, early action to maintain an airway and reduce bleeding could be administered by ambulance personnel, while the next most important prerequisite for survival was to be treated in a hospital offering comprehensive skills and facilities – the regional hospital.

In its early 2003 draft report, the Hanly task force eschewed politics and did not name which hospital should fall into which tier of service. At the time of writing, it remained to be seen whether politics would intervene and cause a dilution of its recommendations or, less probably, whether they would be strengthened and assign a defined status to named hospitals, as in the FitzGerald Report. By admitting the possibility that there might remain a few general hospitals, in regions of very dispersed population, the draft report offered an avenue of escape for the defenders of small hospitals from demotion to "associated" status, which might make ultimate political decisions more difficult. The task force's recommendation of a national plan for hospitals, to be administered by a central agency, drew it into discussions of administrative reform, which were simultaneously under review by the Prospectus and Brennan bodies.

The Prospectus group developed a model of a national health services executive (HSE), in effect a new semi-state body, which would administer the health service at arm's length from the Department of Health. The Minister for Health would appoint its board and its chairman would report to him. The national hospitals' agency, now a national hospitals office (NHO), and four regional health offices (RHOs) would report to the HSE. Like Hanly, Prospectus proposed an empowered national hospitals office, which would plan, commission and fund acute hospital services, manage waiting lists and approve consultant posts, effectively subsuming both the National Treatment Purchase Fund and Comhairle na nOspidéal. The regional health offices would plan, commission and fund services outside hospitals, such as primary and community care.[86]

The political kernel of the proposed Prospectus reforms was that they envisaged the abolition of the existing 11 health boards and, with them, local political representation in health administration. Prospectus considered but ultimately rejected the idea of introducing regional health advisory councils, along the lines proposed by the 1989 Commission on Health Funding.[87] This was a top-down, centralised model of administration. The hospitals would be run as regional networks, with managers of smaller hospitals reporting to managers of the central regional hospitals, who would administer a coherent service for the region and report in turn to the national hospitals office. The separation of a line of command for hospitals from the line of command for the rest of the health service, albeit under the overarching control of the national executive, gave rise to some concerns that primary and community care would remain insufficiently integrated with the hospitals, an acknowledged shortcoming of the existing system.

In early 2003, Prospectus was developing its thinking with a clear mandate from the Department of Health and receiving direction from a steering committee, chaired by the secretary general, Michael Kelly. This report was intended to be the voice of the Department, which already in the 2001 health strategy had acknowledged the inadequacies of the existing system of health administration. Prospectus described a fragmented structure, split into 58 agencies, nearly half of which had been established over the preceding 10 years, in which the Department had nominally ceded the executive role to the health boards but retained many executive functions. Since the Commission on Health Funding had reported, 14 years earlier, it had become even more difficult to discern who was in charge. Prospectus advocated cutting down on the number of agencies and establishing clear lines of accountability to deliver a more responsive service that spent money to better effect. The Department was clearly concerned that, without this reform, it would never secure the investment the service needed.

In its early draft, the Brennan Commission proposed a similar model of executive authority but would retain a reduced number of regional health boards. Charged with improving efficiency in health spending, the Brennan Commission's motivation in advocating this centralisation was to introduce greater financial accountability. It discerned a "management vacuum at the heart of the health service", a consequence of the devolution of management to the health boards. Like Prospectus, it advocated clear lines of financial accountability from top to bottom of the health service, with hospital consultants ultimately accountable for their own budgets.[88] In the spring of 2003, representatives of the Departments of Health and Finance sought to achieve convergence between the two reports' recommendations prior to publication. The Minister for Finance, Charlie McCreevy, was resistant to the proposed executive authority for health, apparently because of a concern that this would remove decisions on health spending too far from the control of the mandarins of Finance.[89]

However, the drift of thinking was clear – centralise, increase managerial accountability and reduce local political input. But what about democratic accountability? Barrington was not alone in her reservations about attempting to take politics out of health. Politicians from a number of parties pointed out that a tendency in the proposals for reform to prefer unelected consumer panels to elected representatives, as a means of involving the local population in decision-making, smacked of tokenism. Yet, if local representatives were to retain their existing power of veto, any attempt at rational planning would fail. The obvious alternative to local democracy as a means of ensuring democratic accountability was to restore control to the Minister for Health, who is part of a government, answerable to the Dáil. If the Department of Health were to set policy and an executive implement it, it should still be the Minister's job, by legislation if necessary, to determine the parameters of policy: the appropriate catchment area for a particular class of hospital, for instance; the appropriate level of training at which a doctor might administer unsupervised care. In a state-funded health service, the spending of society's resources on health and the delivery of health services are decisions for the citizen. In a democracy, the citizen delegates decision-making power to the elected government. A new plan for configuration of hospitals would be a major national decision. It should require a Dáil mandate. This was the path on which Brendan Corish embarked with his plan in the 1970s, when electoral politics intervened. Once a plan had Dáil approval, an executive agency could then be given the freedom to implement it, subject to review by Dáil committees, by the Ombudsman and by, perhaps, the kind of local health councils which the Commission on Health Funding envisaged – with power of delay but not veto.

With some modifications, this was the balance between politics and health proposed in the Department-of-Health-sponsored Prospectus Report, in its early 2003 version. The Department of Health would set policy targets, evaluate outcomes and agree an annual National Service Plan with the HSE. The HSE would then be responsible for delivering the plan by funding, commissioning and overseeing services. "The direct line of political accountability" would run through the Minister for Health and the government "to the Dáil". Politicians might still interfere or, as Prospectus put it, "executive matters" might be pulled "into the political arena". Electoral politics could continue to affect health service planning. But, without electoral politics, there would be no democracy. This system would at least establish an institution with the power to set and pursue consistent national goals, and with the ability to explain to politicians and the electorate the financial consequences of deviating from plan.

In defence of the medical profession's preoccupation with removing politics from health, it should be said that the Medical Council's requirements for training had drawn a line about standards of patient care that the political system had been unprepared to draw. Comhairle na nOspidéal had produced a sensible plan for regional accident and emergency services. In a chaotic and underfunded system, these bodies had fought for standards of care. This professional voice would have to remain an important component of any new dispensation.

Since the publication of the FitzGerald Report in 1968, comprehensive reform of the Irish hospital network to deliver the best care for patients has not taken place. Despite the stated commitment in 2002 of the incoming government to provide 3,000 extra acute beds, delivering and staffing these beds would require the political will to fund sustained investment, if not by this government then by some future government. If this investment were to repay the people of Ireland – throughout the state – with improved health services, better care and better outcomes, the allocation of beds and services was critical. All the experts were agreed that investment should be concentrated on regional centres of excellence. These would never develop without institutional reform. In 2003, three further bodies had explored options for administrative reform, which had the potential to liberate the health service from the stasis in which it had been locked since the FitzGerald Report. The proposed new structures could potentially deliver a much greater coordination between primary and acute services, within a coherent and accountable framework, in which it would be possible at last to answer the question "who is in charge?" Whether the government chose to dilute, suppress, ignore or implement their proposals would be critical for the future of Irish health care. It remained to be seen whether any government or Minister truly wished to be seen to be in charge of the health service.

11

WHEN THE DOCTOR COSTS TOO MUCH

"We have cases where families put off going to the doctor. There isn't a conference of the society which isn't paying out money for doctors' bills every day of the week."
    – John Monaghan, president of the St Vincent de Paul, November 2000.[1]

"Private doctors' fees are way too high. A lot of women who don't work and don't have a medical card don't look after themselves because they can't afford to go to the doctor."
                                                – a woman in her 50s, 2001.[2]

Most Irish families pay for each and every visit to a family doctor. Travellers to Ireland from other European states find this an extraordinarily alien discovery. The most basic level of health care, the initial point of contact with the health service, is not free nor does the state take responsibility for its delivery. In Ireland, general practice is a private enterprise, administered by private contractors who choose where they will set up practice and how much they will charge. The state pays GPs for the care of, approximately, the 30 per cent of the population on the lowest incomes and has paid for the care of all over-70-year-olds since 2001. Those who qualify for coveted medical cards need pay for neither care nor medication. For many others, the cost of general practitioner care is a barrier to access, compounded by the cost of medication.[3] In 2002, one visit to a family doctor cost one-third of the weekly income of an individual earning just above the threshold for a medical card.[4] In 1900, GPs charged proportionately less – one-eighth of the weekly income of a labourer.

    GPs are in a marketplace selling care and are only aware of the needs of the patients who come to their door. There is no register of patients, so GPs cannot decide, for instance, to remind every man of a certain age in their area that he ought to have his cholesterol checked. Consequently, Ireland has virtually no population-wide preventive care.[5] The cost of care causes patients to defer seeking treatment, while their health deteriorates, resulting in hospitals seeing many patients who should have first attended their family doctor.

Because primary medical care is a private enterprise, it has suffered from chronic underinvestment and is insufficiently linked to the rudimentary public health care system. There are too few GPs. They frequently work from their homes, in converted garages, or in small rooms rented over shops. They seldom have the support of nurses or other health professionals. Frequently, they are unavailable after hours. They have few treatment facilities and refer patients onwards for procedures which are within their competence and which they could perform in a well-equipped local surgery. After patients' expensive visits to their GP (and the cost has risen sharply), they may then be referred to hospital, where they join a long queue in accident and emergency for the privilege of being seen and perhaps treated by a junior doctor with far less experience than their GP. The charges for and the deficiencies of primary care increase the stresses on the hospital system, which provides care at relatively little cost to patients (when they can gain access), compared to what it costs the state to supply. This bias in Irish health care away from low cost, preventive care and towards costly, institutional treatment runs counter to received international opinion on the optimal way to run health care systems.[6]

As part of its 2001 health strategy, the government published proposals for substantial investment in primary care teams of GPs and other health care professionals, working from one-stop shops and offering 24-hour cover.[7] This strategy for primary care contained no commitment to extend eligibility for free access to care. Although an early draft of the strategy defined primary care as a "universally accessible" range of services designed to keep people well, by the final draft this had been amended to a "fully accessible" range of services. Universality, with its implication that services would be accessed without financial barriers, had been dropped.[8] At the strategy's launch, Micheál Martin said he planned to extend medical card eligibility to 200,000 extra people, beginning in 2003. This was, however, dependent on "budgetary matters".[9] The 2003 Budget did not extend medical card eligibility. Not only had the government failed to fund improved access to existing GP services, but also the promised investment to implement the primary care strategy seemed unlikely to materialise.

In primary care, as in the hospital system, there remain three central challenges: to improve access; to increase resources; and to address the manner in which doctors work.

Outside the gates

On the November morning in 2001 that Micheál Martin launched the new primary care strategy, Tom O'Dowd was seeing patients in his Jobstown practice. In a downtown Dublin hotel, the Minister admitted to journalists that the government had no plans to extend eligibility for medical cards, either that year or the following year. In the deprived west-Dublin suburb, Tom O'Dowd saw a patient, a young woman with two children, whose income was just above the eligibility threshold for a medical card. "She said 'It's going to be great, doctor, with this new health strategy, we are going to get a medical card.' But she won't," O'Dowd related a little later, as he absorbed the shock of the government's decision.[10]

That O'Dowd should emerge as one of the first critics of this decision was ironic because the TCD professor of general practice was working in the Mary Mercer Health Centre, which government publicists had presented as a model for the Minister's planned primary care one-stop shop. Ideal facilities were of little use to patients who could not afford access, O'Dowd readily appreciated.

Others shared his sense of shock. Audrey Deane, social policy officer of the Catholic charity, the Society of St Vincent de Paul, which had campaigned for free GP care for children, said she was "shocked and incredulous" at this "obscene" decision, which failed to take account of the needs of the most vulnerable members of society. The ICTU, which had sought the extension of medical cards to all workers and their families, said the decision struck at the very foundations of social partnership. The social partners' medical card review group had recommended extended eligibility for medical cards. The Irish Medical Organisation said the decision was unacceptable and would "undermine the health strategy's guiding principles of equity, access and fairness". It estimated that 250,000 people could not now afford treatment. James Reilly, chairman of the IMO's GP committee, had earlier supported a trebling of the income below which people would be eligible for medical cards. Government backbench TDs joined the opposition in expressing their dismay at the decision.[11]

Micheál Martin later defended this government decision on the grounds that extending eligibility for free care would have overwhelmed the existing system. Here was an open admission that behind the financial barrier to access was massive unmet medical need:

> If you flood it [primary care], you are giving access to what is generally agreed from the consultative process to be an inadequate infrastructure, with 50 per cent of GPs not having a secretary or a practice nurse. I think it is important that when we don't have endless resources in any one year, we need to beef up the practice infrastructure first.[12]

Ten months later, at the Adelaide Hospital Society's annual public conference at Tallaght Hospital, Tom O'Dowd erupted from the audience to argue against defenders of the quality of Irish health care:

> A patient of mine has got terminal cancer. He applied for a medical card. He was told he could not have it. This is because discretionary medical cards are not now being issued. He will die in six months in pain, malnutrition and poverty because of the health care system we voted for last May. I work outside the gates of this hospital but I might as well be 1,000 miles away from the health care system you are describing.[13]

Multiple tiers of access to general practitioner care

As an academic, working in the area of general practice, O'Dowd's sense of the medical needs of the excluded was not purely based on anecdotal evidence. In a survey of male patients in their 50s, conducted by his practice, 25 per cent reported that either they or a member of their household were putting off going to see the doctor because of the cost. "These would be a very vulnerable group, men with a high cardiac risk factor," O'Dowd observed.[14]

While some GPs like to compare their service favourably with the two-tier hospitals, pointing out that their medical card and fee-paying patients wait in one queue in their surgeries, there nonetheless exist multiple tiers of access to general practitioner care. There is the tier of patients who are simply invisible because they do not have the financial means to attend the surgery. There is the fluctuating tier of medical card holders whose access may be cut off if family income rises above the eligibility threshold. There are the chronically ill who may receive a "discretionary" medical card on hardship grounds but are by no means guaranteed one.[15]

A further tier is composed of patients who receive an inferior service because there are so few doctors in their area. A study conducted in 1997 found that in areas of Dublin with concentrations of medical card patients and the low paid, there were three times fewer GPs than in middle class areas.[16] Since the study was restricted to GPs in the GMS, the probability was that middle class areas were even better served, since they would also have a population of GPs engaged exclusively in private practice. The "location of practices does not accord with the location of need", an informal working group on primary care, established by the Department of Health, reported.[17] Yet another tier of access was added in 2001, when, following the extension of eligibility for medical cards to all over-70-year-olds, regardless of income, the government struck a deal with the IMO which would pay GPs substantially more for the care of these elderly people than for existing medical card holders.

Doctors respond to the economic incentives of the medical marketplace. In 2002, fee-paying patients were typically paying between €40 and €45 for a single GP visit.[18] This was approximately equal to the capitation payment (€45.44) which GPs would receive for their entire annual care of an adult male medical card patient. On economic grounds alone, there could be no contest between building up a practice in a middle class or working class area. A further extraordinary discrimination was introduced in the deal, which secured the agreement of the IMO to the allocation of medical cards to over-70-year-olds without a means test. While GPs would receive an annual capitation fee of €95 to €171 for treating the lower income, formerly eligible elderly,[19] they would receive €462 for treating the higher income, newly eligible elderly. GPs in middle class areas were thus compensated for the extension of free GP care to their elderly patients, while the more sparsely scattered GPs in working class areas must continue to treat their elderly patients for as little as one-fifth the payment. The incentive to locate practices in wealthier areas was further reinforced.[20]

Within these multiple tiers of GP care, there is precisely the kind of hybrid system of payment of doctors against which Dale Tussing had warned in the 1980s, when arguing for a capitation system of payment to cover all patients.[21] He repeated the warning in 2001, arguing: "When we pay GPs by fee for one group of patients and by capitation for another group, a possible consequence is that GPs will develop a bias, perhaps an unconscious one for treating the fee-for-service patient." Each visit by a fee-for-service patient increases the doctor's income but this does not apply to each visit by a medical card patient, whose treatment is funded by an annual fee from the state. Tussing acknowledged that "when a GP has a waiting room full of patients, he or she is likely to treat them all similarly, without sorting them by remuneration method" but suggested that there should be research on the volume of return visits by each group before dismissing the possibility of "biased GP behaviour".[22]

Since the 1980s, Tussing had advocated a free GP service "to encourage early, routine and preventative care", although by 2001 he considered modernising the GP service a higher priority. Modernising was "a 20th century issue", a free GP service belonged "on the 21st century list".[23]

Senior officials in the Department of Health have not hidden their realisation that charges for GP care are an impediment to meeting health needs. When Micheál Martin was attempting to explain to an incredulous press in November 2001 that he had no immediate plans to extend eligibility for free GP care, he was flanked by his chief medical officer, Jim Kiely, who had proposed that all children should receive free GP care in his 2000 annual report. This argued:

> Specific policy measures which redistribute resources, provide opportunities and services for families with children, especially poor children, will do most to create better child health. For this reason, basic universal health provision, such as free access to primary care for all children, should be considered.[24]

When an informal working group started drafting the primary care element of the government's health strategy, they initially proposed a free primary care system, in which doctors and other professionals could be salaried health board employees. The system would be funded by universal health insurance, which was then being proposed by the opposition but not by government. The small working group, with members from inside and outside the Department of Health, was chaired by Frances Spillane, the Department official who directed the health strategy team.

The group's early draft argued that universal eligibility for primary care would

> remove the current barrier of financial accessibility which arises as a result of the public/private mix in the community. Many people not entitled to medical cards do not attend for services, from which they could benefit, particularly in the area of prevention such as hypertension, asthma and diabetes. While we do not have the information systems, which can indicate the burden that may result in terms of increased

asthma admissions or stroke incidence, it does act as a significant barrier to the emergence of a primary care system, which places appropriate emphasis on prevention. Many people without medical cards cannot get access to other essential primary care services such as physiotherapy and occupational therapy because those services are available in many cases only to those who can pay for them.[25]

This group's radical support for universal eligibility soon met counter-arguments in the Departmental policy-making process. Although a further Departmental working group, with a brief to consider wider issues of eligibility, expressed concern that eligibility for medical cards based on "undue hardship" promoted "a negative attitude towards eligibility, which sees it as a tool to prevent hardship rather than facilitating and promoting the health and social well-being of citizens", it nonetheless advocated an incremental approach to widening eligibility because of "competing priorities" for health spending. It did, however, recommend "generously increasing" medical card thresholds.[26]

While the vision in the early draft of the primary care strategy of universal eligibility for free primary care, funded by an insurance system, did not survive into the eventual document, it reveals that at least some policy-makers shared Tussing's view of the need to make primary care universally accessible, in the interests of early interventions to improve the population's health and to remove pressures on the more expensive hospital system.

Resources for primary care

In 2001, there were 2,200 general practitioners in active practice in Ireland, of whom 1,650 were participating in the General Medical Services scheme with contracts to treat medical card patients. There were 1,600 practices in all.[27] This meant that Ireland had approximately 6 GPs for every 10,000 people – the same ratio as the UK, and well below the 10 per 10,000 in Germany or 15 per 10,000 in France.[28] Since Irish private patients were believed to visit their doctor less frequently than the average European, with a free GP scheme "you could suddenly find 70 per cent of the population doubling their visiting rate", according to Richard Brennan, chairman of the Irish College of General Practitioners (ICGP).[29]

In a presentation to the cabinet in May 2001, deputy secretary Tom Mooney described primary health care as "patchy" and "overloaded", with an unrealised "capacity to make a major contribution to health". There was "unanimity" among policy-makers that the way forward for the health service was to develop primary care but this required a major increase in staff, clinics and equipment. Half the state's 2,200 GPs were working single-handed, often for over 80 hours a week. There were fewer than 1,000 practice secretaries and under 500 practice nurses.[30] Small wonder that 25 per cent of GPs, surveyed by the IMO in 2000, would not choose medicine were they to start their careers again.[31] While, in 2001, the majority of existing GPs were male and over 45 years old, 80 per cent of trainees were female.[32] In 2002, the ICGP feared an imminent staffing crisis in general practice, because younger doctors – both male and female – were unwilling to put in the long, unsupported hours of the traditional Irish GP.[33]

The government's primary care strategy envisaged the eventual development of up to 1,000 primary care teams. Delivering two-thirds of the teams would require an additional 500 GPs and 2,000 nurses over a ten-year period, with similar large increases in the number of other professionals and support staff. While primary care had been traditionally provided by GPs and public health nurses working in an uncoordinated manner, this new model of team-working would bring them together with other professionals. The cost of housing and staffing these teams would be €1,270 million in capital investment and €615 million in annual pay, at 2001 prices, the Department of Health estimated.[34]

The logic for this development was endorsed in the 2003 Hanly report on medical staffing, which recommended a complete reorganisation of the hospital network to offer better quality care at regional centres of excellence. Since hospitals would therefore no longer offer acute care in every county, the report envisaged that primary care must develop to its full potential, so that patients might access diagnostic and treatment facilities at local health clinics which they formerly sought in their local hospitals. Local hospitals and primary care teams should have close links.[35] The Department-of-Health-sponsored Prospectus Report observed that to shift the balance from care to prevention, an objective which was "still in its infancy", primary care should be at the core of health service delivery structures.[36]

Why not a free GP service?

The continuum in the politics of health care is nowhere more evident than in primary care. Not since Noel Browne resigned in 1951 has any Minister for Health attempted to introduce anything approaching universal, European-style access to free primary medical care. After the trauma to the body politic of the comprehensive defeat of the Mother-and-Child scheme, for over fifty years Ministers of each of the major political parties have presided over a health care system in which access to general practitioner care remains largely dependent on income. Ministers' reforming efforts have been directed at improving access to hospital care. When there have been funds for political empire-building in health, they have been devoted to hospital-building, as efficacious in securing votes as locating a new factory in a constituency. Primary care has remained a neglected service, in the hands of private practitioners and expensive to access, despite its potential to prevent many patients from ever needing to visit a hospital.

Governments have been distinguished by the generosity or parsimony with which they have disbursed medical cards, for which eligibility has a notorious element of discretion, an open door to local politicians' representations on behalf of their constituents. A cynical view is occasionally advanced that politicians resist the introduction of free GP care because they would lose the potential for this form of parochial political patronage. Governments' failures to index medical card eligibility thresholds to rising incomes have significantly reduced the proportion of the population who are eligible for free care.[37] Eligibility peaked at 38.6 per cent of the population in 1977. It remained close to or above 35 per cent of the population until, under the 1997–2002 Fianna Fáil/Progressive Democrat coalition, it fell from 36 per cent in 1996 to 31 per cent in 2001, despite its extension to include all over-70-year-olds. This explains the level of outrage at the government's failure to increase the income thresholds for eligibility in 2001.[38]

GPs are not indifferent to the inaccessibility and inadequacies of their care. Faced by the needs of patients, many may waive their fees. Although often more progressive than other doctors, GPs have not, however, campaigned as a group for universal access to their care because of the implications for their independence and manner of payment. They are an alienated body, who distrust government because of its failure to invest in their service and to value it and them, in contrast to the value placed on hospital care and their consultant colleagues. GPs recall past state efforts to discipline them for "over-visiting" and the state's refusal to fund preventive care under the GMS.

A central issue for GPs is how they are paid and for whom they work: whether they remain self-employed or become employees. In the UK, GPs are self-employed but, in effect, work under contract to the state and are paid by a mixture of capitation, fees and allowances. Sweden and Spain, whose national health services were placed by the WHO amid the top five countries worldwide, have almost entirely salaried general practitioners.[39] In Germany and France, GPs generally receive fees through the health insurance system but their rates of pay are highly regulated by government. Methods of payment vary greatly in systems which, nonetheless, share the attribute of offering free care to patients.

GPs who object to the state controlling their working conditions and their level of remuneration sometimes argue that patients must continue to pay fees out of pocket rather than access care free at the point of delivery. These doctors would defend their continued self-employed status even if it prevents their fellow citizens from choosing to develop a universally accessible primary care system. Those who take this stance repeat the arguments of their predecessors who opposed the Mother and Child scheme. Opponents of a universal system frequently focus on the failings of the UK's NHS and do not take into account that the NHS is attempting to meet the demands of a freely accessible service with as few GPs per head of population as Ireland. Irish GPs appear to do better in meeting patient demand because financial barriers to access leave great numbers of people with unmet, unmeasured demand for care. In a free system, as Micheál Martin admitted, they would be swamped. It may be the case that the UK's service might benefit from a greater element of fee payment to encourage greater productivity, which is quite another matter from adducing its failings as evidence that Irish patients should continue to pay fees out-of-pocket, rather than access medical care free at the point of delivery.

The determination of doctors to defend their independent, private fee-earning status was central to the defeat of efforts to extend access to free primary medical care in the 1940s and 1950s. Some contemporary critics of the failings of primary care assume that reforms that threatened the private income and status of doctors would meet equally formidable medical opposition today. The Deloitte and Touche 2001 value-for-money audit of the health service listed the failings of the existing system of general practice, and then observed that, although the "self-employed status of GPs" made their integration with acute or community services unlikely, it was "well established in Ireland and it is likely to be difficult to change". The management consultants did not advocate a free GP service and remarked, "to achieve this may in any event be complex given the self-employed nature of general practitioners and the financial rewards associated with private patient income".[40]

The informal working group that worked on the government's primary care strategy predicted that doctors would perceive the free primary care system proposed in their early draft as a threat to their income and would object to losing their independence and becoming employees. They might regard it as "too big a change". However, the group pointed out that new trainees were unwilling to work in single-handed, rural general practices.[41] Rises in property prices have also made it difficult for young GPs to start up practices in the cities.

In its refusal to endorse the group's early work and seek universal eligibility, the Department of Health was ignoring the advice of its own appointed panel of international experts[42] that "European analysis suggested there was a strong case for free primary health care". This panel observed that Irish political debate tended to over-emphasise the issue of hospital waiting lists and failed to understand the potential impact of the primary care system on referrals for hospital services. They suggested that it was "imperative" to "find a way to make health status (as opposed to health services) an important issue both in the public eye and politically".[43]

The unwillingness of the Department to pursue a free primary health care system may have reflected concerns about professional opposition; it may have reflected a lack of conviction within the Department about the desirability of universal provision; or it may have been based on the assumption that, with a tax-cutting government in power, the Department of Finance would not support the financing of free GP care, either through taxation or insurance. However, after the Labour Party began promoting the idea of free GP care within an insurance-based system, there was evidence in 2002 of growing openness within the medical profession to universal provision. This was despite the VHI's failure in 2000 to achieve agreement with GPs in the IMO on an insurance scheme that would cover VHI members for primary care and pay GPs by a mixture of capitation and fees.[44] In 2002, the VHI instead introduced a limited scheme to reimburse a proportion of patients' payments to GPs.

Although GPs voted against a motion proposing a national GP system at the IMO's annual general meeting in April 2002, this narrow defeat at a debate attended by some 60 of the 1,825 GPs in the union masked a sea change in doctors' views of a universal service.[45] Cyril Daly, a Dublin GP and veteran *Irish Medical Times* columnist, who proposed the motion in an annual testing of opinion, later commented that the climate of opinion among doctors had "hugely" changed. A "sense of inevitability" had developed about the eventual introduction of a universal system, despite "strong pockets of resistance". If all GPs were balloted on a concrete government proposal for free GP care, he thought it would be accepted. "Obviously it would depend on the terms but I think it would have a very, very good innings." He contrasted his narrow defeat in Killarney with a "packed and passionate" extraordinary general meeting of the IMO in Portlaoise in 1997, when his proposals for a free GP service were "thrown out totally".

A measure of the change in opinion among GPs was that Daly now had the support of a former key opponent. That bell-wether of medical opinion, Cormac MacNamara, afterwards explained that in 1997 he had thought the timing wrong, that "we could not call for extension of a scheme which we thought inadequate". In 2002, he supported Daly's motion "in the context of the primary care strategy". He said:

> If there was a comprehensive national health service, provided it was adequately funded, the vast majority would be happy to subscribe to it. For me personally and, I suspect, for the majority of doctors in the IMO, in principle a free GP service would hold no fear. Our priority is to have a system with properly trained doctors with appropriate resources. I have always agreed with Cyril.[46]

MacNamara's read of the politics was supported by the IMO's treasurer and negotiator on its GP committee, Martin Daly, who observed that "if a government had a serious radical proposal, that guarantees and improves quality of care and breadth of access, the IMO would have to look seriously at it". The vote at the AGM should not discourage "a serious politician". "There were no very strongly held views that we should not get involved with the state." The AGM had passed a motion calling for an immediate trebling of the income eligibility limits for the GMS.

The IMO's chief executive officer and its principal full-time official, George McNeice, who in 2002 remained a staunch defender of private practice rights for hospital consultants, showed much greater openness to the possibility that general practitioners would accept a unified primary care system.

> GPs are very open-minded. At the moment GPs' costs are going through the roof – insurance, buildings, staff – and GPs' fees are getting higher and higher and higher. You may get to the point where there is bigger demand from people to have a state-sponsored system or an insurance-based system. GPs are always open to looking at new systems but they

are not going to give up their independent contractor status easily. All they have to do is look at the other employees of the health services, who are seriously demotivated.[47]

For GPs to become employees, at least 80 per cent, if not 100 per cent, of the population would have to be eligible for free GP care, he believed.

The IMO has frequently been regarded as an obstacle to extended access to free GP care because in 1989, when capitation payments were introduced for the GMS, the trade union's agreement with the state on rates of pay only covered the treatment of up to 40 per cent of the population on lower incomes. It was subsequently widely assumed that the IMO would oppose extension of eligibility beyond this level. McNeice, who had been with the IMO since 1984, insisted in 2002 that this was a misunderstanding of the union's position. The union had agreed to fund up to 40 per cent at existing capitation rates but would be prepared to negotiate a rate for extending eligibility to higher earners, as it had done for over-70-year-olds.[48] However, this requirement for fresh negotiation had the effect during the 1990s of discouraging the Department of Health from attempting to introduce incremental increases to the scheme's coverage.[49]

The ICGP has been more vocal than the IMO in defending private practice. Although the two bodies produced a joint strategy proposal for general practice in 2001, which insisted "practice income should not be reliant upon a single payer and the public/private mix of funding practice should be maintained",[50] the IMO has been more open than the academic ICGP to a potential state service.

Cyril Daly had reached the view in 2002 that it "would bother very few GPs now if they were salaried". Cormac MacNamara concurred that GPs were coming to see their method of payment as less important than its adequacy, although he believed their income should retain some recognition of productivity.[51] MacNamara was the principal IMO author of the IMO/ICGP policy, which appeared so wedded to the public/private mix. In contrast, its principal ICGP author, Michael Boland, argued strongly against a salaried and free GP service: "Irish general practice combines the fee for service with capitation payments and allowances. This balanced system has been shown to work best. Salaried systems do not encourage optimal performance." While accepting that more people should be eligible for medical cards and that some preventive services should be free, he insisted that "giving medical cards to the whole population in an NHS-style service is unnecessary on grounds of equity, wasteful in terms of cost-effectiveness and damaging to quality. Our health services should be deregulated not nationalised."[52]

Despite its insistence on retaining private fee income, the ICGP/IMO published policy confirmed MacNamara's view of a professional group who were more concerned about the level of their income and of investment in their practices than the source of either. The policy argued for a "new package of income and benefits" for rural doctors, for "parity of income with other specialists" (that is, hospital consultants) for all GPs, and for investment in all practices, even those which were not within the state service. It must have been apparent to the authors that achieving these objectives was incompatible with continued independent contractor status, although perhaps they were encouraged in their ambitions by the ability of hospital consultants to retain many of the freedoms of the self-employed while receiving a state salary and using state facilities for private practice.

Whatever their public posturing, there seems little doubt that GPs' acceptance of employment in a state system could be achieved – for a price. "If you went to GPs and offered them a consultant's salary for a basic nine-to-five service, the IMO would bite off your hand," predicted one influential policy-maker.[53] It seems that an Irish politician, who sought to achieve free GP care, could adopt Aneurin Bevan's approach to winning hospital consultants over to the introduction of the NHS, when he "stuffed their mouths with gold".[54]

"Many GPs would be happy to be put on the salary of a consultant in full-time public practice," James Reilly, chairman of the IMO's GP committee, acknowledged but added that the IMO would oppose state employment as GPs' only option, since some GPs feared that as state employees they would lose their freedom to be "patient advocates". He favoured an insurance-based system, since the involvement of insurance companies in a state-funded system would avoid the state being the "sole payer".

The issues of how GPs should be paid and by whom they would be employed were typically ducked in the 2001 primary care strategy. Responding to questions at its launch, Micheál Martin obscurely allowed that GPs "will not have to become state employees" but added "there could be the option".[55]

The future of primary care

Despite the IMO's disappointment about the government's failure to extend eligibility for free GP care, its 2001 primary care strategy was greeted with enthusiasm by some GPs, who hoped that primary care might at last receive attention and investment and that the bias towards hospital care might finally be redressed. Their enthusiasm was not shared by all their colleagues. The ICGP and the IMO, who had harboured doubts about the government's approach during the drafting of the strategy, remained sceptical after its publication. "They turned up with their glossy document and they were surprised that GPs didn't drop everything? They are seeking to undo 30 years of isolation. A major bridge-building exercise is required," were some representative comments from influential representatives of the group. Since the government had published a strategy not just for general practitioner care but for primary care, which was by no means synonymous and encompassed both medical and social services, the bridge-building exercise would have to coax GPs into a whole new way of seeing their role. Although GPs had been consulted during the process of drawing up the strategy, they considered the consultation "perfunctory", in the words of the ICGP chairman, Richard Brennan.[56]

The Minister established a taskforce to "deliver" the strategy reforms and report to a wider steering group, representing professional groups and participants in social partnership.[57] Although scepticism set in among steering group members when health cutbacks succeeded the 2002 general election, Martin proceeded to announce ten primary care teams, to include GPs, nurses and midwives, health care assistants, home helps, occupational therapists, physiotherapists, social workers and administrative personnel.

The Minister had yet to overcome the reservations of the medical organisations although Michael Kelly, the secretary general of the Department, told the strategy's critics "there is no other show in town".[58] Some GPs feared a loss of the virtues of their traditional care in this new broad primary care model. They objected that they had not designed the system and were not central to it. The strategy's rationale for the primary care approach, for combining health and social services, was that a primary care team working together could not only treat illness but also support people to care for themselves and their families "from a health and social well-being perspective". Thus, when a patient presented with a medical complaint, the broader social and psychological needs, which might underlie the condition, might also be addressed.[59] Early drafts of the primary care strategy had envisaged that the primary care teams might be led by any one of a number of health professionals – by a nurse or social worker, for instance, rather than by a GP – and that patients would be permitted to self-refer, that is to phone up and seek an appointment with any of the professionals who seemed relevant to their query, rather than to go through a GP in the first instance.[60]

The final strategy document retained the reference to self-referral but did not address the issue of who would lead the teams. This, explained the Minister, was yet to be "worked out" and would involve discussion with the IMO and ICGP.[61] George McNeice of the IMO was still insisting nearly a year later that, while GPs recognised that there should be better developed community services, GPs would wish to be "leading the system".[62] Tom O'Dowd concurred:

> At the moment, the GP has to be the team leader, other people may emerge but there is an authority that it needs in its early days. The strategy does not acknowledge the strengths of general practice. They've got general practice confused with general practitioners, who can be awkward, but actually their practice of medicine is very popular and very successful. I think they have to build the strategy around general practice – and it will change general practice enormously.[63]

Cormac MacNamara, on the other hand, was an enthusiastic supporter of the strategy and pointed out that, while his practice was the largest group practice in the country, it was still incomplete without the input of a wider range of other professionals:

> There is no doubt that over the next 10 to 20 years, this is what society will demand – a more integrated approach. While many GPs will wish to have the lead role in the diagnosis and treatment of illness, with regard to a whole range of other activities they may not. There is nothing to suggest that the majority of GPs will particularly want to become involved in management and administration.[64]

The new primary care teams, announced by Micheál Martin, were entering uncharted territory. They must reconcile GPs' independent status with team working and the general practice approach to care with the broader vision of primary care. At a purely financial level, it remained the case that the majority of GPs still had significant private earnings. Having borrowed to invest in their own practices, GPs wondered how they would now be incorporated into this new state system. If they were not to lead the primary care teams, at a mercenary level, they faced the alarming prospect that they might discover their private patients being referred to other professionals without their input – or fee.

However, for GPs to seek to be the central pivot of a state-funded and state-run system, while retaining their status as independent contractors with large private practices, was patently a nonsense. It was clear that between the lines of the government's ambitious strategy for primary care was an assumption, unspoken but transparent, that this must lead in time to a state system. While Cormac MacNamara appeared predisposed to accept this, the ICGP was not. The strategy was "written by people who were very much influenced by qualifying in public health in an NHS-style system. It hasn't taken into account that we have a mixed payer system, a public/private mix and that the Commission on Health Funding recommended maintaining that *status quo*," Richard Brennan objected. He identified a feeling among GPs that "if everybody bides their time, this will die a death". Coupled with that feeling (or hope), however, was an anxiety that, if the primary care teams began to get off the ground around the country, "two-tier general practice" might emerge – not for patients this time, but for GPs – because the new primary care teams would have access to dieticians, physiotherapists and diagnostic equipment, which would not be on offer in other practices.

Brennan's fear might be the Department's hope – that patients would vote with their feet and GPs would find themselves forced into the state system, since they could no longer survive outside it. After decades of confrontational industrial relations between the Department of Health and GPs, it might be that the Department could perceive no other way of gaining GPs' participation in a state system. However, if the Department were intent on implementing its strategy, it would eventually have to address GPs' role and win their acceptance of its vision. And it could not do this without also addressing the intertwined issues of how they should be paid and how patients should access their care. For the primary care strategy to become a reality, some government, some Minister would have to take up where Noel Browne left off and legislate for universally accessible primary care.

Campaigning in the 2002 general election, Fine Gael promised greatly increased eligibility for medical cards and Labour free GP care for all, which provoked the outspoken opposition of Michael McDowell, Attorney General and Progressive Democrat candidate. While Fianna Fáil was careful not to rubbish such a potentially vote-winning concept, and concentrated its artillery on questioning Labour's costings, McDowell attacked the idea itself. Free GP care for all was a "crazy, loony Left" proposal, he said. The "disastrous" British NHS experiment showed that a universal free GP service simply did not work. "The predictable result for millions of patients in the UK has been the introduction of appointment waiting lists to see GPs … The Labour election bribe would wreck the GP service."[65]

McDowell was competing with Fine Gael for a middle class vote in a middle class constituency. The existence of financial barriers to accessing GP care was perhaps an abstract concept for this wealthy senior counsel and his electorate. His knowledge of health care systems did not apparently extend beyond the English Channel. Labour, perhaps foolishly, decided not to give his attack the oxygen of further publicity. They might have been better advised to use the opportunity to widen the audience for their reform proposals.

Free primary health care is the norm throughout the EU in states where health outcomes are demonstrably superior to Ireland's. That McDowell could characterise it as a "loony Left idea" and that, in 2002, it was only advocated by a minority political party, reveals how far to the right of the European political spectrum is the centre of Irish politics. The concept of universal provision is not accepted in Ireland. That access to health care should be a right, that it should not be a marketable commodity, is an alien proposition. In its place, reigns the 19th century concept that the individual should provide for himself and his family and the state supply the needy with means-tested, lower quality access. While doctors have had their own reasons for resisting universal provision of health care, they have found support in middle class resistance to higher taxation. Universal provision of the same quality of service would mean better access for the poorer to better-funded services, which would inevitably require redistribution. That every member of society would benefit from *all* having good health is a proposition which is seldom put to the Irish people.

Unfortunately, discussion of free GP care in Ireland tends to begin and end with disparaging references to the UK's NHS, an even more underfunded system[66] but at least one which offers universal access. With greater travel, however, awareness has grown that other EU states have overcome the obstacles to a quality, comprehensive health system. Ironically, while doctors' opposition was an important obstacle to reform 50 years ago, now their self-interest may force change. Today's young doctors, many of them women, are not prepared to work the long hours required to build up a single-handed practice. General practice will face a staffing crisis if the state does not step in to offer structured employment.

At the intersection between medicine and politics, the issue of how GPs are paid and employed is entangled with the issue of how patients should access the health care system. While some proponents of the public/private mix in general practice insist that its retention is in the public interest, the mix has not facilitated the development of a primary care system which values health. The absence of preventive care is testimony to that. The mix has survived because of GPs' concerns about their income and status; health officials' concerns about GPs' productivity; the state's unwillingness to invest in health care; and ideological resistance to universal provision.

Primary care in Ireland is rudimentary, an important recognition in the 2001 government primary care strategy. Remedying this would require committed investment in people, equipment and premises. If delivered, this would overturn the imbalance in the health care system, the equation of hospital services with health care and the assumption that more hospitals mean better health. It was unfortunate that the government did not publish the views of its advisory panel of international experts – their belief in the potential of primary care to improve health and reduce referrals to hospital, and their urging that failure to improve health should be as political an issue as hospital waiting lists. On the evidence, it would appear that there is support within the Department of Health for an eventual free service. Realising this ambition will require its adoption by a government with a belief in and electoral mandate for reform.

A state-funded system of primary care, without financial barriers to access, whether tax or insurance-based, has the potential to revolutionise Irish health care. Within that system, it would not require genius to devise a method of payment which would motivate GPs. GPs would have to be assured of a predictable income with some payment for productivity. Reforming primary care would require very large investment and significant behavioural change among professionals. It would take time – 20 years, perhaps, rather than the 10 years that the primary care strategy envisaged. The pay-off for the state and for Irish society for this investment in primary care would come in greatly improved health and quality of life and in reduced demands on the hospital service. Whether Ireland decides to go this route will depend much more on public opinion expressed in the ballot box than on medical opinion.

PART FOUR
OPTIONS FOR REFORM

12

Health spending and the black hole

"It is not a case of throwing money into a black hole."
– Minister for Health, Micheál Martin.

"Spending has been quadrupled since 1992, '93. I don't think the Irish people are that much more ill in that period of time."
– Minister for Finance, Charlie McCreevy.

"If a superior system is demanded by the public (and there is much evidence to believe this to be the case), then, as taxpayers, the financial implications of addressing the current health service deficits need to be accepted."
– Deloitte and Touche, Value for Money Audit of the Irish Health System.

The failures of Irish health care are not confined to inequity, inaccessibility, inappropriate staffing or inadequate systems of administration. They also reflect decades of underfunding, so that, despite recent increases in spending, the health service requires many further years of sustained investment. This realisation has brought arguments about health spending back into the centre of political discourse, where they are intimately interlinked with arguments about how the health care system might be reformed. It is the thesis of this book that the two must come together – sustained investment and reform – to deliver an acceptable, modern health care system.

By the year 2000, it had become abundantly clear that the health service was failing to deliver adequate care. That summer, 95 per cent of the population wanted the government to spend more on health to reduce waiting lists.[1] The following spring, 74 per cent of voters said they would sacrifice tax cuts for a better health service and 65 per cent included health care in the top three issues that would influence their vote in the next general election.[2] Health re-emerged as a political priority. Labour launched a discussion document with detailed proposals for a universal health insurance system in April 2000.[3] Fine Gael followed in November with a similar "health plan".[4] A year later, the Fianna Fáil/Progressive Democrat government published its health strategy.

While chronic underfunding and the discriminatory treatment of public patients had not sufficed to make health care an issue of general public concern in the mid- to late 1990s, by the end of the decade many other factors had combined to produce a sense of crisis. The population increased by 8 per cent from 1996 to 2002[5] yet there remained fewer hospital beds in 2001 than in 1992. Despite increased recruitment, hospitals suffered staff shortages. The shortage of nurses reflected reduced training places in the 1990s, their more time-consuming academic courses, the competing attractions of private employment and the soaring cost of living in Dublin. The shortage of doctors was provoked by the requirement that junior doctors from outside the EU should meet more exacting standards. All contributed to logjams in hospitals' accident and emergency departments, which were particularly politically sensitive for there the middle class shared public patients' experience of long delays and low standards of care.

As the overstretched service struggled to cope, doctors expressed growing disillusionment, medical reformers like Muiris FitzGerald campaigned for change and nurses took industrial action, in the interest of patients, to demand that over-crowding should be addressed. Perhaps most significantly, in this booming economy a more educated, wealthier and more widely travelled public was no longer prepared to accept public squalor beside private affluence and demanded better standards, influenced by models of care in other states.

Among all these reasons for the public's sense of the need for reform and investment in health care, it would be heartening to include greater egalitarianism and to suggest that, at the turn of the new century, a consensus had developed that the two-tier system must end. That, however, was not the case. Despite the vigorous debate that developed about options for reform, the two-tier system survived into 2003, when concern about the level of health spending began to eclipse more fundamental reform arguments. In truth, the two concerns were sides of the one coin. Reform was necessary to deliver efficacious health spending and investment was essential to deliver a reformed health service. Answering the many contemporary questions about the adequacy and efficacy of investment in health care becomes central, therefore, to making the case for reform.

"It doesn't seem to make any difference how much money goes into the area",[6] Rory O'Hanlon, the chairman of the Fianna Fáil parliamentary party, said of health spending in 1998. Over the following four years, in coalition with the Progressive Democrats, his party more than doubled day-to-day public spending on health.[7] Yet hardly a day passed without a report of dissatisfaction with some aspect of the health services: waiting lists, bed shortages, inadequate services for the disabled, the mentally ill. The government had increased health spending at a time of economic boom, when it could also reduce taxes without provoking fiscal crisis. But now the boom was over. Further significant increases in health spending would require increased taxes. That realisation produced many converts to the O'Hanlon view of health spending, not least the Minister for Finance, Charlie McCreevy. Yet Fianna Fáil and the Progressive Democrats had been re-elected to government in 2002, with a commitment to funding a €13 billion health strategy. How would they fund it? How could they explain their failure to do so to the electorate? And even were they to deliver it, would there ever be any end to public dissatisfaction with the health service? "Health will bring down this government," predicted an insider.[8]

Scepticism about the value of health spending was not confined to the government. The public too asked: had health spending been wasted? Where had the increases gone? Was there any point in spending more? The unresolved issue of how to fund health has become a symbol of a deeper debate about the direction of a wealthier, yet still unequal society, where higher disposable incomes have been valued more than public services or social solidarity.

Health spending – the facts

How much does Ireland spend on health?

In 2002, public spending on health was €8.3 billion.[9] Health accounted for nearly a quarter of government day-to-day spending.[10]

Spending on health had experienced a rapid catch-up. Public health spending per capita had been below the EU average for decades, having reached its nadir of 57 per cent in 1989, after the cutbacks of the late 1980s. In 2001, health spending exceeded the EU average for the first time, both in terms of spending per capita (see Figure 12.1) and as a percentage of national income. Total health spending, both public and private and excluding spending on social services, increased from 7.4

per cent of national income in 1998 to 9.6 per cent in 2002, compared to an EU average of approximately 8 per cent.[11] Ireland was now spending close to the same proportion of national income on health as France, although still somewhat less in per capita terms.[12]

Figure 12.1 Total health spending in Ireland compared with EU average 1990–200(

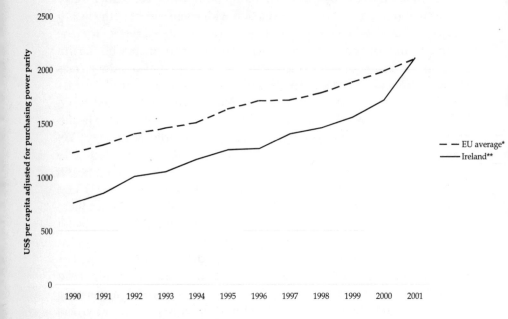

Source: Quality and Fairness, Department of Health, 2001, p.43.
*EU average excludes Irish spending.
**Irish figure excludes spending on personal social services.

If Ireland is now spending above the EU average on health, why continue to increase health spending?

In 2001, the year health spending first exceeded the EU average, the secretary-general of the Department of Health, Michael Kelly, advanced a powerful case for further increases at a special meeting of the cabinet convened to discuss health.[13] "Under-investment has been endemic in our health system: despite recent increases, serious capacity deficits remain," Kelly told ministers at the meeting in Ballymascanlon, Co Louth.

His officials explained that recent rapid increases in health spending had not obliterated the effect of decades of neglect. Neglected generations of people were now sicker and more needy than they should be. Life expectancy, while rising, had fallen further behind the EU average. Health needed more beds, clinics, equipment and staff. Social services funded through Health were also seriously deficient.

The Department's description of the cumulative effect of underfunding is supported by international comparison. In 2001, Ireland had on average 3 acute hospital beds for every 1,000 people, compared to over 4 in France, over 6 in Germany and an EU average of 4.1.[14] More importantly, many beds were in the wrong places delivering the wrong kind of care. The Eastern region had 2.45 beds for every 1,000 people, when inflows of patients from all over the state were taken into account. In 2002, Ireland had 20 doctors for every 10,000 people compared to 30 in France, 36 in Germany and an EU average of 33.[15]

A series of official studies had revealed a pressing need for additional facilities for the intellectually disabled, the mentally ill and the elderly. There were 27,000 people with intellectual disabilities in 1999, 60 per cent of whom had moderate to profound disabilities and over 800 of whom were still inappropriately placed in psychiatric hospitals. To address immediate need over the years to 2004, it would be necessary to provide over 1,000 more residential places and nearly 1,000 more day places – and, of course, providing places meant providing staff as well as buildings.[16] In 1999, community facilities for the mentally ill were so inadequate that people in need of community care occupied over half of hospitals' psychiatric beds, which could not therefore be used for people in need of acute psychiatric care.[17] A review of facilities for the elderly in the late 1990s had disclosed that no health board had the recommended norm of 2.5 assessment beds per 1,000 elderly people and only two had sufficient rehabilitation beds.[18]

On paper at least, the Department won the argument at Ballymascanlon. The government's November 2001 health strategy assessed that the health services needed a further €7.6 billion in capital investment over the ten years to 2011, on top of €2.5 billion already allocated in the national development plan.[19] By 2011, current spending would need to have risen by €5 billion annually to fund the new developments planned in the strategy. Subsequent detailed analysis of the implications of these spending increases suggested that health spending would rise to approximately 12 per cent of GNP by 2007, if the strategy were implemented, and would then remain close to that proportion. The share of national income going to health would exceed that of all other developed states except the United States, although in the UK too it had been forecast that health spending might need to rise to over 12 per cent of national income to meet the needs of an ageing population. The government greeted the publication of this analysis, shortly before the 2002 election,[20] as welcome evidence that it had already increased health spending above the EU average, but the more significant implication that the health strategy could not be funded without a substantial reallocation of national resources to health and social services was ignored. How a health system could continue to perform so badly, while consuming so much of national income, was a further avenue of enquiry, which on the eve of an election, the government parties preferred not to explore. Before pursuing that issue, the question arises as to how the Department proposed to allocate these additional funds.

What could more money buy? Hospital beds

"The average number of patients waiting for a bed in my institution every morning is now 17. Patients, whom consultants recommend for admission, regularly spend two or three days in hospital casualty departments."

– *Stephen Cusack, consultant in emergency medicine at Cork University Hospital and secretary of the Irish Association of Emergency Medicine, November 2001.*[21]

"After suffering a stroke, she waited eight hours in casualty before seeing a doctor and then spent a horrendous night on a makeshift trolley until a bed became available."

– *Dermot McGrath describing his mother's experience in Tallaght Hospital, July 2000.*[22]

The number of hospital beds was dramatically reduced during the cutbacks of the late 1980s and early 1990s. Despite population growth, the number of beds remained virtually unchanged through the 1990s – from 11,809 in 1993 to 11,985 in 2001.[23] The consequence was extreme pressure on the acute hospital system, manifest in waiting lists for elective surgery and in appalling bottlenecks in accident and emergency, where patients awaited care. If the 2001 health strategy was in reality a wish list, its greatest wish was for more hospital beds. The strategy identified a need for 3,000 extra beds in acute hospitals, which, the government promised, "will be added to the system" over a 10-year period. That would be a 25 per cent increase, the "largest ever concentrated expansion of acute hospital capacity in Ireland".[24]

The strategy's target was based on a study of hospital bed requirements, largely the work of a clinical epidemiologist, Mary Codd, who had informed the cabinet at its Ballymascanlon meeting that

Ireland had the highest bed occupancy level in the OECD, and that was "unacceptably high". The study confirmed the public's sense of a health system in crisis.

"Acute hospitals in Ireland are experiencing significant difficulties in the delivery of services at this time. There are capacity issues, staffing and resource issues and dissatisfaction among patients and the general public." Inadequate capacity – too few beds – was leading to long delays in A & E, delays in admission, cancellation of elective procedures and long waiting lists. Shortages of staff and other resources compounded the problem but beds were "the cornerstone of service provision in the acute hospital and the resource to which all other resources are mapped".[25]

While the cabinet had heard at Ballymascanlon that 4,800 additional acute beds could be required to meet the needs of the health service to 2011, in its published study the Department later reduced this estimate of need to 4,335. It suggested this could be further reduced to 2,840 additional acute inpatient beds and 190 additional acute day beds, provided a number of measures were taken to lessen demands on the acute hospital system. These included greater use of day procedures; ensuring that private patients did not exceed the 20 per cent of beds allocated to them; and providing care elsewhere for those elderly and convalescent patients who were remaining too long in acute hospitals because they had nowhere else to go. The corollary was that, if the government was to provide "only" 3,000 acute beds, it must compensate by providing many more convalescent and geriatric beds. At Ballymascanlon, the cabinet had heard that a total of 4,700 extra beds would be needed in assessment and rehabilitation units, in community nursing units, for palliative care and for the mentally infirm. Yet the strategy specifically committed itself only to a reduced target of 1,370 assessment and rehabilitation beds, 600 day beds and 800 community nursing care places.[26]

The Department's study was a wake-up call. Health spending had increased, health staffing had increased and, most importantly, from the mid-1990s population had increased dramatically, but the number of beds in hospitals had not risen.[27] The ratio of acute beds to 1,000 population, which cutbacks had reduced from 5.1 in 1981 to 3.3 in 1993, with rising population had continued to fall to 3 by 2000.[28] In the EU in the 1990s, the average number of acute beds per 1,000 population had remained at around 4.1 – 25 per cent more beds than in Ireland. The Codd study reported that 23 hospitals had occupancy levels above the internationally accepted measure of full occupancy of

85 per cent. Their occupancy ranged from 85 to 123 per cent, presumably reflecting patients sleeping on trolleys.[29]

The number of acute beds is not necessarily an accurate measure of a health system's capacity to provide care. Canada delivers superior care with 3.3 acute beds per 1,000 population.[30] With changing medical technology and growth in day procedures, it is possible to treat many more patients while reducing bed numbers, as Ireland indeed achieved in the 1990s. If all Ireland's existing acute beds were in top-class hospitals, which were capable of delivering efficient acute services, then the Codd study's assessment of need in 2001 might have been considerably lower. However, the reality was that many of Ireland's so-called acute beds were in sub-standard hospitals of sub-optimal size, which in 2003 the Hanly task force recommended should cease to offer many aspects of acute care. The true count of acute beds in hospitals with the capability to deliver comprehensive care was probably closer to the Eastern region's 2.45 per 1,000 people. The sub-text of the Codd study's numbers was that the state needed to provide thousands more beds – but in the right places and delivering the right kind of care.

Underlying the Department's forecasts of future bed needs was the expectation that population would continue to rise and that it would simultaneously age. In 2000, people over 65 years of age constituted 11 per cent of the population, 27 per cent of hospital patients and accounted for 46 per cent of hospital bed days. People over 65 were expected to constitute over 16 per cent of the population by 2026.

Whatever way you looked at the numbers, the implications for investment in health care – whether in acute hospitals, geriatric homes or the community – were enormous. Management consultants Deloitte and Touche, who independently assessed value for money in the health services, forecast that the level of investment in facilities for the elderly was "likely to be of a very significant magnitude" and "the historically low investment and service base" during the 1980s and well into the 1990s "makes this challenge more difficult".[31]

Although this analysis was available to the government before the May 2001 Ballymascanlon meeting, it took until January 2002 – four months before the general election – for an announcement that 709 additional beds would be provided that year. Funding was eventually provided for 520 of these beds in 2002 and, by November, fewer than half had opened, having been squeezed into existing hospitals all over the state. The total count of acute beds available that month was 12,191 – just 200 up on 2001.[32] In their programme for government, the re-elected Fianna Fáil/Progressive Democrat coalition had promised again to provide 3,000 extra hospital beds but, despite a commitment to implementing the health strategy, had not specified how many equally essential convalescent and geriatric beds it would provide.[33] Then six months later, in November 2002, the Minister for Finance, Charlie McCreevy, announced that funding for the strategy "cannot be addressed at this particular time, and won't be addressed next year or the year after".[34] The Department secured funding in 2003 for the remainder of the promised 709 beds but for no more.

What else could more money buy?

The health strategy provided a comprehensive list of the other needs of an expanded health service: for many more staff, for the development of primary care, of community care and of care for the disabled. Implementing the strategy would require increasing the numbers of doctors, nurses and therapists in training, enticing emigrants and those who had left the workforce to return and recruiting more generally abroad. The strategy proposed that 10,000 nurses should be trained over its lifetime and thousands more therapists. Substantial but unspecified increases in consultant numbers were also proposed.[35] The development of a new model of primary care, involving teams and GP cooperatives, was priced in the separate primary care strategy.

The published health strategy shared less information with the general public about the needs of the health service than the cabinet had heard at Ballymascanlon. Although the strategy document outlined general development targets, costed and itemised details were missing. At Ballymascanlon, Frances Spillane, director of the health strategy project team, had explained how over the next five years mental health services would need £340 million (€432 million); services for the physically disabled would require £500 million (€635 million) to supply 3,400 day places, 1,000 residential places, home helps, therapy and other services; expansion of child protection services – foster and residential care and aid for the homeless – would require £225 million (€286 million); travellers' health required £6 million (€7.6 million). There was increased demand for residential, day and respite services for the intellectually disabled and for specialist support services for children with behavioural problems and autism. The strategy lacked this detail.

Nor did the strategy enumerate how many health staff would be required. Medical staffing requirements would depend on how discussions developed on the medical hierarchy and the consultants' contract. Nurse staffing – one-third of health service employment – was considered in a subsequent report, which also failed to calculate how many nurses might be needed but concluded that an ageing, growing population with fewer community supports and with more surviving disabled would need so many more nurses that, even with increased nurse training, it would be critical to retain the nurses already in the workforce.[36] Yet the Irish Nurses' Organisation (INO) was rebuffed when it pursued extra pay for nurses in Dublin, in late 2002.[37] At Ballymascanlon, officials had argued that an additional 1,500 nurses must be recruited each year for current needs, and more should be recruited if the service were expanded.

Although the strategy's wish list was long and its price high, it neglected the psychiatric service, advocates argued, despite its acknowledgment that existing services were "inadequate" and few health boards had "completed the process" of shifting from institutional- to community-based care.[38] In 2000, there were 4,000 patients in Irish psychiatric hospitals compared to over 20,000 in 1960.[39] Sufficient community facilities to replace the old psychiatric hospitals had simply not materialised, Kate Ganter, a child and adolescent psychiatrist and president of the Irish Medical Organisation, charged in 2002. "The resources just aren't there: intermediate hostels, long-term, high-support hostels, rehabilitation programmes. These involve huge human resources: a lot of nursing staff, one-to-one care of people."[40] Agencies for the homeless estimated that 40 to 50 per cent of homeless people suffered from mental illness. The agencies regarded their presence on the streets as a direct consequence of the closure of psychiatric beds and insufficient investment in community support.[41]

Ganter pointed out that the government's bed capacity review excluded mental health beds.[42] "Child and adolescent psychiatry never gets a look in because we are mainly community based, with very few beds. We need more beds but not a huge number." And since mentally ill young people were seen as outpatients, their wait for services was not even registered in waiting lists and their treatment did not qualify for waiting list initiative funding. The level of need had not even been measured. "The treatment process in mental health is the skills of the team. When resources are scarce, it's people that you can't get. There are insufficient clinical psychologists, psychiatric social workers, psychotherapists, counsellors and child care workers."

How could it be that, when health spending exceeded the EU average, the health service had so many remaining needs – beds, hostels, convalescent care, people? This question has exercised many people inside and outside politics. Where has all the money gone? Is health spending a black hole?

Where has all the money gone?

Health care is a labour intensive business. Health service employment grew from 58,738 in 1990 to 92,996 in 2001 – a 58 per cent increase.[43] The number of hospital consultants increased from 1,122 in 1990 to 1,731 at the beginning of 2003 – a 54 per cent rise. The number of NCHDs increased from 2,193 in 1990 to 3,932 in 2002 – a 79 per cent rise.[44] Nurses in the public health service increased from 24,574 in 1990 to 31,429 in 2001 – a 28 per cent rise. The number of nurses in the voluntary hospitals increased by only 8 per cent, however.[45] Voluntary hospitals are concentrated in Dublin, where the problem of nurse retention has been most extreme. Had all their nurse vacancies been filled, these hospitals would have employed 16 per cent more nurses in 2001 than in 1990.[46]

Of the increase in health spending from 1996 to 2001, 65 per cent was taken up with paying salaries.[47] Health service workers received the normal national pay increases and nurses, junior doctors, consultants and other staff secured additional pay increases. While during the 1990s extra staff were recruited to provide new services, they were also needed to maintain services: to make up for junior doctors' reduced hours; to replace trainee nurses who went into full-time education and ceased staffing wards; to avoid sole rostering, where staff might be vulnerable to accusations of abuse; and to replace the dwindling religious, who frequently worked unpaid overtime or took no salary.[48]

Hospitals may not have gained beds but they treated many more patients. Between 1997 and 2002, the number of patients treated in acute hospitals increased by 23 per cent – almost a quarter.[49] Additional consultants, junior doctors and nurses were treating additional patients. Hospitals achieved this increase despite their static bed numbers because productivity increased dramatically during the 1990s. Many more procedures were performed as day cases and patients remained in hospital for shorter periods. Between 1995 and 2000 a patient's average length of stay in hospital decreased from 7.2 to 6.9 days; and the number of day cases rose by 68 per cent, to nearly 40 per cent of all hospital activity compared to 2 per cent in 1980.[50]

Health spending rises even when there is no increase in services because the wages of health care workers rise and because of other inflationary pressures that are common internationally. Prices in medicine rise above general prices reflecting new, expensive drugs, surgical treatments and technologies – such as the synthetic products which replaced plasma-derived blood products, following the infection of patients by contaminated blood.[51]

Day-to-day or current public spending on health almost doubled in money terms between 1997 and 2001. After adjusting for price inflation, spending still increased by over 50 per cent.[52] Most of this extra spending went to maintaining existing services, meeting rising wage costs or increased demand in areas like drug payment schemes. Of the 40 per cent available for the development of services,[53] over half was devoted to community services – the homeless, the addicted, children at risk, the intellectually and physically disabled, the elderly. Primary care received about 20 per cent and the acute hospitals only 26 per cent of these development funds. Dublin's academic teaching hospitals argued in 2001 that, when they excluded funding for development of new services, the financing of their core activities had in fact been decreasing.[54]

The destination of the bulk of development funds illustrates an often-ignored aspect of Irish health spending. Much so-called health spending is in fact much-needed social spending.[55] For much of its early life the Department of Health was wedded to the Department of Social Welfare – the same Minister had responsibility for both departments. Health retained responsibility for the administration of many social services, even when Social Welfare acquired a separate Minister.[56] From 1997, Health was given responsibility for implementing child care legislation and became known as the Department of Health and Children. It should more appropriately be titled the Department of Health and Social Services. Because the Health budget funds social services, the Department excludes 10 per cent of its budget when it compares health spending in Ireland with other states. It could arguably exclude more.[57]

It is instructive to observe how often health board officials must attend court to explain deficiencies in social services, which must be made good from the health budget. This arose most strikingly during the crusade of Mr Justice Peter Kelly of the High Court to force the health authorities to provide special care and high support units for children at risk. Largely due to his efforts, the number of secure care places rose from 17 to 93 between 1997 and 2001. Childcare workers were offered increased salaries. The units cost £30 million (€38 million) in capital investment and £135 million (€171 million) in current spending.[58]

The health boards are also responsible for the young homeless. In 2000, it emerged that a 16-year-old girl, who had been raped and tortured by her father, was homeless. Donal O'Shea, the chief executive of the Eastern Regional Health Authority, acknowledged that the authority could not "be satisfied with the current arrangements for dealing with the young homeless".[59] Later that year it was announced that the Meath Hospital, which had been closed in Dublin in 1998, would be partially reopened as emergency accommodation for homeless children. The health boards provide medical and other support services for the adult homeless, who are the responsibility of local authorities. The boards provide an accommodation placement service and administer a rent supplement scheme. While these costs are reimbursed to the boards, personnel administering these schemes are counted as employees of the health service. Victims of sexual assault and abuse also come under the umbrella of the health boards.

In their audit of the health services, Deloitte and Touche came to the defence of the Department of Health in its stewardship of social services.

> The many deficiencies and issues surrounding the organisation and delivery of community care are continually brought to the attention of the public through media reports on such prominent issues as childcare, drug abuse and the elderly. While these issues are certainly real and need to be addressed, the Department of Health and Children and the health boards are now in many respects unrealistically expected to have a quality service in place despite having only recently received the funds to do so.[60]

Developments in community services between 1997 and 2001 included a 70 per cent increase in respite care places for the intellectually disabled – an extra 1,650 residential places and 2,300 day places; and 400 extra day places and 150 residential respite places for the physically disabled. For the elderly, there were 400 extra beds in community nursing units and over 1,000 new day places in 10 new centres with 880 new staff.[61] One of the explanations for the popular impression that investment in health care has failed to produce results is that services have been so deficient that even when investment provides improved care for some, the persistence of unmet needs for many others eclipses that achievement. Investment in facilities for the disabled, the elderly and children at risk, and in training and recruiting staff to care for them has been long overdue. That much more needs to be done does not negate its value.

While it is clear then that there have been many competing demands for health spending and remain many deficiencies to address, the quest for a black hole in health spending has continued – motivated in part by concern at the level of spending and also by a hostility among politicians with a tax-cutting agenda to the apparently inexhaustible demands of health.

Is health spending a black hole?

The revelation that implementing the 2001 Health Strategy would increase health spending as a proportion of national income to a level approaching that of the US inevitably raised questions about the efficacy of health spending. Two bodies have gone in search of a black hole of misspent funds.

Deloitte and Touche were commissioned by the Department of Health to study value for money in the health service and reported in 2001. The Progressive Democrats had advocated such a study during the 1997 general election campaign. For the management consultants, evaluating value for money in health spending involved not just assessing economy and efficiency but also investigating the effect of spending on the health of the population.[62] This they found difficult since, in Ireland as in most other states, patients' outcomes were not systematically assessed.[63]

Once they reported, Deloitte and Touche were suspected of having gone native in Health. Not only did they fail to find a black hole in health spending, they recommended increased spending – and increased taxation to fund it:

> The issue for government is that a demand led health service with a growing public expectation as to standards of service and care is capable of absorbing a more or less unlimited amount of funding. This report points to deficits and limitations across the system; in primary and community care, the mental health services, services for the elderly, childcare, and the acute hospital sector. By any analysis, the level of incremental funding required to address the service gaps and the other investment requirements outlined in this report, is very significant. We come from a position where the per capita spending on health in Ireland has been low by international standards. As a nation we need to decide what type of health service we require. If a superior system is demanded by the public (and there is much evidence to believe this to be the case), then, as taxpayers, the financial implications of addressing the current health service deficits need to be accepted.[64]

The report essentially concluded that, compared to other countries, Ireland had spent little on health over time; the health service needed big investment to catch up from the "often traumatic"[65] effects of the cutbacks in the 1980s, which should be committed in advance over three-year cycles; and the state needed to monitor and evaluate the spending of that money. While there might not be a black hole, not all spending delivered good value: the large number of smaller acute hospitals in rural areas raised "questions of quality of care and value for money".[66] One yawning chasm identified in the report was the absence of explicit values at the heart of the Irish health care system:

> What we are trying to achieve through our particular system is not clear. The principles of equity and access ... are not sufficient in themselves ... Access, equity and quality are important but the value system must set out what is or is not acceptable in terms of Health Care service provision.[67]

The Minister for Finance, Charlie McCreevy, was not pleased with the report nor were the Progressive Democrats – all ideologically committed to low taxation. So the Minister sent a further group in search of the black hole. This was the Brennan Commission, and an early draft of the Brennan Report forms the basis of this discussion. Less ambitious than the massive Deloitte and Touche study, it rapidly moved from assessing health spending to advocating reorganisation of the administration of the health service. Its sceptical tone, however, provided useful ammunition for Finance in its increasingly adversarial relationship with Health.[68]

The question remained – was there a smoking gun? Where in these studies, or outside them, was there evidence of poor health spending in Ireland? Neither study stated what any reader of the earlier analysis of the two-tier system will by now have realised: that an inequitable health care system cannot be considered to deliver value for money – if that is to be measured in terms of health outcomes. If the patients who are most in need are not treated first or at all and patients with lesser need are treated before them, health spending is inefficient. This persistent inequity in access to care remains the most glaring example of poor value in the Irish health service.

The experience of other states suggests that higher spending unaccompanied by equity produces poor results. Ireland has been spending more per capita on health than the UK since 1999 yet had much longer hospital waiting lists in 2002. Although the US has the world's highest health spending, nearly 16 per cent of the US population remained uninsured in 2000 and life expectancy for both men and women remained lower than the European average. The lesson is clear: how a state spends is as important as how much.

If the length of time that patients remain on waiting lists were considered the measure of a health system's success, then quite simply introducing a common waiting list would improve Ireland's performance. Although private patients would wait longer, public patients would be treated sooner and the average waiting time would drop – a levelling down, which would accomplish the prior treatment of patients with greater need. Better measures of the success of a health system are improved patient outcomes: higher life expectancy, better health. Delayed care for public patients means their health deteriorates and their life expectancy may be reduced. Such patients may eventually require costlier treatments, like the patients with arthritis who wait so long to see a rheumatologist that they require surgery or the children awaiting tonsillectomies who eventually need speech therapy because their hearing has been impaired.

Under the current system, privately insured patients with ready access to state-subsidised care may, however, indulge in "worried well" behaviour, pressurising their GP for specialist referrals and seeking second opinions, which specialists are happy to provide for a fee. These patients may be prescribed expensive medications, the cost of which the state reimburses if it exceeds a monthly threshold. Yet the sick poor may not even get as far as their GP, whose fee they may find prohibitively expensive. They may be unable to afford preventive medication, like asthma inhalers, or to contemplate spending sufficient on medication to reach the threshold for reimbursement. The insured may consume health care as a commodity, while the poor may continue to fall through the net and suffer preventable ill-health, despite the state's investment in health. If efficacious health spending is spending which makes the population healthier, then prioritising the care of the less ill and neglecting the more ill is an inefficient use of resources. Only when all citizens can access adequately resourced primary care and when hospitals treat the most ill first can Irish life expectancy and health be expected to improve significantly relative to other EU states'.

Neither of the government-commissioned diviners of the entrails of the Irish health system returned with evidence of a gaping black hole. Management consultants and accountants can be relied upon to spot failures in accounting, information and management systems – as indeed they did. Deloitte and Touche criticised the Irish system for failing to evaluate value for money systematically but observed that this failing was not unique to Ireland. Controlling the growth of demand for health care was difficult and not particularly well-conducted in other states. Only in the US were health information systems sufficiently developed to allow "rapid, regular and low cost monitoring of care".[69] The Brennan Commission criticised the absence at national level of anyone with explicit responsibility for managing and evaluating the service, and health boards' failures to meet accounting deadlines and instances of unauthorised expenditure.[70] Although these administrative failures reinforced the case for health system reform, none was, in itself, proof of misspending.

Deloitte and Touche concluded that some areas provided value for money, such as general practitioners' £51 (€65) average annual payment for GMS (medical card) patients in 2001.[71] Given the scarcity of GPs in areas where many medical card patients live, this might be regarded as a failure not a success of health care. The Brennan Commission, however, found increased GMS costs "alarming". Their concern appeared to be primarily focused on the rapidly escalating cost of prescribed medicines for medical card holders, which partially reflected rising drug costs but also reflected the inclusion of all over-70-year-olds in the GMS. The Department of Health under-estimated the cost of their inclusion because they miscalculated the number of eligible patients – evidence of poor information rather than misspending. However, the rates paid to GPs for the care of these patients were unusually high. The fault here was political and lay at the door of the Minister for Finance, who had announced the initiative prior to its negotiation, gifting the IMO a position of strength.[72] In so far as the Brennan Commission's draft report instanced other smoking guns, these occurred in the payment of GPs for dead patients and the costly method of remunerating pharmacists under the scheme for reimbursing the drug costs of non-GMS patients – unquestionably areas where savings could be made. Although escalating expenditure on drugs perennially concerns all governments, Ireland's per capita spending on pharmaceuticals has however been consistently below the EU average.[73]

If the Brennan Commission showed a tendency to equate accounting and information failures with misspent funds, Deloitte and Touche's shortcoming was a confusion of underinvestment with value for money. The replacement of inpatient psychiatric beds by other care suggested "improved value for money",[74] yet inadequate substitute services had in fact offered inadequate care. The consultants concluded that acute hospitals appeared to offer good value for money, given their high utilisation of capacity,[75] but contradictorily acknowledged that, with occupancy rates frequently exceeding 100 per cent, the Dublin acute hospitals "working at such levels of activity, will invariably compromise service quality, suffer from huge pressures on diagnostic facilities, and potentially cause consultants to protect beds" and increase patients' length of stay.[76]

Although the Department-of-Health-commissioned Prospectus study had not been mandated to seek black holes, its parallel assessment of the deficiencies in the system of health administration suggested areas where the quality of spending could improve: by reducing the number of agencies with overlapping briefs; by ensuring systematic evaluation of the outcomes from spending, hitherto only statutorily required of the ERHA; and by having clear lines of accountability for spending. It observed that, although the GMS Payments Board was responsible for processing payments, it was unclear where accountability for the level of spending under the GMS payments scheme lay. While a new system of administration might deliver more effective overall health spending, Prospectus did not appear wholly convinced that it would reduce administrative costs. Productivity gains might save some €140 million per annum but investment in information technology could rapidly eat that up.

Even though Prospectus proposed the abolition of the health boards, this was motivated by a search for a more accountable and less politicised system of health management, rather than by any considered view that the system suffered from over-management or over-recruitment of administrators. Both Brennan and Deloitte and Touche dismissed the notion that the health service had recruited too many administrators, a popular IHCA slogan. Managers and administrators increased from 11 per cent to 15 per cent of the health workforce between 1990 and 2000, when they totalled 12,366 compared to 5,698 doctors and dentists.[77] Yet, when the government decided not to fill 800 primarily management and administration posts following the 2002 election, the IMO immediately protested that consultants already had too little administrative back-up; accident and emergency, radiography and laboratories could not afford to lose posts; and the cuts would impact on the expansion of outpatient clinics and surgery proposed in the health strategy.[78] In 2001, one hospital manager had asked consultants to see fewer patients because of a shortage of clerical staff to retrieve files![79]

The reality was that, despite the IHCA's vision of an expanding army of grey bureaucrats, the "managers and administrators" identified in the health service personnel census were disparate employees, working in diverse health and social services. They included child care workers, workshop managers, librarians and computer operators. Nearly two-thirds of them were directly supplying services to patients as community welfare officers, ward clerks, secretaries to consultants or nurse managers, telephonists, or as personnel in outpatients, A & E departments, admissions and medical records. Other categories of so-called managerial employee were in areas such as payroll, human resources and information technology. Actual senior service managers – the people who might legitimately be called managers – accounted for 3 per cent of the total.[80]

Deloitte and Touche advocated increased recruitment, higher pay and investment in many areas of health service administration and management, particularly information technology, finance and human resources.[81] Between 1990 and 1999, the most significant increases in pay had been awarded to health professionals: when adjusted for inflation, the average pay of doctors and dentists increased by 77 per cent, compared to 66 per cent for nurses and paramedical staff, and 32 per cent for management and administration staff.[82] In 2000, 70 per cent of the management and administration category were low-paid clerical officers. CEOs of health boards remained on a salary scale, which was lower than the salary for consultants' public commitment alone.

Although both the Deloitte and Touche and Brennan investigations highlighted areas of health service spending where savings could be made, they failed to make the central connection between inequity and misdirected health spending. The Brennan Commission's limited brief – to examine financial management and control systems – did not deter it from recommending changes to the consultants' contract and favouring an eventual separation of public and private medicine in its draft report, but its analysis was piecemeal. Although written over a year after the publication of the health strategy, it did not pursue the question of how health spending might become sufficiently efficacious to permit the delivery of the health strategy at reduced cost nor did it address the feasibility of the strategy. If Deloitte and Touche expressed a Department of Health viewpoint, Brennan read like the voice of the Department of Finance, which had never been convinced of the merits of the strategy and was more preoccupied with emasculating Health than funding the strategy. In 2002, a Finance-sponsored assessment of Health's spending plans had concluded "there is a growing recognition that shortage of funding may no longer be the key issue in the health services".[83] Recognition by whom? Certainly not the authors of the health strategy, to which the government had committed itself six months earlier. What the Department of Health strategists perceived, as expressed by the Prospectus draft report, was "a generally held view among the public that additional investment in the Irish health system alone is not the answer and that radical structural reform is required".[84] Health was arguing for reform and investment; Finance for reform as a substitute for investment.

Although each of these studies, published or in draft, cast light on some of the system's failings and some of the necessary elements of reform, none offered a coherent challenge to the status quo. None simply stated the obvious: that the many distortions in the health care system – the preferential treatment of private patients, the over-emphasis on hospital care at the expense of primary care, the financial barriers to availing of primary care, the dispersed hospital network and the peculiar medical hierarchy – guaranteed that additional health spending would not deliver the improvements to health that it should. More compelling evidence of misspending was provided by the work of the Hanly task force on medical staffing: failure to rationalise the rural hospital network and the related issue of failure to reform how hospital doctors work have cost the health service dearly.

Here are the smoking guns in health spending, where the state invests funds for inadequate return: staffing small hospitals to deliver sub-optimal care; consequently paying an army of junior doctors large sums in overtime to cover hospitals which may see very few patients; paying the average registrar more than some consultants' public salary;[85] having multiple tiers of junior doctors on-call, who refer patients up the line to progressively more senior doctors, until someone can take responsibility for treatment; paying consultants for a contract which does not require their availability to public patients; subsidising preferential access to care for less-ill patients; and, most importantly, spending billions on these services in expensive institutions, while failing to develop relatively low-cost primary care, accessible to all without financial barriers, and therefore leaving illness untreated and preventive care neglected.

Rapid, politically motivated increases in health spending in pursuit of instant results have fostered expensive sticking-plaster solutions. One such was the Treatment Purchase Fund, which, while offering welcome and overdue treatment for the patients who had waited longest, was an expensive way of purchasing procedures that could have been delivered by increasing capacity in the public system. It was a "peculiarity", the National Economic and Social Forum observed, that "the government is turning to private suppliers to provide capacity for public patients, while dedicating some 20 per cent of existing public capacity to private patients".[86] Prior to the creation of the Fund, Miriam Wiley of the ESRI had commented that "the State is paying twice over for the provision of certain types of services" by subsidising both private patients' treatment in public hospitals and the displaced public patients' treatment in private hospitals.[87]

Paradoxically, failure to invest has caused wastage of resources. In 2002, the pressures for admission of medical patients was so great that elective surgery was cancelled in many hospitals, leaving expensive surgical and anaesthetic teams idle. Only more beds – either in the hospitals or for convalescent care in the community – could unblock this impasse. Deloitte and Touche argued that lack of investment in equipment was affecting value for money "where existing equipment is not fully functional".[88]

Any assessment of the impact of the massive increases in health spending from the late 1990s should have commented on the economic environment in which they took place. The 1997–2002 government's attempts to please everyone in the years prior to the election – to lower taxes, increase spending and keep every constituency happy – undoubtedly lessened the impact of additional health spending. Deloitte and Touche noted that, even though the health service badly needed extra funding, the "sheer pace" of additional funding injections was producing pressures to spend rapidly rather than effectively.[89] The largest increases took place from 1999 to 2002, years of tax-cutting budgets, high consumer spending, spiralling house and construction prices and an increasingly over-inflated economy. With labour in short supply, incomes rose generally. Hospitals' costs were driven up as they recruited nurses from overseas and competed to hire agency nurses. New facilities remained idle because health authorities could not recruit sufficient staff. Construction inflation rose steeply as developers of hospitals competed for construction workers. In 2001, 40 per cent of the value of investment in health under the National Development Plan had been eroded by inflation.[90] The price of new construction in the health sector rose by 50 per cent from 1997 to 2002.[91] The Brennan Commission objected that the rates paid to child care workers had caused knock-on wage rises in the health service[92] but the health boards were under immense pressure from the courts to rescue and care for children at risk, and had been forced to seek care workers at a time of labour shortages.

In the year 2001–2002, Ireland had the highest rate of inflation and third highest health costs in the eurozone. In a study of price changes during the changeover to the euro, doctors' fees showed an "unusual" 7.6 per cent increase over a six-month period, in excess of health and national inflation.[93] The IMO argued that GPs' costs had been "going through the roof".[94] VHI premium levels rose by 18 per cent from September 2002, an increase which the VHI attributed to wage increases for health care workers, rapid increases in the cost and number of procedures, much greater use of expensive drugs and high-tech diagnostic tools such as MRI scans, upgrading of facilities and increased charges for private patients in public hospitals,[95] which still contributed less than half the actual bed costs.[96]

The conclusion that to avoid inflation and prevent deterioration in the public finances government and society must choose between better public services and a low tax economy, metaphorically between building hospitals and holiday homes, invited a decision about priorities and values which the outgoing government was not prepared to make. Rapid pre-election injections of cash into an unreformed health service, at a time of high inflation and labour shortages, had indeed produced poor value for money – a more complex and more politically unpalatable argument than uncovering a black hole or discovering a smoking gun for which health administrators would take the blame. The rapid investment had been driven by electoral concerns. The failure to reform was a political, not an administrative, failure and one that it would be unfair to lay solely at Micheál Martin's door: he was following in his party's tradition of unexamined support for the public/private mix and unwillingness to confront the local supporters of small county hospitals. His paramount critic, the Minister for Finance, was no challenger of state support for private medicine, having unilaterally introduced tax subsidies for private, for-profit hospitals.

Health spending – the politics

Discussion of health spending – its level, its efficacy – cannot be divorced from politics. Spending decisions are political decisions, often opportunist, frequently with redistributive consequences and driven by undeclared ideologies.

The return to cutbacks

When the 2002 election returned Fianna Fáil and the Progressive Democrats, it appeared questionable whether this government would ever fund its health strategy. Growth had slowed. Since mid-2001, the economy had been feeling the effect of the high technology slowdown, followed by the impact of September 11th. The public finances were in crisis. Taxes had been so reduced that the government could no longer fund improved public services without breaching EU fiscal requirements. During the election no politician, either in government or opposition, wanted to break the news to the electorate that this was now the morning after the night before, that the boom-time years of apparently limitless possibility were over and that hard choices must be made. All the parties' election manifesto costings were based on the false premise that the outgoing government's budgetary forecasts were accurate, when in fact revenues were falling behind target and spending massively overshooting. Shortly after the election, the Central Bank warned "the public will have to be satisfied with a more modest provision of public services or will have to be called on to pay for these through charges or fees or through higher taxes".[97]

The new government chose to act by making access to health care more difficult for the working poor. Although all parties and the public[98] agreed that health was the main issue in the election and although Fianna Fáil had pledged that health spending would be its "number one priority", even in a downturn,[99] the new government announced successive reductions in state subsidies for the purchase of drugs, increased hospital charges[100] and failed to increase the income eligibility level for medical cards. In 2002, one visit to a family doctor and buying prescribed medications could cost over 20 per cent of the monthly income of a patient who failed to qualify for free medical care.[101] A substantial increase in hospital charges for patients who attended accident and emergency departments without a referral from their doctor, while designed to reduce inappropriate hospital attendance, removed for poor patients this hitherto cheaper route to care.[102] The overnight charge for patients admitted to hospital was also increased. Patients, who were too poor to purchase health insurance but not poor enough to qualify for a medical card now might have to pay up to €360 – over 60 per cent of their monthly income – if they were unfortunate enough to require ten days' hospital care.[103] The package of cutbacks, albeit in the context of an overall annual increase in health spending, included leaving approved posts unfilled and increasing charges for private accommodation in public hospitals which, nonetheless, remained heavily state subsidised.

In 2001, an official of the Department of Health had eagerly anticipated that, such was Ireland's wealth, such was the will to reform the health service, "we have a chance now to do for health what Donogh O'Malley did for education" – to remove income as a barrier to access.[104] His optimism had been misplaced.

Although Health fared well relative to other departments in spending allocations for 2003, with a planned 10 per cent nominal increase in current spending, this was its lowest increase since 1998.[105] The budget for hospitals increased by 8.5 per cent, which was below health cost inflation and, barring the unlikely possibility that significant wastage would be identified and rapidly eliminated, insufficient to maintain existing services. The government had neither provided funds to implement the health strategy nor had any immediate plans to do so, as the Minister for Finance made abundantly clear.[106] Planned capital investment in health was €515 million, 3 per cent lower than in 2002,[107] and just over half the investment which would have been required to implement the strategy at the pace originally envisaged by the Department of Health.[108]

The Department of Finance placed a ceiling of 96,000 on employment[109] in the health service in 2003, only 3,000 above the 2001 level and below its 2002 peak.[110] Health boards and hospitals insisted they could not live within budget, left vacancies unfilled, banned the hiring of agency nurses and forecast job cuts, reduced services and bed closures.[111] Hospitals cancelled elective operations because of insufficient convalescent beds for patients ready for discharge.[112] The incoming CEO of the ERHA, Michael Lyons, confirmed that the number of elective operations would have to be capped.[113] The Department of Finance questioned the use of synthetic blood products for haemophiliacs, an avenue of inquiry which suggested a rash venture into false economy.[114] Compensation costs for victims of infected blood were budgeted at over €100 million in 2003, 1 per cent of the health budget[115] and approximating to the funding deficit which major Dublin hospitals feared they faced at the end of 2002.

The government was reverting to the all too familiar pattern of stop-start health funding. Its pessimism about the impact of earlier investments might prove self-fulfilling. Providing training for more nurses and therapists would prove of little benefit if they graduated to discover no jobs, or insufficient beds to accommodate patients. A contrasting approach to the long-term funding of health care was adopted by the UK government, which in 2002 announced a five-year programme of investment, to be funded from increased social insurance contributions from employers and employees[116] and paced to avoid "input price inflation". The British Chancellor, Gordon Brown, observed that decisions about health funding over the next decade would "determine not only the long-term future of the health service but the character of our country."[117]

Health and ideology – the Boston versus Berlin debate

Now that the fiscal crunch had come, the dominant ideology of the Fianna Fáil/Progressive Democrat partnership was no longer sympathetic to the needs of the health care system. Their 1997–2002 government had always regarded tax cutting as an overriding imperative. In the year preceding the election, in response to opinion poll evidence of concern about health, some Damascan conversions had occurred in cabinet, but they were to prove short-lived. The Tánaiste and Progressive Democrat leader, Mary Harney, who had accused the Labour Party of "tax and spend"[118] policies when they proposed an end to tax cutting in favour of spending on services like health, said in the summer of 2001 that health spending must come before tax cuts in the next Budget.[119] Charlie McCreevy, who had been hostile to Health's arguments for extra spending at the Ballymascanlon cabinet meeting in May, decided in July that the next Budget should be about quality of life issues like health.[120] The Ministers were responding to the popular mood. The *Sunday Independent*, from the newspaper group which had championed tax cuts, announcing "payback time" prior to the 1997 general election,[121] concluded in August 2001 that "Health, not tax, is the priority".[122]

Harney's Progressive Democrats had been fervent supporters of tax cutting since their foundation as a party of former Fianna Fáil dissidents in 1986. Influenced by the ideology of Reagan in the US and Thatcher in the UK, they embraced supply side economics, the belief that removing disincentives (like tax) to the supply of labour or capital was the key to economic success. Considerations of redistribution and equity or the consequences for the public good of eviscerated public services were secondary. The market would provide. In coalition with Fianna Fáil, they found an ideological ally in McCreevy, with whom they dominated the 1997–2002 government, under the leadership of Bertie Ahern, the ultimate Fianna Fáil pragmatist. When, on its re-election, the government turned its back on its health strategy, this reflected the recanting of the earlier Damascan conversions and the re-emergence of divisions in the cabinet, which had been papered over during the election. McCreevy and the Progressive Democrats had been openly sceptical about health spending for most of the government's first term. The Minister for Finance was an accountant with a taste for gambling, elected by the heartland of the bloodstock industry, who represented the Tory wing of Fianna Fáil, while the earnest Micheál Martin, who had once described himself as a social democrat and "left of centre", had a lonelier job on its liberal wing. Fianna Fáil's chameleon qualities could dictate victory for either man depending on prevailing circumstances.

The divisions in cabinet mirrored a broader debate about the character of the country, in Gordon Brown's phrase, in which health came to be viewed as a defining issue.

Mary Harney supplied its title – the "Boston versus Berlin" debate – when, in 2000, she told American lawyers in Dublin: "Geographically we are closer to Berlin than Boston. Spiritually we are probably a lot closer to Boston than Berlin." The American economic model, she suggested, was based on enterprise, incentive, individual effort and limited government intervention. "The European way" was "built on a strong concern for social harmony and social inclusion, with governments being prepared to intervene strongly through the tax and regulatory systems to achieve their desired outcomes." The government favoured the former and had "a clear tax-cutting agenda ... This model works."[123]

In the ensuing debate, "Boston" came to represent the option of continuing on the path of a low-tax, low-state-spending society, in which the market would to a large extent be depended upon to provide for needs like health care, housing and child care. They would be primarily private goods. Proponents of the "Berlin" model advocated that health care was a social good to be provided as an equal right to all citizens. While "Bostonians" believed that the economic success of the 1990s was a consequence of the unleashing of private enterprise by lower taxes, which remained a prerequisite for continued success, "Berliners" saw Ireland's expansionary period as the payback for the introduction of free secondary education, for the strategy of wooing foreign investment in industry and, crucially, as the consequence of Ireland's membership of the EU,[124] all state-driven policies and, in the case of education and industry, very much state-investment driven. Fine Gael, like Fianna Fáil and the Progressive Democrats, belonged in the ranks of the Bostonians, sharing the belief that low taxes must be sustained.[125] The Labour Party were Berliners, but approached the topic of increased taxation with caution. In the 2002 election, they proposed increased capital taxation to fund income tax relief for the low-paid and increased employers' social insurance contributions to fund child care.

During the term of the 1997–2002 government, McCreevy had defied warnings that to continue cutting tax rates at a time of unprecedented growth was to run the danger of over-inflating the economy, provoking recession and so reducing the tax base that in less affluent times, there would be insufficient revenue to fund services. His approach to tax and spending was dictated by an accountant's rather than an economist's understanding of the economic cycle – "when you have the money, you should spend it, and when you haven't, you should stop".[126] If McCreevy blamed Martin for spending without results, the Finance Minister had authorised the spending in accordance with this counter-Keynesian belief. McCreevy derided critics of his tax reductions as "left-wing pinkos",[127] and fuelled the boom by generous tax concessions to the wealthy, although property prices were spiralling out of sight of the average citizen and deficiencies in infrastructure – social housing, hospitals, roads, schools – were increasingly manifest.

With Budget giveaways overwhelmingly favouring the rich, government revenue fell to 41 per cent of national income in 2002, nearly 5 percentage points below the EU average of 45.7 per cent. Government spending was 42 per cent of national income, compared to an EU average of 47.6 per cent. France, Denmark and Sweden, states with enviable social provision, spent close to or above 54 per cent.[128] The Department of Finance quibbled that Ireland's actual relative spending was 4 rather than nearly 6 percentage points below the EU average, since its debt repayments were lower than the average.[129] But Ireland still needed to acquire many social assets, such as hospitals, hostels, convalescent homes and health clinics, which these other states possessed and might have borrowed to acquire. The Department could be accused of the smugness of the outright owner of a hut, who points out that his neighbour in a mansion must repay a mortgage. These cross-country comparisons additionally failed to distinguish the nature of governments' spending, which might favour the poor or the rich. While the government made health care more expensive for the poor after its re-election, it resolutely refused to revisit a generous incentive scheme for savers which was anticipated to cost over €500 million a year, sufficient to fund free GP care for the entire population, by the Labour Party's estimate.[130]

The health battle in the cabinet

The contest between McCreevy and Martin had never been an explicit argument about tax and spending. Martin played the traditional role of a spending Minister, seeking greater funds, McCreevy the role of the Finance sceptic, in a Department which had so honed the skill of paring expenditure that it proved incapable of administering coherent plans for social and capital investment at a time of plenty. When, after the election, the government's focus shifted to concerns about administrative reform and efficiency in health spending, the resurgent Tory wing had a wider agenda. If they could convince the electorate of the Department of Finance's belief that shortage of funding was not an issue in the health service, that, to paraphrase Rory O'Hanlon, it didn't matter how much you spent, then perhaps health might once again retreat as an issue and tax increases to fund health spending might be avoided. Despite his Department's sanction for large increases in health spending, McCreevy had always belonged to the O'Hanlon school of thought. "Spending has been quadrupled since 1992, '93. I don't think the Irish people are that much more ill in that period of time."[131]

The Ministers' disagreements had become public on more than one occasion. When the cabinet assembled for its meeting on the health services in the scenic Ballymascanlon Hotel in May 2001, this had been intended as a public relations exercise, an opportunity to show concern for the health of the nation while providing a boost to tourism in County Louth. Instead, it had become the occasion for a public airing of the split within the cabinet on the issue of health spending and raised public awareness of the needs of the health service.

The agenda for the meeting had been extensively reported in advance. Martin spoke to newspapers and radio about the needs of a health service in which some hospitals were "stretched to capacity". Extra funds would go to increased services and facilities. "It is not a case of throwing money into a black hole ... It is at the Taoiseach's initiative that we are having this cabinet meeting tomorrow. He is of the view that it is a key issue that society needs to address."[132]

The television news that Monday showed the Minister in his shirt-sleeves, a business-like image, as he greeted the Taoiseach and other cabinet colleagues on their morning arrival at the hotel. He looked very different that night on television. The gala event had become the occasion for a public rebuff. Visibly shaken, he attempted the impossible: to avoid criticising colleagues, who had refused to hear his pleas for extra funding, and still defend his government's record on health. The first grenade had been lobbed by the Taoiseach who, on his way into the meeting, told reporters that the health service was "excellent" and "well-resourced", a direct contradiction of his Minister's description, but an understandably defensive posture for the man who had governed the country for the previous four years.[133] The *coup de grâce* was delivered by McCreevy, who emerged from the meeting to state that the Department of Health would have to join the queue for extra funding in the Budget. He reiterated his dissatisfaction with how "enormous" sums had been spent on health care. "I am not happy with how it's being spent."[134]

No announcement had been made of new plans for the health service, not even a statement of intent. Martin's interviews had raised expectations that the cabinet would at the very least endorse his view that money spent so far had been put to good use and support his planning for the future, in broad outline if not in detail. Instead the Minister had had his stewardship of the health services questioned in public by his colleague in Finance. Within the cabinet meeting, Martin had found few allies. Ministers of other spending departments saw his plans as a threat and potential rivals for the future leadership of Fianna Fáil were only too happy to see him disappointed.

"Government sources say relations between Health and Finance have turned 'nasty'," wrote the *Sunday Tribune*. The cabinet meeting had been a "PR shambles" and "just what a beleaguered opposition needed and guaranteed, if such guarantees were necessary, that health would be a major issue come the next general election".[135] Serious enough that the ministers should disagree, bad that they should do so in public but worse was to come. Ten days later, *The Irish Times* reported what health officials had told the cabinet at Ballymascanlon. Bertie Ahern's excellent, well-resourced system suffered from "endemic" under-investment, "overloaded" primary care and "serious deficiencies" in hospitals. The gap between life expectancy in Ireland and the EU was widening.

Although in autumn 2001, McCreevy allocated Martin significantly increased funds for 2002, this did not signify cabinet unity. To the eve of the health strategy's publication that November, Martin and McCreevy disagreed about its spending implications. McCreevy warned Martin not to publish his strategy until finalisation of the 2002 Budget, a caution which Martin apparently chose to ignore. The Minister for Finance then wrote to Martin:

> I understand that you are proceeding with the printing of the Health Strategy. You are well aware of my views in the matter, particularly in relation to the financing position. I wish to make it clear that initiatives contained in the Strategy involving expenditure implications for 2002 are included without my approval and carry no commitment on my part to the allocation of any particular sums to your Department in the Budget … I am copying this letter to the Taoiseach and the Tánaiste.[136]

Twelve days later, following a temporary truce, Martin launched the health strategy, which Fianna Fáil pledged to fund in the 2002 election campaign, and McCreevy again disowned in the 2003 Budget.

The paradox of health as an issue in the May 2002 election campaign

During the 2002 election campaign, political commentators grappled with the paradox that, although opinion polls and virtually every interview with a voter suggested that health was the major issue, this was not reflected in debate between the parties. That was Fianna Fáil's achievement and the opposition's failure. Fianna Fáil's strategists had conducted detailed research prior to the election which revealed that middle Ireland was happy with the wealth delivered in the boom years and while voters professed concern about health and other "quality of life" issues, they were susceptible to arguments that radical reform and expensive social programmes might jeopardise their newfound affluence. The party concentrated on questioning the costings of the opposition parties' platforms and successfully prevented debate on health service reform – on access to health care – from emerging as the central issue of the election. That the government parties were late converts to the need for investment in health care and that their tax cuts had so eroded the tax base as to make their own strategy unfundable were arguments which never gained mainstream currency. The election was dominated by a conspiracy of silence between the political parties to avoid taking from the electorate the cherished belief that it is possible to pay very little tax and also enjoy the level of public services offered by more highly taxed societies. It returned 15 independent TDs, of whom 5 had run on health issues. In all, 22 independent candidates had campaigned on health, including a hospital consultant, GPs, a psychiatric nurse and a psychologist. An alliance of eight candidates sought services as of right for people with disabilities and included people with disabilities, parents of disabled children and campaigners for the disabled.[137]

The catch-up in health spending in the late 1990s and to the year 2002 was necessary but poorly executed. Driven by electoral concerns, these too rapid increases, at a time of high inflation and labour shortages, were channelled into an inequitable and poorly organised system. Without reform, they would not deliver the only kind of value for money that makes sense in health spending: a significantly healthier population. Concern for value for money, in itself legitimate, and the consequent and overdue rediscovery of the need for reform in the system of health administration, became in 2002 a political smokescreen to distract attention from the government's extraordinary reneging on its commitment to fund the investment needs it had itself identified for the health service.

While investing in an inequitable system would never deliver optimal health outcomes, the large spending increases of this period were not wasted in the more obvious ways, which some seekers for a black hole appeared to anticipate. Two investigations of value for money failed to unearth evidence of vanity projects or featherbedding by bureaucrats. Hospitals had treated more patients. Many necessary services had been developed – for the elderly, the disabled, the mentally ill. If achievements had been insufficient, this was largely because the level of need was so great, so much more remained to be done and so much had been attempted in such a short time. The Department of Health had at last been given the resources to begin remedying some of the effect of the decades of neglect: to provide appropriate care for the many people who had formerly been consigned to psychiatric hospitals and county homes and, after they closed, had been abandoned to the care of their families or the streets. It would take time and sustained investment in facilities and staff before Irish society would have satisfactory services for the disabled, the mentally ill and an ageing population.

It was striking that, despite the abundance of bodies enquiring into aspects of the health system and its funding, no one in officialdom apparently saw fit to attempt to model the implications of implementing the health strategy, which a simple, private calculation had suggested could drive health spending up to 12 per cent of GNP. If misspending were accepted – and, depending on one's views of the health service, varying instances of misspending readily sprang to mind, inequity topping the list – then surely the next logical step was for a government, which believed in the needs identified in the strategy, to assess how these misspent funds might be reallocated, to explore different scenarios, different priorities and the consequences of different rates of investment. In the UK, the Wanless Report on NHS funding attempted just that, looking as far forward as 2022.[138] But the political reality was that Fianna Fáil and the Progressive Democrats had never been wholeheartedly committed to the health strategy. Micheál Martin had supplied an electable platform – nothing more. A government motivated by concern for health outcomes would as a priority have sought to ensure that no citizen faced financial barriers to care, especially primary care. A government which failed to increase the eligibility level for medical card holders manifestly was not so motivated.

A commitment to raising tax to fund health care, a commitment to genuine reform to achieve an equitable, efficient service, would have required Fianna Fáil to rediscover the radicalism which it abandoned in the 1960s. In 2002, as in 1987, 1989 and 1992, health care issues loomed large in a general election. Won with false promises, the election was a missed opportunity. The failure to debate how health care should be funded – and reformed – reflected a deeper failure to resolve the "Boston versus Berlin" debate about the values and future direction of Irish society. If the government's approach to health defined the future character of the country, the outlook was bleak.

13

REFORM WITHOUT EQUITY

"We are concerned that no specific commitment is made to ensure that all admissions to public hospitals – whether public or private – should be prioritised in accordance with medical need."
– National Economic and Social Forum comment on 2001 government health strategy.

"We will use all of our influence to make sure nobody takes it and it doesn't become a reality."
– Finbarr Fitzpatrick of the IHCA on the strategy's proposed public-only contract for new consultants.

The 2001 health strategy was not just a plan for spending and investment but also constituted the Fianna Fáil/Progressive Democrat government's response to growing demands for reform. The strategists evolved views on whether underfunding or inequity was the central problem of the service; explored and proposed changes to the system of bed designation; planned greater involvement for the private sector in the treatment of both public and private patients; and proposed changes to the consultants' contract and in how hospital consultants would work, in the interests of improving public patients' access to care. Ultimately, however, the strategy was founded on the politically tenuous assumption that spending enough would banish scarcity and end rationing for public patients. It left standing the edifice of two-tier access.

Despite the limited nature of the government's reform proposals, they met a hostile response from defenders of the interests of the privately insured and provoked threats of militant resistance from the IHCA to any attempt to impose a public-only contract on consultants in their early years. Negotiations on a revised consultants' contract were delayed to await the report in 2003 of the Hanly task force on medical staffing, which in its early drafts contained far-reaching proposals for improved patient care, to be delivered by consultants rather than junior doctors. This report, like the strategy, appeared to envisage a continued mix of public and private care in public hospitals, yet, were it to be implemented, it would so revolutionise the delivery of care and the work of consultants that it was difficult to reconcile with the continuation of the two-tier system.

Underfunding versus inequity – a debate about cause and effect

"We live in a low taxation, low public-spending economy by European standards. That's by choice of the Irish community. The fact that we have an under-invested health system is no excuse for the two-tier system that's in place at the moment. The mood now is for investment, development and growth. Change must go along with that."
– *Michael Kelly, secretary-general of the Department of Health, February 2001.*[1]

The problems of underfunding have for so long been apparent in the health service that for many people – health professionals and politicians – they have masked the significance of inequity in access to care. In reality, the service has had multiple problems, has been simultaneously underfunded, inequitable and poorly organised, all of which Michael Kelly, newly appointed to the most senior civil servant post in the Department of Health, was well-placed to appreciate. Kelly was a career civil servant, who had come up through the ranks in Health and was fortunate to have been on a temporary posting in the Department of Justice during the worst of the fall-out from the blood scandals in the late 1990s. His appointment in 2000 was greeted with enthusiasm by his colleagues, who respected his abilities. The secretary-general volunteered his assessment that underinvestment was no excuse for the two-tier system at a debate in 2001 organised by physicians in the lions' den itself, the hallowed halls of the Royal College of Physicians in Dublin's Kildare Street.

When he argued for a complex understanding of the problems facing the health service, he sought and found support from consultants in the audience who, while responding loquaciously about the problems of working in an underfunded service, dispersed between too many small hospitals, which politicians refused to rationalise, also recognised the unacceptability of the two-tier system, which they described as "embarrassing" and "shaming". It was "totally and utterly wrong", contributed Shaun McCann, professor of pathology at St James's Hospital in Dublin. Yet not all hospital consultants had shown such willingness to accept that the two-tier system required reform. A central division of opinion had become apparent between some doctors, who saw the problems of the health service as primarily under-resourcing coupled with poor management; and others, including some general practitioners and medical academics, who believed that the two-tier nature of the system and the role in it of consultants' work practices could not be ignored.

In a debate in *The Irish Times* in 2000, preceding Michael Kelly's intervention, Peter Kelly, the IHCA activist and consultant pathologist, had argued "the basic problem of the Irish health care system is underfunding".[2] Physicians in Dublin's Beaumont Hospital wrote that "appalling delays waiting for emergency treatment and for ward admission" were due to a shortage of beds and staff. "It is difficult to see how these problems relate to the consultants' contract of employment."[3]

Noel Rice, a general practitioner from Mayo, countered that while Peter Kelly was right "that underfunding is the basic problem in our health care system", he was

> wrong in trying to absolve hospital consultants of the blame. Yes, the vast amount of them may fulfil their contractual requirements, but what about moral requirements? It has long been obvious, to anyone prepared to accept it, that private patients are subsidised at the expense of public patients in public hospitals. As with justice, treatment delayed is treatment denied. Consultants have the power to change this overnight: one waiting list determined by condition of health, not that of bank account. Other changes, such as staffing levels must come, but first we must end our two-tier system.[4]

Garret FitzGerald, professor of pharmacology at the University of Pennsylvania and formerly a consultant and professor of medicine at Dublin's Mater Hospital, recognised the coexistence of "the erosion of structural investment by government" and "conflicts of interest that beset practitioners of private and public medicine". The "consultants' cartel system" would "make Hugo Chavez blush".[5]

While the contention that the health system suffered from both underfunding and inequity, and that both should be remedied, has gradually gained greater currency, differences of emphasis have persisted, which critically determine the nature of prescribed remedies. Deloitte and Touche described it as

> a facile analysis ... to point to the existence of private practice in public hospitals as the reasons for the problems in the acute sector ... The public/private mix, while a fair issue for debate, should not be used to mask the more fundamental issue creating pressures and inequities in the hospital system, namely the recurring lack of investment and inadequate physical capacity of the public health system.[6]

However, when the Department of Health's working group on the public/private mix sat down to consider strategic options, with Michael Kelly as a participant, it advocated immediate action to address inequity, since building capacity would take time. The resources existed "to remove the current inequities in the system", the group reported, but since "there are no simple solutions to this problem in the absence of increased capacity; therefore, a set of targeted, radical and intensive interim measures are necessary, if equity is to be meaningfully addressed in the near-term."[7] The 2001 strategy failed to deliver on this analysis.

Delivering equity: the health strategy proposals and the backlash they provoked

"A hospital may be directed to suspend admission of private patients."
– the health strategy inches towards equity.[8]

"The middle classes, once again, are the big baddies."
– a taste of backlash in the Sunday Independent.[9]

Despite the Department's concern about inequity, in their proposals for reform neither the government nor its Departmental advisers were prepared to contemplate abandoning the system of designating private beds in public hospitals. Although only in operation since 1991, this system, with its intrinsic institutionalisation of two-tier access, was now apparently sacrosanct. Yet, as earlier analysis has made clear, the operation of bed designation was incompatible with an equitable system of access to public hospitals. In an equitable system – one with a common waiting list for public and private patients, for instance – access to public hospital beds would be governed by medical need not by patient status. A private patient could still gain more rapid treatment in a private hospital but, at one stroke, over 20 per cent more beds would be available in the public system to clear waiting lists.

In 2001, this was still apparently too radical a measure for policy-makers to contemplate. Instead, as one of its targeted measures to improve equity, the Department working group proposed a dilution of the bed designation system to redress some of the discrimination against public patients. It proposed that the 80/20 ratio of public to private beds should be "strictly enforced in all hospitals"; that in Dublin, where the private hospital supply was greatest and waiting lists longest, the ratio might be reduced so that only 5 to 10 per cent of beds in public hospitals would be private; that the ratio should be adjusted in any area where waiting times for public patients exceeded 6 months; and that, where the waiting list for a specific specialty exceeded 12 months, private admissions for that specialty should be temporarily suspended.[10]

Following ten years of stasis in public policy on equitable access to care, these proposals with their implicit threat to consultants' private earnings, showed evidence of a renewed interest in and appetite for reform within the Department. However, they were only adopted in part in the strategy, which implicitly envisaged that the designated ratio would change in favour of public patients, since all additional beds funded under the strategy would be designated "solely for public patients".[11] When the strategy was launched, Micheál Martin elaborated that the addition of 3,000 new public beds "would get the balance to 84/16", which would indeed be the approximate arithmetic consequence for the public/private bed designation, were his government to deliver the promised beds.[12]

Most controversially for insured patients accustomed to preferential access to public hospitals, the strategy suggested that "a hospital may be directed to suspend admission of private patients for elective procedures in a specialty until the waiting time for public patients is restored to within the target period of time". This was followed by the qualification that "this directive can be set aside if hospital management and the consultants can agree on alternative means of restoring the target waiting time",[13] a rider which was interpreted by some senior health service managers as indicating that the threat of temporary suspension of private elective admissions, and consequently temporary reduction of consultants' private income, was intended to coerce consultants into greater public sector productivity but its enaction would be avoided if at all possible.

This then was the distance the government was willing to go to improve access for public patients. The traditional, complicated fencing between consultants and management, the elaborate measuring of who was in what bed when, in short the apparently untouchable public/private mix, would continue. The most radical proposal, evidenced in the working group's paper trail, was put to the group by its chairwoman, Maureen Lynott. In early discussions, she suggested that the public/private ratio in public hospitals could be altered to 90/10 for an interim period until increased bed supply was in place, in order "to address the current unacceptable situation and inequity in access to non-emergency hospital care". She pointed out that private hospitals did not have "material waiting list or access issues" and were benefiting from investment incentives in the Finance Bill. This "interim alteration" would be "linked to negotiation of changes in the Common Contract to address the longer-term issues in the public-private mix arising from potentially 3,000 additional beds and 1,500 additional consultants".[14] Although Lynott's proposal proved too radical for either the working group or the government, it too still stopped well short of proposing equitable access to state-funded public hospitals.

The immediate reaction to the strategy proposals for temporary suspension of private elective admissions was an eloquent reminder to the government and politicians in general that they would disturb the interests of the middle class at their peril. The government received a taste of the backlash from the private health insurance industry and media defenders of private patients' preferential access, which would accompany any efforts to achieve equity for public patients. Temporary suspension of private elective admissions was immediately described as "not workable" by the chief executive of the VHI, Vincent Sheridan. "Private insurers must be in a position to deliver the benefits they contract for and need certainty with regard to the resources available to them and not have these resources subject to events completely outside their control," he argued.[15] Martin O'Rourke, managing director of BUPA Ireland, weighed in: "What the private side will have great difficulty in adjusting to is a start-stop situation, where the monopoly supplier can arbitrarily decide that beds are going to be closed off."[16]

Some media commentary showed a poor grasp of the realities of private patients' preferential access to public hospitals, their ready access to private hospitals, or, indeed, of their relatively healthy, wealthy status. Mairead Carey wrote in *Magill* magazine that, unless waiting lists were reduced, hospitals

> must put a freeze on treating any more private patients, about half of whom are "outrageously" taking up beds in public hospitals ... In their haste to vilify the private patient, the Government seems to have forgotten that over half [sic] the population of the country

have health insurance. Far from sponging off the poor, they pay double for an appalling health service.[17]

When Carey wrote, under half (46 per cent) of the population had private health insurance but, it could safely be assumed, a majority of media commentators were insured. Her illusion that the insured constituted the majority was shared by Patricia Redlich of the *Sunday Independent*, who believed that more than 60 per cent of the population had private health insurance. "The middle classes, once again, are the big baddies," she wrote, in response to the health strategy. She did not define where she discerned an attack on "the middle classes", but accused "sections of the Government" and the Labour Party of implying that the middle classes were the reason for hospital waiting lists. While she didn't say so, it appeared that she too objected to the possible suspension of private elective admissions in favour of public patients. "The so-called two-tier system is a symptom, not the cause, of our ailing health service. And the middle classes are most definitely not to blame."[18]

In the same issue of the *Sunday Independent*, Alan Ruddock, who wrote with a broader understanding, conceded that a better service for the insured "is certainly unfair on those who cannot afford insurance, and it creates without doubt a two-tier system". But, he argued, "that is certainly not the fault of the insurance-paying class. Threatening to diminish their chances of quality health care in favour of the less fortunate may sound fair, but it could backfire as spectacularly as the postponement of medical cards."[19]

So, even this timid attempt at reducing discrimination against public patients provoked a strong response. In contrast, the members of the National Economic and Social Forum (NESF), who had been engaged in a study of equity of access to hospital care, immediately discerned the timidity of the strategy's approach. The NESF insisted that "at a minimum, access to public hospitals should be on the basis of a common waiting list". "Past experiences should have taught us that repeating the piecemeal pragmatic approaches of the past will again be self-defeating as long as the structural problems of the system are not adequately addressed." While supporting the proposal to suspend private elective admissions to give priority to public patients, the forum objected "we are concerned that no specific commitment is made to ensure that all admissions to public hospitals – whether public or private – should be prioritised in accordance with medical need and not that of ability to pay". It observed that the strategy's proposals for "increased capacity and efficiency and increased emphasis on the needs of public patients, however welcome, may not suffice to bring about equity in access to hospital care".[20] NESF reports must be seen by government before they are released. Given its trenchant criticism of the health strategy, although this report went to the government well before the May 2002 general election, it unsurprisingly did not make its way into print until the following July, after the electorate had made its choice.

The initial response from the medical profession to the possibility of a change in the ratio of public to private beds and the suspension of private electives was relatively muted. The profession tends to keep its powder dry for contract negotiations. George McNeice, chief executive of the IMO, questioned whether suspending private electives in response to the length of public waiting lists was legal. "Do you have a right to health care?"[21] It might have been more pertinent for him to have enquired whether a citizen in lesser need had a right to care before a citizen in greater need.

Finbarr Fitzpatrick, secretary-general of the IHCA, maintained that the government could implement these proposals – for a price. Consultants could offer no objection to altered bed designations, the temporary suspension of private elective surgery or even to a common waiting list:

> The decision with regard to waiting lists rests with the Department. It is national policy. If they decide in the common interest to change the regulations, there's nothing we can do about it legally or contractually. We can and we would argue that we would be entitled to compensation for it salary-wise but that's a consequence of the change. We are recognising the reality that the Minister of the day can decide national policy, in the so-called common good or common interest, and we can't stop him doing it.

The IHCA would not, therefore, resist a change in bed designations. "In the same way as the government changed eligibility over our heads in 1991, they can do it again, with the stroke of a pen."[22]

Fitzpatrick was, of course, aware that the government was not in fact proposing a common waiting list and that its strategy took as its point of departure that consultants retained the right to private practice in public hospitals. "Consultants have a contractual right to carry out private practice in public hospitals. The challenge is to ensure that a fair balance is achieved," the strategy stated.[23] Notwithstanding this concern for balance, the inherent contradictions of the public/private mix remained in the strategy. To maintain private practice, private patients would require preferential access. Consequently, although the strategy incorporated some of the targeted measures to reduce inequity, which the Departmental working group had advocated, it did not propose to dismantle two-tier access. Essentially, it relied on additional public capacity – more public beds – to improve access for public patients. It assumed that spending enough would banish scarcity and end rationing for public patients – an heroic assumption. To address inequity by extra capacity presupposed that the capacity would be delivered notwithstanding the vicissitudes in the public finances. A system which depended on the generosity of the Department of Finance to deliver equitable access would always be vulnerable.

Even were the increased capacity to materialise, the strategy did not promise that this would mean equitable access. The privately insured would retain fast-track access to at least one-sixth of the beds in public hospitals. And with public hospital managers still vying with the private sector to retain the services and presence of their publicly salaried consultants, some might still allow the proportion of private beds to creep upwards. Were the government to suspend private elective admissions to reduce numbers on public waiting lists, public patients would still be obliged to wait before this measure would be triggered. The clarity and ethos of a medically rather than financially determined system of access – one waiting list determined by need – was still absent. At its core, the strategy failed to accept the case which Michael Kelly had advanced that, however inadequate health care resources, the sickest should be treated first.

The small foretaste of middle class wrath, which the proposed suspension of private electives provoked, was evidence enough of why the government preferred to opt for increasing capacity rather than more equitably distributing scarcity. As the Departmental working group report had privately recognised, altering the public/private bed ratio in response to long public waiting lists could lead to "waiting lists for private hospitals and an increase in health insurers' costs",[24] until the private sector provided more beds. In other words, immediate equity would mean levelling down, a solution which would provoke the anger of the articulate and influential – the people who wrote newspaper columns, the people who were more likely to vote – even though it would deliver better care for the less influential (and sicker) majority. Better by far, for this canniest of governments, to promise equity in the future, when public capacity would materialise – perhaps. A government which desired to lead, reform and truly deliver a first class health service might have been swayed by a political counter-argument:

that to level down would ensure that the middle class would acquire a stake in the public health service, in place of their current ability to parasitise it, that they would then accept the argument for adequate funding and then, and only then, would it be possible to level up.

Targeting waiting lists ... again: the Treatment Purchase Fund

While the government ducked the fundamental challenge of addressing inequity in access, a simpler approach to addressing public patients' exclusion recommended itself to the junior partners in the coalition, the Progressive Democrats. Although waiting lists were only one facet of the inferior care received by public patients, they were the visible tip of the iceberg and reducing them would deliver political dividends. In September 2001, when the draft strategy was already under consideration by a cabinet sub-committee, the Progressive Democrats decided that, with an election imminent, it was time to make the public aware that Fianna Fáil had no monopoly of wisdom on health policy. With maximum publicity, they announced a proposal for the establishment of a "treatment guarantee fund", which would finance the treatment privately or abroad of public patients on waiting lists. "Any patient, who has waited three months, will be offered a definite appointment date as a private patient instead of simply being put on a public waiting list as at present," the Tánaiste and Progressive Democrat leader, Mary Harney explained.[25]

Now coming to the end of a prolonged and inclusive process of consultation in preparation for the health strategy, Micheál Martin diplomatically pointed out to these late arrivals in the vineyard that already, under the Waiting List Initiative, health boards were permitted to contract beds from the private sector and some patients had been sent abroad for operations.[26] Privately, the Department of Health was incensed at the Progressive Democrats' opportunism. The Department was especially unenthused about their proposal that consultants would be paid by fee-for-service for public patients who were treated privately.[27] It was apparent to anyone familiar with the dangers of the hybrid system of paying consultants that this proposal might further bias the system against the treatment of public patients by consultants in their salaried hours. Unless the consultants' contract were changed, the Treatment Purchase Fund could offer an incentive for public hospital consultants to devote less time to working for public patients in public hospitals and more time to the private sector, where they might now receive additional fees to treat both public and private patients. In subsequent discussions with Health, the Progressive Democrats eventually agreed to drop the reference to fee-per-item payment "for self-referral by consultants from public to private practice"[28] but official concerns remained about the potentially distorting effect of the Fund. The Department of Finance later queried how the proposed National Treatment Purchase Team would "prevent consultants manipulating the system to their own advantage".[29] Health responded "the Treatment Purchase Team will monitor the number of public patients each consultant will treat in private practice. If there is evidence of any otherwise unexplained increases from a consultant's present level of cases, the Team will have to review the position."[30] When subsequently the Fund adopted as a principle of operation that no consultant, to whom public patients were referred for treatment, should "predominantly treat patients from his or her own public list", this contributed to consultants' reluctance to cooperate with the Fund.

Although the Progressive Democrats' interjection was greeted with some scepticism by the IMO, which questioned whether there was sufficient private capacity, either beds or manpower, to deliver the guaranteed treatment,[31] it was a gift to the owners of private hospitals, who were campaigning for tax reliefs. The Independent Hospitals Association of Ireland informed the government that, were they to receive tax incentives to help them to expand, they could treat a further 5,000 to 7,000 public patients a year.[32]

Since, in the *realpolitik* of the coalition, a means had to be found to assuage the Progressive Democrats' electoral anxieties, the health strategy incorporated a "new ear-marked Treatment Purchase Fund". However, the proposed "guarantee" of treatment within a specific timescale had been replaced by a "target" that, by the end of 2004, all public patients would be treated within a maximum of three months of referral from an outpatients' department.[33] Later, during the 2002 election campaign, both government parties promised to eliminate waiting lists within two years.

The first treatments of patients from public waiting lists began in Dublin private hospitals in June 2002. The Fund proposed to concentrate on long waiters: adults who had waited over a year and children who had waited longer than six months.[34] By December 2002, the Fund had arranged the treatment of 1,920 patients and hoped to increase its throughput by encouraging more referrals for treatment in England.[35]

The National Treatment Purchase Team's latitude to purchase care outside the state and the pressure it could bring to bear on hospital consultants to refer their patients onward gave it superior clout to the still coexisting Waiting List Initiative. For patients who had virtually given up hope of ever reaching the top of the list, the Progressive Democrats' initiative was bringing tangible change to their experience of the health care system. This was pragmatic populism at its best. It still fell far short of its initial billing, when Mary Harney suggested it would help to "transform the Irish public health system" and implied that it would end two-tier treatment.[36] A waiting list guarantee which meant something would undoubtedly have been a good idea, as was flying patients abroad for treatment, if necessary. Other states, with equitable health systems, had had recourse to such measures to expedite patients' access to care. However, the PDs failed to convince their colleagues in government that they should commit themselves to a guarantee and this initiative, grafted onto the two-tier system of public hospital care, did not deliver equity. Public patients could still wait years to see a consultant before they were ever referred for treatment or counted as "waiting". The Fund had no role to play for patients whose condition had not even been assessed. Even were the government to achieve its target of treatment for public patients within three months of referral, there was no guarantee that private patients with lesser need might not receive faster access to public hospital care. Nor would this initiative change the reality that, within public hospitals, public and private patients would continue to have different experiences of treatment.

Only if the government's promised investment in public hospital capacity were to materialise, and if access to public hospital care were to be based on need, would the Fund cease to find a market for its services. "As public capacity grows, the need for this safety mechanism to guard against lengthy waiting lists will decrease," the Progressive Democrats suggested, when arguing with the Department of Health for their approach,[37] echoing Brendan Howlin, who had envisaged that his 1994 Waiting List Initiative would be short term.

The PDs differed from Howlin in their willingness to encourage the private sector to supply beds, on the assumption that they would do so more rapidly than the state sector. If the government's investment in expanding the public sector were not to materialise, the possibility now existed that the state would, through the Fund, funnel public patients into an expanding and state-subsidised private system, still primarily staffed by public hospital doctors. These doctors and private hospital developers would gain from this state investment, and meanwhile the impoverished public system would continue to accord preferential access to private patients. State resources would have been used to better effect had the government decided to grant priority in state-funded institutions to those in greater need, to end state subsidies for private care and to purchase care in private hospitals only if, having been granted access in accordance with need, public patients could not be accommodated in public hospitals.

The common contract revisited

Although the health strategy retained the bed designation system and recognised consultants' contractual right to carry out private practice in public hospitals, it made clear that the Department wished to renegotiate the terms of the consultants' contract to deliver better care for public patients. "Greater equity for public patients will be sought in a revised contract for hospital consultants," the strategy stated. "It will be proposed that newly-appointed consultants would work exclusively for public patients for a specified number of years. This would mean that consultants would concentrate on treating public patients in the early years of their contract, but would be in a position to develop private practice at a later stage where their contract so permits."[38] The strategy's language was tentative – to seek equity is not to achieve it. If this government planned to take on the consultants on the issue of private practice rights, it was starting out in a timorous manner.

This timidity extended to the government's advisors. Civil servants are not recruited for their crusading zeal, although they may prove more radical than their ministers. However, on the issue of confronting hospital consultants, memories are long and appetite slight in the Department of Health. During the 1997 common contract negotiations, consultants in the IHCA had threatened to cause chaos by withdrawing their cooperation with policy-making and administration in hospitals, and consultants in the IMO had warned of possible industrial action. In its private deliberations in 2001, the Department working group on the public/private mix observed "any near-term measures that would attempt to unilaterally remove the right and extent of private practice is likely to be met with the strongest opposition. Amending the terms of the contract can only be achieved through a process of negotiation and agreement."[39] Officials of the Department were continuing to show undue respect for the industrial muscle of consultants and, consequently, according them too powerful a role in determining the shape of the health service and too great a proprietorship in a service which rightfully belongs to the citizens of the state. The working group members echoed their predecessors, who advised Barry Desmond in 1984 that, if an extension of eligibility for hospital services were attempted, "strong opposition could be anticipated from the consultants who would probably see a threat to their incomes from private practice."

When, in 2001, a Department sub-group proposed that consultants should be given productivity targets for the treatment of public patients which, if not met, should trigger restrictions in their right to private practice,[40] the full working group demurred. "Monitoring of waiting times with productivity targets for individual consultants ... may be too confrontational to engender cooperation with more strategic change in regard to equity".[41]

Yet the group considered it "vital to improvement" of public patients' access that "a programme of change relating to equity of access ... should form the central part of the negotiating agenda for changes to the current contract". This programme would include a monitoring system where consultants were not complying with existing features of the common contract; paying consultants fees only where private patients were in or awaiting private beds; when a public bed was occupied by a fee-paying patient, supplying a private bed to a public patient to compensate; requiring insurers to furnish lists of patients for whom claims for consultant fees had been accepted; and concentrating new beds where they would deliver greater access.[42] The Department appeared unwilling to learn the obvious lessons from its previous failures to devise an adequate monitoring system – that the existing public/private mix could not be reconciled with equity, which would only be delivered by a common waiting list governed by need and a common system of payment for consultants. The Department's detailed negotiating agenda was unsurprisingly not disclosed in the published strategy, which took refuge in euphemisms.

The Department was not, however, overstating the potential opposition from consultants to the reduction or ending of opportunities for private practice. With varying degrees of hostility, the IMO and the IHCA opposed the proposed imposition of a public-only contract for newly appointed consultants for a specified number of years. Although they had sought the restoration of a voluntary public-only contract, withdrawn in 1997 because of the Department's desire to promote private practice as a source of hospital revenue, this mandatory contract was quite another matter.

Interestingly, the IMO's president in 2002, consultant psychiatrist Kate Ganter, engaged only in public practice. The first woman to lead the profession since the foundation of the IMA in 1839, she was not untypical of growing numbers of women doctors who opted not to undertake private practice for quality of life reasons. Women were the majority of medical school graduates and 37 per cent of new consultants appointed in 2002.[43] Representing this changing face of the profession, Ganter anticipated that the two-tier system would disappear because the soaring cost of professional indemnity insurance would force many doctors out of private practice.[44]

Yet the IMO was not prepared to accept fundamental change in the contract without a battle. George McNeice, its chief executive, unconsciously repeated Rory O'Hanlon's defence of two-tier medicine in 1991, asserting: "The public/private mix has served the country very well. Where you have a public-only service, the quality of the service goes down."[45] If, however, a government were to legislate to end private practice in public hospitals, McNeice accepted "we can't stop the legislation. They would have to negotiate the change and pay compensation to people to buy out their contracts, the same as you would in any other walk of life." While the profession had a right to defend its interests, "that doesn't mean the profession is saying to anyone 'unless we get our way, you can't change anything'. We have never said that."

This trade union pragmatism was not shared by the IHCA. Finbarr Fitzpatrick predicted confidently that his association would defeat the government's efforts to introduce a public-only, salaried contract for newly appointed consultants. Although he accepted that the Minister had the power to introduce this contract for new appointees, who would not be "in a good negotiating position", Fitzpatrick asserted "if he wants to get the agreement of the IHCA, I can tell you now that he won't". The IHCA would never strike, he said, but, "notwithstanding our lack of industrial muscle", if the Minister did not accept that the contract should be optional, "then we will use all of our influence to make sure nobody takes it and it doesn't become a reality. We might fail but I am confident we won't."

Fitzpatrick's militant defence of private practice rights was in apparent contradiction with his acceptance of the Minister's right to change the waiting list or bed designation systems and his general insistence that consultants were unfairly viewed as obstacles to equity.

> There is an inconsistency in the Department's thinking. On the one hand they want the income from private practice. On the other hand, they preach *ad nauseam* about equity and access. The socialists of this world would say that a single common waiting list is the solution to equity. That's the decision of the Minister for Health. It requires a stroke of a pen to do it. If Micheál Martin comes out in the morning and says there will

271

be a common waiting list, what are we going to do about it? They want
the bloody money. Why won't they be honest with people? The number
of beds in any hospital and their designation as public or private is not
decided by the consultant.[46]

While there was some justice in Fitzpatrick's charge of inconsistency
on the part of the Department in simultaneously seeking equity and
wanting to protect private income for public hospitals, he and his
association were equally exposed to the same charge. To threaten
resolute resistance to the Minister's attempts to hire new consultants
with a full-time commitment to public patients, while maintaining a
neutral stance on a common waiting list, which would inevitably reduce
demand for private practice, appeared utterly inconsistent. The key to
the IHCA's position, however, was the distinction between on-site and
off-site private practice. A common waiting list, changes to bed
designations or suspended private electives would diminish
opportunities for private practice on-site in public hospitals and trigger
demands for higher public salaries. But, critically, consultants might still
supplement their private income by working off-site. On the other hand,
a mandatory public-only contract would remove the opportunity for all
private practice, off and on-site. New public consultants would no
longer be able to staff private hospitals. They would be entirely salaried
employees of the state and this the IHCA appeared willing to resist to
the death. Despite Fitzpatrick's professed neutrality on a common
waiting list, by insisting on public consultants' right to engage in private
practice, the IHCA remained an obstacle to the dismantling of the two-
tier hospital system. In contrast to Kate Ganter, who anticipated that the
cost of medical indemnity would eventually kill private practice,
members of the IHCA hoped that the government would assist
consultants in paying for professional indemnity insurance for off-site
private practice, possibly as part of a deal to cement a new consultants'
contract, or even without that trade-off. As the government was
subsidising the development of private hospitals, for it to subsidise
further the off-site private practice of consultants would not be
inconceivable, however ill-conceived.

The strategy's agenda for contract negotiations between the
Department and the medical organisations was delayed to await the
publication of the report of the Hanly task force on medical staffing.
Meanwhile, in 2003 in its review of the system of health administration,
an unpublished draft of the Prospectus Report proposed that the
contract should be revised to achieve "flexible provision of clinical

services" and "co-operation with clinical audit and with management" – minimalist targets.[47] In its critique of the health strategy, the NESF observed that "the Irish arrangement, where private practice is part of hospital consultants' public contracts and carried out within the public hospital seems to be very unusual". Comparing international models of care, the NESF found that most states did not provide private services in public hospitals. Even in a state such as Australia, where private patients were admitted to public hospitals, there was a single waiting list for elective surgery and patients were treated on the basis of clinical need. Irish practice remained "exceptional". "The scope for 'two tiers' in terms of access is much greater here than in, for example, our European Union partners."[48]

The NESF, unfortunately, did not pursue the logic of its analysis in its recommendations, presumably reflecting the very wide coalition of interests represented on the forum. While critical of the strategy's shortcomings and advocating a common waiting list "at a minimum", it put forward no suggestion for how the consultants' contract should be changed. On the other hand, the Department-of-Finance-sponsored Brennan Commission, in its 2003 draft report, baldly recommended that all new public consultant posts should be exclusively for public sector work, observing that the public/private mix caused a "conflict of interest for consultants" between their public obligations and the treatment of private patients "for gain". Almost as an aside in a discussion of financial accountability, the Commission had in effect advocated the phased ending of the public/private mix in public hospitals. The Commission was apparently either unaware of the political implications of its recommendation or had chosen to disregard them. It did not explore the consequences of its recommendation for the system of bed designation. Although a sketchy and unworked-through proposal, this was a significant break with the conventional wisdom. The public/private mix had indeed existed since the foundation of the state, had been defended by the 1989 Commission on Health Funding, in the 1998 Government White Paper and had survived in the 2001 strategy. The Department of Health had been outflanked and, if the Brennan Commission were to prove influential, the medical organisations might face even tougher negotiations than they envisaged.

The differing stances of Fitzpatrick, McNeice and Ganter illustrate that a government with a clear sense of its reform objectives might not face united opposition from consultants and their representatives. While the IHCA has traditionally defended private practice rights, consultants with divergent views have become more vocal. When Fine

Gael held a conference on health policy in Ennis, County Clare in November 2001, it was electrified by a contribution from the floor from John Barton, a consultant cardiologist from Ballinasloe in County Galway, who, professing himself to be "altruistic and dedicated to my profession", passionately disowned the two-tier system, echoing his colleagues at the Royal Academy of Medicine debate earlier that year. Barton said:

> I am fed up to the teeth with patients saying "if it's money, I have VHI". I am fed up with getting calls from nurses saying "Doctor, your private patient is admitted". The system is that private patients are superior. It's disgusting, immoral, amoral and it has to change. I also worked in the Canadian health care system. It's a magnificent system, it's beautiful. All patients are the same. I get fed up with patients coming into my rooms and saying "Doctor, what's your fee?" It's got to change. We have to take cash out of the relationship between doctor and patient.

Ending the winner-takes-all medical model

When the government formulated its strategy, it had the benefit of considerable analysis of the dependence of the hospital system on junior doctors and its consequences for patient care. While all parties in a forum on medical manpower had not agreed on precisely how the system of medical staffing should change, there was a consensus that much more care should be provided directly by consultants and, consequently, that many more consultants must be employed and correspondingly fewer junior doctors. However, this general support for a consultant-provided service met resistance from the Department of Finance, who questioned its cost.

The strategy, therefore, espoused no view on this key issue of whether public patients would receive the same quality of care as private patients. Nor did the strategy disclose how many new consultants might be appointed. It merely neutrally observed that the 2001 Report of the Medical Manpower Forum and the 1993 Tierney Report "saw considerable advantages in such a move".[49] Having refused to endorse the Medical Manpower Forum's recommendation of a consultant-provided service,[50] which Micheál Martin continued to support in public,[51] the government then established the Hanly task force on medical staffing, which was requested "to quantify the resource requirements and costs that would arise if a consultant-delivered hospital service were developed in place of the existing consultant-led system".

Represented on the task force, the Department of Finance attempted without success to overturn the consensus about the need for a consultant-provided service. Michael Kelly responded to Finance reservations with some acerbity:

> Every analysis to date comes back to the same key point: service provision in the Irish hospital system is over-dependent on doctors who, while still in training, are required to provide 24-hour, 7-day medical care. While this care is formally under the supervision of individual consultants, their presence on site is in the main limited to 33 hours per week provided between 9 am–5 pm Monday–Friday. Patients therefore have limited access to appropriate levels of senior clinical decision making, with inherent implications for safety of diagnosis and treatment on the one hand and efficiency and cost-effectiveness on the other.[52]

The task force attempted to avoid the politics of the Medical Manpower Forum. The forum had been established by Brian Cowen in 1998, with a membership of medical professionals and health administrators, when it became apparent that, if junior doctors were to work shorter hours and receive proper training, hospitals could no longer depend so much on this form of cheap labour, patients could no longer be subjected to their unsupervised care and the old medical hierarchical system could no longer function. In the forum, the Department pursued the agenda of the Tierney Report, which had advocated appointing more consultants and retaining only sufficient NCHDs, engaged in genuine training of shorter duration, to meet future needs for trained personnel. Consultants would change their work practices to become directly involved in emergency services, public patient care and training their juniors. The ratio of consultants to NCHDs would increase from 1:2 to 1:1.[53] In 2002, despite the appointment of more consultants than Tierney had envisaged, the army of juniors had grown to an even greater degree, so that the ratio of consultants to NCHDs had fallen to 1:2.29 – 1,718 consultants to 3,932 NCHDs.[54]

In its interventions in the Medical Manpower Forum, it had been apparent that the Department shared the analysis of the shortcomings of the hospital hierarchy which had been advanced by Muiris FitzGerald. Simply adding extra consultants, who were allowed unlimited private practice, "would merely consolidate what the public perceives as a two-tier system of medicine", the UCD dean of medicine had argued.[55] The Association of Hospital Chief Executives agreed, arguing in its submission to the forum that increasing consultant numbers without a revised contract "would not achieve significant improvements in public patients being diagnosed and treated by fully trained doctors".[56]

FitzGerald had proposed that, instead of appointing consultants as traditionally understood, there should be "specialists", who would be appointed at an earlier age in a system of career progression based on achievement. At the forum, the Department tried to move in this direction, variously proposing a FitzGerald-style "specialist"; or a new contract for all public hospital consultants, which would roster them to work shifts, including routine weekend and night work, not merely on call but on the premises; or a new category of public hospital consultant, where only new appointees would work the rostered shifts. The medical organisations were not enthused. They professed willingness to negotiate rostered shift working, "where necessary", for certain specialties.[57] They were hostile to a new category of consultant.

Peter Kelly, chairman of the IHCA committees on the common contract and manpower, argued that "such appointees would be wide open to being exploited by hospital managers and other consultants". He quoted a survey of IHCA membership, which showed "overwhelming" rejection of this new category of consultant, yet support for flexibility in permitting routine availability of consultants outside conventional working hours.[58] Finbarr Fitzpatrick maintained the IHCA did not object to "around-the-clock working in certain specialties. If they want to talk about certain specialties having a much larger presence, we are open to persuasion, negotiation and discussion."[59]

Consultants had concrete reasons to resist change. Older consultants, who had come up the hard way, did not want to go back to night work. Some feared that the new category of rostered consultant, proposed by the Department and now referred to as Category Three, would harvest private patients admitted while on his shift, patients whom the NCHDs would have previously treated, while the "on call" consultant at home received the fee. Perhaps most importantly, the cohort of consultants, who had just returned from their onerous exile to take up consultant posts in Ireland, having just reached the pinnacle of the hierarchy would resist diminution of their status and earning power, or easier access to either, for the next generation.

Not represented in the forum discussions was the voice of those doctors who might be attracted by the concept of working on a roster, with a graduated career structure. A macho lifestyle, working long hours for huge rewards, might not necessarily suit the many women doctors, nor men with ambitions to participate in family life. Change would also be welcome to many consultants in hospitals outside Dublin, with fewer opportunities for private practice, who found it harder to attract good junior staff and must work tougher rotas. "Once it was not seen as a sub-consultant and, if the salary was right, people would jump at a contract which allows them not to be on call to private patients all the time," a registrar at a Dublin teaching hospital commented.[60] A postal survey of 104 trainee paediatricians disclosed that, while three-quarters would prefer a consultant grade if given a choice, 85 per cent expressed interest in a new non-consultant specialist grade and 54 per cent, including substantial numbers of men, would opt for a part-time consultant or job-sharing position, if available.[61]

The IMO and IHCA achieved the shelving of proposals for a new category of consultant. The final version of the forum's much-leaked report noted that this option was "not acceptable to the medical organisations".[62] The forum instead adopted as its "preferred option" the negotiation of a revised contract for all consultants, which would provide changed work patterns, flexible rostering and clinicians working together in teams. The report stated that consultants should "have an entitlement to on-site private practice".[63]

It was significant that the report recorded but did not endorse the medical bodies' rejection of the new consultant option. When the 2001 health strategy proposed that newly appointed consultants should work exclusively for public patients, medical organisations saw their apparent victory slipping away. "The Department of Health never accepted the results of the Manpower Forum. They used the strategy to float this idea of a public-only appointment in the first seven years, as a refinement of the sub-consultant grade," commented George McNeice of the IMO.

After this history of antagonism and disagreement, the Hanly task force explicitly decided to set aside industrial relations issues.[64] In its recommendations for medical staffing, as in its prescriptions for the hospital network, the task force set out with a blank sheet to design an ideal system. In its ideal world, every junior doctor would be in training in a post which would eventually lead to a career appointment in Ireland. The "chronic imbalance" between training and career posts, which had led to "inappropriate large scale importing of overseas doctors", would cease. Patient care would be provided by consultants working in teams with trainees and other staff. The present tiered on-call system of "serial failure", in which patients were referred up the line for diagnosis through ranks of junior doctors, would also cease. Consultants would be either first or second on-call. Nurses, an increasingly well-qualified profession, would take on tasks which had formerly been performed by NCHDs and would in turn delegate duties to clerical staff or health care assistants. The task force's recommendations for medical staffing were designed to ensure that all hospitals, within its proposed regional structure, would be predominantly staffed by fully trained doctors, who would have a regional contract, rather than a contract with an individual hospital.

The task force calculated that to staff hospitals in this way, the number of consultants must double to 3,497 by 2011. The number of NCHDs would almost halve to 2,164. The ratio of consultants to NCHDs would be 1:0.6. These calculations, which did not take into account the demands placed on the service by growing population, assumed a marginal fall in the total complement of hospital doctors. But this new workforce would be dominated by consultants, the hitherto highly paid élite. The task force attempted to reach an estimate of the cost of this change, which would eventually depend on how much consultants and NCHDs were paid, an industrial relations issue. Without drawing the obvious conclusions, in its draft report the task force examined medical staffing in Finland, where there were two specialists for every trainee, and where the average salary of a specialist in the public sector was €45,000 compared to €154,000 in Ireland.[65] The implications did not need to be stated. More consultants would have to mean cheaper consultants.

The task force examined and rejected alternatives to consultant-provided care. If EU requirements for reduced working hours for NCHDs were to be met purely by employing more NCHDs, their number would have to increase by a further 2,500, reducing the ratio of consultants to NCHDs to 1:4 or 1:5. Even if all these NCHDs could be found, "the treatment of patients would increasingly be delivered by doctors not yet sufficiently qualified or experienced in their work". The task force concluded that a consultant-provided service was "the only feasible, safe system of care which genuinely places the patient at the centre".

Clearly, the consultants' contract would have to change. The task force recommended that consultants should structure their time in a defined division between clinical, training, evaluative, research and management activities. A specialty within a hospital should be organised as a "clinical directorate", like a "small business unit", with a clinical director, nominated by the relevant consultants and appointed by the chief executive of the hospital for a defined period, and with a nurse and business manager. How this model would ensure smooth functioning as a team of the formerly independent consultant gods, accustomed to occupying the apex of the medical hierarchy, was not entirely clear. Like the forum, the task force refused to contemplate a system of graduated career progression for fully qualified specialists, as Muiris FitzGerald had suggested. Its flat model of staffing did not, for instance, appear to countenance any recognition for seniority or superior skills among consultants on teams. The task force necessarily addressed the issue of consultants' rostered availability, recommending that it should vary, ranging from a 24-hour on-site consultant presence for some specialties, to extended hours with limited on-call, to traditional daytime availability with rare on-call.

The topic of private practice was evidently far too hot for the task force to handle. While somewhat opaquely recommending that the role of consultants should be redefined, to promote equity of access, "by clarifying the circumstances in which private practice is structured so as to avoid any potential disadvantage for public patients", the task force did not address issues such as public-only contracts, a common waiting list or the desirability of the public/private mix. If its conclusions were implemented, it was clear that the public/private mix could not continue in its present form. Without an army of juniors, consultants would no longer be able to delegate their public patient care. In fact, the entire Hanly system was predicated on the assumption that such delegation would now be determined by patient need not patient status, that NCHDs should only treat less serious conditions, consultants the more complex cases. In addition, consultants working in rostered shifts as members of teams would find it much harder to pursue off-site private practice.

The logic of the Hanly draft report was that the public system should now be so resourced and organised that two-tier access and care would become a thing of the past, and that public hospital consultants should restrict their work to public hospitals. How it would translate into real politics was another matter. Its logic might yet be defeated. Private patients might be permitted continued preferential access to these new consultant teams. Newly appointed public consultants might be permitted to build up private practice in private hospitals, particularly if public hospital capacity did not grow adequately. If either were to occur, the investment of public funds in recruiting this new army of specialists would have been money ill-spent.

The challenge for the government – divided already on the desirability of investing more in health – and indeed for any successor government, was that to realise the Hanly recommendations would require confronting local interests, in order to reorganise the hospitals; confronting the medical organisations, in order to rewrite the consultants' contract; and confronting the contradiction at the heart of traditional policy on the two-tier system, the incompatibility of permitting some patients to purchase superior access to care, while purporting to support equity.

The approach to reform of the 1997–2002 government was inconsistent. Although the internal deliberations of the Department of Health revealed that it wished to promote equity, its proposals for reform fell short of achieving that, even before they were emasculated in the 2001 strategy. Unwilling to challenge the central contradiction of the public/private mix, the strategy retained the system of bed designation, which necessarily meant that preferential access would continue. If additional public beds were provided, an increasingly shaky assumption, and if the Department were to achieve a public-only commitment from new consultant appointees in their early years, the position of public patients would certainly improve, but the two-tier system would remain.

The Department's willingness in the strategy to go so far but no further in pursuit of an equitable system appeared to be dictated by a respect for hospital consultants' industrial power, which consultants themselves shared. The government's failure to pursue equitable reform was entirely consistent with Fianna Fáil's record since the 1960s. A catch-all party, it favoured the line of least resistance in public policy. It had last confronted hospital consultants in 1953 and wished to alienate neither them nor middle class voters.

This timidity on the public/private mix was at odds with the Department of Health's growing willingness in 2003 to contemplate a complete overhaul of the system and structures of health administration, driven in part by the need to placate Department of Finance concerns about the efficacy of health spending. The Department's continued wary incrementalism on the public/private mix contrasted with its apparent support for sweeping changes in administrative reform, proposed by Prospectus, and in hospital networks and medical staffing, formulated by the Hanly task force. Michael Kelly's belief in the need for equity was a matter of public record. While, under his leadership, the Department appeared willing to contemplate considerable reforms, it had yet to offer a coherent blueprint for an accessible and equitable modern health care system.

14

PRIVATE SECTOR SOLUTIONS

"Minister [for Finance] is under pressure from James Sheehan to concede tax incentives for the project."
— *internal Department of Health memo 2001.*

Consistency in health policy was not furthered by the introduction in 2001 of tax subsidies for the developers of private hospitals. The Minister for Finance pursued this significant U-turn in state policy, formerly directed towards reducing state subsidy for private medicine, despite sustained objections from the Department of Health. The Minister introduced these tax concessions in response to lobbying by Jimmy Sheehan, the founder of the Blackrock Clinic, who identified McCreevy as an ideological ally, unlike Barry Desmond who had resisted his promotion of private medicine in the 1980s. Initially limited to hospitals run as charities, the tax concessions were then extended to developers of for-profit hospitals in 2002, when they provoked an upsurge of interest from investors, ranging from property speculators to large international health care consortia. Government policy had opened the door to the development of a significant for-profit hospital sector.

The Ministers for Health and Finance were once more in disagreement, this time about the appropriate role for private hospitals in the health service. While Micheál Martin battled to increase state investment in public health, McCreevy was providing state funds for private health. As on the broader issue of health spending, the disagreement between the Ministers reflected ideological differences within Fianna Fáil, with McCreevy welcoming market solutions to shortcomings in social provision which might otherwise require increased taxation.[1]

The potential effect on the health service of the development of unplanned, private, for-profit hospitals, subsidised by the state, provoked reservations in the Department of Finance and great disquiet in the Department of Health, which was nonetheless forced to accept the McCreevy policy and to attempt to reconcile it with its health strategy. This state encouragement of private medicine was grafted onto a system in which private hospitals were primarily staffed by hospital consultants on public salaries. Of the 790 consultants staffing private hospitals and clinics in January 2003, 75 per cent held public contracts.[2] Without a change in the consultants' public contract, new private hospitals would be a further drain on the staffing and expertise of the public hospital system.

The Progressive Democrats had also championed an increased role for the private sector, when they promoted the Treatment Purchase Fund to purchase care for waiting list patients in private hospitals and abroad. This turning to the private sector to solve the problems of public health care was a new development, poorly thought through and at odds with other objectives of health care policy. It raised serious concerns in the VHI, whose members would be expected to fund the new private hospitals.

Not only were developers now to be encouraged to run hospitals for profit, but also the government was prepared to contemplate a further commercialisation of health care – the development of a for-profit health insurance sector. In 2002, the government was actively considering the privatisation of the state-controlled VHI. For-profit hospitals and for-profit health insurance would change the face of Irish health care. Market forces would increasingly dictate the quality of care. Although it seldom emerged in public debate, government policy on health care was effectively in disarray, with the Department of Health pursuing an agenda of state investment in improved public care, while the Department of Finance pursued market provision of private care.

The making of public policy on private hospitals

"The private sector in medicine has a case to answer. With a few exceptions it does not invest in the university training of doctors nor is it, in most cases, capable of training future medical specialists. It has not even taken part in the routine collection of activity data that is important in planning future services. It excels at providing comfortable facilities

for common procedures with predictable outcomes. The public system drives our specialists, sometimes easily, into a private sector that helps itself to their hard-won skills and international networks."
– Tom O'Dowd, TCD professor of general practice.[3]

"Private hospitals piggyback on cash-strapped state-funded institutions as they rely hugely on consultants from the public sector."
– Joint Oireachtas Committee on Health and Children, January 2001.[4]

"Private hospitals cherry-pick. No private hospital has a casualty department. Why don't they take AIDS patients, haemophiliacs, bone marrow transplants, or engage in chemotherapy or dialysis in the true sense? What about when their patients end up in our intensive care, when things don't work out quite right?"
– a view of the private sector from the chief executive of a large public hospital, 2002.[5]

The introduction of tax reliefs for the developers of private hospitals was a radical and virtually undebated departure in state policy on the private hospital sector. The measure was inserted in the 2001 Finance Bill at a late stage and only briefly debated in the Seanad. The 2001 Finance Act provided for a generous scheme of tax allowances for capital expenditure on constructing or refurbishing private hospital buildings. A requirement that the hospital must be operated by a charitable body was dropped the following year. The hospital was required to provide a minimum of 100 inpatient beds (lowered to 70 the following year) and to offer outpatient services, operating theatres, on-site diagnostic and therapeutic services and at least five specialist services, ranging from accident and emergency to oncology and cardiology. The state required that 20 per cent of the bed capacity should be available for public patients at a discount of at least 10 per cent of the private rate.[6]

These tax reliefs, in their entirety, were the work of the Department of Finance, over the objections of the Department of Health. They were essentially the brain-child of the Minister for Finance, some of whose own officials had reservations. McCreevy's solo run in promoting the building of private, for-profit hospitals ran counter to the traditional policy stance in the Department of Health. The Department's unpublished 1984 Green Paper had expressed concern at the "proliferation of private hospitals" and observed that "the notion of hospitals being established as business entities, in which their owners' sole motivation is the generation of commercial profit, would mark a new departure in hospital care in Ireland". A "two-tier system of hospital care" could develop "with the wealthy being treated in different hospitals, by different staff and with a higher standard of care than the less well off". "Scarce skills and expertise" could gravitate to the private sector. The 1999 *White Paper on Private Health Insurance*, the work of McCreevy's colleague Brian Cowen, had proposed to reduce state subsidy for private care in public hospitals. Active state promotion and subsidy of private hospitals represented a major policy change and, disturbingly, slipped through the Dáil, as a legislative afterthought.

Labour Senator Joe Costello pointed out at the time that such a measure "would have benefited from a wide ranging discussion on the matter prior to it being introduced as a late amendment to the Finance Bill". He expressed concern that it would "further increase the two tier hospital system" and would "have long-term implications because there will be very little return to the state, other than 20 per cent of the hospital beds, and there will be a very substantial outgoing from the state".[7]

The introduction of this tax relief was the direct consequence of lobbying by Jimmy Sheehan, the founder of the Blackrock Clinic. Sixty-three years old in 2002, Sheehan remained a crusader for private – he preferred the term "independent" – medicine and had plans for a private hospital empire. As a supporter of Catholic health care, he regretted that during the 1990s declining numbers of religious had led to the sale or closure of some religious-run private hospitals and a drop in the number of private beds.[8] Armed with these new tax incentives, he intended to replicate the Blackrock Clinic, with some modifications, across the country and in 2002 turned the first sod for a 101-bed private hospital in the west, just outside Galway. He had plans for a further five such clinics.

When Sheehan launched his Galway project, he was enthusiastic about the potential for charitable hospitals and outspokenly critical of for-profit medicine. While he took credit for the new tax reliefs for charitable hospitals and made no secret of his political influence, he regretted that they had proven a Trojan horse for the for-profit sector, when they were extended in 2002. "I would hate to see for-profit hospitals encouraged in this country. It is not appropriate to our health care needs." Eventually, however, he too adopted a for-profit structure in Galway.

Sheehan had hoped that Galway would be a not-for-profit venture but, as he had discovered when he founded Blackrock, he could not secure bank finance on those terms. He had always been disappointed that Blackrock became a commercial enterprise to care for the rich. While many VHI members attended consultants' private outpatient clinics in Blackrock, less than 5 per cent of the population held the more expensive insurance policies that would cover them for treatment at the private hospital. Blackrock operated "commercial medicine" and must provide a return to shareholders, which would not be reinvested in the hospital. Sheehan, who had "grown to dislike the concept of any profit", initially planned that his new hospitals would be "charitable foundations", which he pictured as benevolent institutions, in which profits would be reinvested, voluntarism would thrive and the state would receive its return through the treatment of public patients on waiting lists. He intended that Galway would not share Blackrock's élitist image.

However, when he sought partners to fund his new hospital ventures – investors, attracted by the tax incentives on offer from government, who would lease the hospital to the foundation at a favourable rent, achievable because of the tax subsidies – he discovered an outstanding problem. Motivated by tax incentives not benevolence, these investors would eventually want to unlock their investment and were not prepared to carry risk. His charitable vision collapsed when he was forced to enlist equity investors, who would assist him in putting up seed capital for his Galway hospital, "on an investor basis".[9]

So despite his objection to for-profit medicine and although he believed that doctors, like insurance companies, should not invest in hospitals – in their case because of a conflict of interest between their caring and investing roles – he would again be a major shareholder in a private, for-profit hospital. His fellow founding shareholders, in this instance, were not doctors but "people of high net worth".[10] The shareholders would control the hospital, sitting on its board with some medical representatives.

Sheehan was undoubtedly driven by something other than the profit motive. He ascribed his motivation for developing his hospitals to "a burning desire, and an obligation, to improve health care". Others considered control a primary motivation. "Blackrock didn't work out the way he wanted because he didn't have control or power," commented one medical observer of his *modus operandi*. In Galway, without BUPA's controlling stake, Sheehan might hope to exert greater control than in Blackrock. He proposed to remain in an organising role in the hospital, "for a minimum of five years". No matter how disinterested his own motivation, it remained the case that he was founding a for-profit hospital, whose shareholders would want to see a return on their money.

Sheehan prevails; Health and Finance fail

Whatever Sheehan's vision, his influence on the direction of public policy provoked considerable concern in the Departments of Finance and Health. Quite apart from the contradiction in introducing this state subsidy when the government's policy was to reduce subsidies to private care, the proposed private hospitals were too small to be considered centres of excellence, might crop up anywhere (defeating state efforts to make sense of the hospital network), would seduce more state-salaried consultants away from their public hospital commitments and were a costly way of delivering public beds. Sheehan anticipated that two-thirds of the consultants who staffed his Galway hospital would be salaried consultants from the neighbouring public hospitals. The state subsidy for Sheehan's Galway hospital alone was estimated at £16 million (€20 million) over a 7-year period[11] and would deliver some 20 public beds – at an average cost of €1 million per bed.[12] In contrast in 2002, the state was funding 520 additional public beds for €65 million – at an average cost of €125,000.[13]

Sheehan's pivotal role in securing this new tax relief for private hospitals emerged in Departmental files.[14] In November 2000, he wrote to the Minister for Finance asking for "tax incentives" for his planned new Galway facility, to be run as a charitable foundation, "so that there are no profits distributed and any profits are re-invested in health care", and which could treat public patients on waiting lists. He invoked the support of two local Fianna Fáil TDs, Frank Fahey and Éamon Ó Cuív, who had been "very helpful with the planners and general advice with this project".[15]

By the following February, Department of Health assistant secretary, Dermot Smyth, noted to a colleague: "Minister [McCreevy] is under pressure from James Sheehan to concede tax incentives for the project."[16] Within days, an official of the Department of Finance observed in an e-mail to the Department of Health: "the Minister is inclined to extend the tax relief sought by Mr Sheehan".[17] A series of communicated objections from Health to Finance failed to shake the Minister's resolve. In March, McCreevy was presenting the measure to the Seanad as government policy.

Sheehan had not been the first supplicant for tax relief for private hospitals but it was he who succeeded in bringing political pressure to bear. In February 2000, another applicant, whose name Finance would not release for "commercial" reasons, had also sought tax relief. In exchanges over the following year, officials of Finance and Health rehearsed their objections in principle to such a relief. "It would be difficult to secure the orderly development of hospital facilities in appropriate locations within each region if the relief were open-ended," wrote Finance.[18] Such a scheme "might also create excess capacity which could be inflationary from the point of view of private health insurers", wrote Health.[19] Finance advised its Minister:

> A proliferation of hospitals might occur. Hospitals must have a significant volume of patients if they are to meet medical safety and quality standards and therefore small hospitals should not be encouraged ... The Department of Health and Children have commented that a 100 bed acute hospital would be very small indeed. Of 55 acute public or voluntary hospitals in the State only 14 have 100 beds or less.
> The granting of capital allowances will involve a significant cost to the Exchequer ... A discount of 10 per cent of a price that is not yet set for state funded patients seems low considering the capital allowances will cost the state 42 per cent of the cost of construction and fitting out of the hospitals.[20]

Health reminded Finance that "the overall thrust of Government policy is ... to remove or significantly reduce public subsidisation of the private health sector". As a consequence of the proposed tax incentives, "the private hospital's continued viability" would be dependent on the health board purchasing services at 90 per cent of the going private rate.[21]

McCreevy nonetheless achieved government backing for the scheme. The Taoiseach, Bertie Ahern, permitted him to steamroll through this tax incentive, even though its consequences would be so at variance with the overall direction of health policy. On March 2nd 2001, McCreevy wrote to Micheál Martin "As you know, the Government have agreed" to the tax incentive scheme. He then proceeded to dictate to his colleague how its benefit "will be captured for the public health system". Where a private hospital brought added private beds to a particular health board area, he announced, "you will designate as public beds a similar number of beds in the public hospital system which, prior to the provision of the new beds, has been designated as private. In this way, the legislation will result in an increase in public hospital beds."[22]

In characteristically gung-ho fashion, the Minister for Finance was now dictating to the Minister for Health how the public/private mix should operate in public hospitals. In order to make this tax incentive more palatable to critics of state subsidy for private medicine, and to make its cost to the exchequer more defensible,[23] he was requiring that private practice in public hospitals should be reduced. McCreevy was proceeding in apparently blissful ignorance of the fact that hospital consultants were currently working under a contract which permitted them to engage in private practice in public hospitals, in proportion to the designated ratio of private beds. Reduce the number of beds and you would reduce their opportunities for private practice in the hospital, where they were salaried to work. Accompany that with the establishment of a private hospital right down the road and, unless they were willing to accept a reduction in income, you would reduce their presence in the public hospital and make it all the more likely that public patients would be treated by unsupervised juniors. And thanks to Jimmy Sheehan and to McCreevy's tax incentives, the opportunity to practice medicine in this manner would no longer be geographically restricted since, aided by state subsidy, small private hospitals might spring up all over the state.

Health was aware of all these arguments. Officials drafted a letter for the Minister to sign, pointing out that to do as the Minister for Finance suggested would reduce the number of private beds in public hospitals from the present 20 per cent, "and we can anticipate vocal resistance to a selective change in this ratio". It was

> preferable from a service point of view to have consultants operating on-site rather than off-site … Based on experience elsewhere re-location of private practice from the public hospital to a private hospital will reduce the availability of consultants to the public hospital … Under the terms of the Consultants Common Contract, consultants have a right to engage in private practice within the hospital/hospitals in which they are employed. Any proposal which would attempt to unilaterally remove this right is likely to be met with the strongest opposition and possible legal challenge by the medical organisations … [It would also] possibly undermine the success of negotiations to amend the contract in other respects which I would hope to obtain the approval of the Government to commence shortly.[24]

Either events overtook the Department of Health or Micheál Martin decided that there was no percentage in fighting this particular battle any further. Although submitted for his signature, this letter was never sent. Dermot Smyth observed in a note on the file copy of the letter "as the Bill has now been passed into law, I have advised ... not to issue the letter now".[25]

Reducing the number of private beds in public hospitals in proportion to the creation of private beds in private hospitals had become government policy. On March 28th, Charlie McCreevy told the Seanad that the relief would "reduce the pressure on public hospital beds" because "the Minister for Health and Children will designate a similar number of beds in public hospitals as public beds but which prior to the provision of the new beds in the private hospital would have been designated as private".[26] The Finance Act became law two days later and confirmed that there would be tax relief for the construction of private hospitals of 100 beds or more, which must make 20 per cent of their beds available to public patients at not more than 90 per cent of the private rate.

The Department of Health now had to attempt to come to terms with this unasked-for policy. Having fought the proliferation of private hospitals, the Department now accepted them as a datum. Its working group on the public/private mix, which reported in July 2001, was prepared to contemplate a system, in which private patients would be channelled towards private hospitals, in a potential deepening of the schism in hospital care. This was a profound philosophical shift for the Department, which, in Desmond's era, had warned against creating "a separate and two-tier system of hospital care". The working group anticipated that private hospitals would now treat private patients to a much greater extent. Its report argued that private hospitals would face greater demands, if its recommendations for improved access for public patients to public hospitals were implemented. This would force private patients to turn to private hospitals, and, "while private hospital capacity is being developed and the Finance Bill incentivises this", waiting lists for private hospital care and increased insurance costs were "likely". This might result in a falling off in membership of insurance schemes but "the private system, favoured by the economy and its demographics, should be able to sustain increases and assertively negotiate with suppliers".[27]

This was a wholly new language from health policy-makers. Now patients who chose to insure themselves for private care might have to depend on the market to supply their care. Traditionally, the privately insured had been secure in the knowledge that their insurance would buy them preferential access to public hospital care. And for really serious conditions, most patients would prefer to be treated in large, well-resourced public hospitals. The logic of this new policy was that the middle class would be presented with a choice between taking their place in the queue for public hospitals or paying for care in small, private hospitals, too small to be regarded as centres of excellence, establishments whose location and development was driven by entrepreneurial logic. Of course, the staff from local public centres of excellence might treat private hospital patients in their uncontracted hours, a reassurance for private patients and a continued undermining of the public hospital system.

The 2001 health strategy did not make this logic explicit. It did not mention the new requirement to reduce private beds in public hospitals in response to the growth of private hospitals, in its discussion of bed designations or the consultants' contract, nor did it acknowledge that private patients would be driven into private hospitals as a consequence of government policy. As with all awkward topics on which the government found itself unable to provide leadership, the strategy proposed that a forum would be created to discuss the role of the private sector. The extra beds promised in the strategy for public patients would be provided by "a strategic partnership" involving public and private providers, to be "progressed by setting up a Forum under the aegis of the new National Hospitals Agency".[28] It remained an inescapable reality that the government had created a legislative framework designed to foster the private market, which had the potential to deepen the two-tier divide in hospital care. Although Health was clearly aware of these dangers, the issue was kicked into limbo.

Worse was to come. The 2002 Finance Act then extended the relief to for-profit hospitals and reduced the required hospital size from 100 to 70 beds.[29] The lobbyist on this occasion had been Michael Heavey, chief executive of the Independent Hospital Association of Ireland, who objected on behalf of hospitals that were not charities:

> Why should these hospitals not qualify for relief, in the event of capital expenditure being incurred, when their activities are just as valuable to the government's stated goal of increasing bed capacity? Where an existing hospital does not have 100 in-patient beds at the moment, but meets the other criteria, will it receive allowances in the event that it expands its existing facility to encompass the requisite bed numbers?[30]

Heavey opened his lobbying efforts with a letter to Health, which evidently wanted nothing further to do with this measure. An internal memo observed that the tax relief "was conceived and driven by Finance with minimum input from this Department".[31] Health redirected Heavey's enquiries to Finance and the Revenue Commissioners.[32] While Health's exasperation with Finance's unilateral interference in health policy was understandable, giving up the ghost at this stage on the critical issue of state support for for-profit hospitals was indefensible. In Finance, where Heavey now directed his efforts, the concept of state subsidy for for-profit health care apparently rang no alarm bells whatsoever. An official memo to the Minister observed that the "abolition of charities condition" would "not present any difficulty".[33]

The Department of Finance was undoubtedly motivated by a desire to reduce the demands on the public purse from the voracious Department of Health, with its wish list for 3,000 new acute hospital beds. Finance saw merits in part-funding the private provision of beds through tax foregone. If Finance had simply proposed to encourage private providers of beds for rental or lease to the public sector, a strategy pursued in the UK, assessing the merit of this approach would have been a straightforward cost-benefit analysis. If the government were short of capital in the short-term, then the long-term higher costs of providing a return to a private sector provider of beds might be worthwhile. But this was not what this tax incentive was designed to achieve. What Finance was fostering was an alternative health care system for private patients, which would remove them from public hospitals into an uncontrolled and unplanned network of care, but which would still be staffed by public hospital consultants. Health reportedly regarded the Finance approach as "simplistic".[34]

Proliferation of for-profit hospitals

In speculative, boom-time Ireland, following the passage of this legislation, for-profit hospitals had now become just another venture which developers would pencil in on their planning applications. Alongside shopping centres and exclusive leisure clubs, why not an exclusive clinic? The property pages of the newspapers reported on planned hospital developments. International health care groups began to investigate the potential of Ireland. Within a few months of the 2002 Finance Act, at least eight private hospital groups had expressed an interest in developing hospitals in Ireland, including the giant HCA healthcare corporation from the US, the Australian Ramsay Healthcare group, Hospital Corporation of Australia, BUPA and Nuffield from the UK and the Swedish Capio group.

While Sheehan proceeded with construction in Galway, other

existing private hospitals passed from religious ownership to the hands of lay for-profit operators. Michael Heavey, who as chief executive of the Independent Hospital Association of Ireland had lobbied for the extension of tax reliefs to for-profit hospitals, subsequently left the association and, in partnership with a cardiologist, John Clarke, negotiated to purchase the 104-bed Aut Even hospital in Kilkenny from the Sisters of St John of God. Heavey proposed to run the hospital as a for-profit concern. Its purchase would not incur tax relief but refurbishment or extension would.

The management of the Mater private hospital had bought the hospital from the Sisters of Mercy. Jimmy Sheehan publicly criticised the sale because, although contingent on the hospital retaining a Catholic ethos, it did not require it to operate as a charity.[35] The Mercy order responded that it would invest the greater part of the proceeds of the sale in facilities for the public hospital, which would not otherwise be funded by the state, and the profits of the now independent private hospital would go to servicing its debts for at least 20 years.[36]

In this new climate of government support for private medicine, like the phoenix from the ashes, the project of a private hospital on the site of Dublin's Beaumont public hospital was resurrected. Barry Desmond had denied Beaumont consultants a private hospital on the site in the 1980s, when he argued that permitting consultants to invest in a for-profit hospital would give them an incentive to increase their private practice at the expense of their public patients, an argument that had lost none of its relevance.

Hospital consultants at Beaumont initially entered into negotiations with the stock-market quoted Australian Ramsay Healthcare group. The consultants proposed to take a stake in a 150-to-170-bed private hospital on the public hospital site. Reports of their discussions provoked representations to the Department of Health from the Independent Hospital Association of Ireland, seeking an assurance that this private development on the publicly owned campus would be open to tender by its members.[37] The Department responded that there was "no question of a 'done deal' with any particular party", others would be permitted to make submissions and "given its status as a publicly owned institution, the hospital will be consulting with this Department and the ERHA before any final decisions are taken".[38]

Beaumont consultants formed a private limited company, Beaumont Private Hospital Ltd., with a management committee of seven consultants, chaired by radiologist Frank McGrath. The board of Beaumont agreed in principle to the development of a private hospital on the public hospital's site. The consultants' company then began a tendering process for an international partner and received expressions of interest from a number of large, international for-profit and not-for-profit hospital operators: from France, the UK and the US, including the University of Pittsburgh.

A dam against the flood – the VHI defies the government

Every one of the potential private hospital developers beat a path to the door of Vincent Sheridan, chief executive of the VHI. Sheridan reported an "unprecedented interest" from would-be developers of private hospitals in 2002. Without VHI cover for its members' treatment in these hospitals, many developers thought there would be little point in going ahead. Sheehan and the Beaumont consultants, however, were apparently determined to proceed, on the assumption that they would be able to generate such political pressure that the VHI would be forced to cover their enterprises or, failing that, that BUPA or another insurer would do so and force the VHI to follow suit. During 2002, other developers held off to await the outcome of a VHI review of future demand for private medicine, which would guide Sheridan's approach. Sheridan commissioned the review because he was concerned that, should he agree to cover his members for many new private facilities, this would drive up premium rates and lead to a fall off in membership. Conversely, he argued, if the VHI's membership was satisfied with the existing service, there was no need for extra supply.

Sheehan took the diametrically opposite view. He argued that "the cost of private insurance is too low", reflecting his assessment of the appropriate cost of care in an ideal, cutting-edge private hospital. Private insurance should be more expensive and purchased by a smaller proportion of the population, as it had been ten years previously, he maintained. The majority of the population should remain public patients, whom the state would fund for treatment in his private hospitals.

The VHI review by PricewaterhouseCoopers was complete in the spring of 2002 but was not released until after the May election. It reached some surprising conclusions. The report forecast that the number of privately insured would fall, reflecting rises in the cost of insurance, which would be required to "retain profitability against large increases in the cost of health care".[39] Within months, the Minister for Health sanctioned an 18 per cent increase in premiums. The report further concluded that there was no need for more private hospitals. It identified a small future deficit in private beds in Dublin but Vincent Sheridan took the view that the supply was sufficient "to give timely and adequate treatment to our members in the medium term".[40]

As he explained in letters to the Department of Health and the Minister, the VHI's "current stance based on the PWC report is to discourage the creation of additional private beds". "Our approach to those who are considering the development of additional private bed capacity is to emphasise that it is their decision not ours."[41] The proliferation of private hospitals, which seemed inevitable after the passage of the legislation, was slowed but by no means halted by the VHI's stance. The continued construction of Sheehan's Galway hospital and the enthusiastic efforts of consultants at Beaumont to develop their private hospital ensured that the VHI would face sustained pressure to cover its members for treatment in these hospitals.

Sheridan was erecting a dam against the flood of would-be hospital developers and, in the process, working against government policy by thwarting the intent of McCreevy's new tax incentives. The PWC report argued in turn against each of the planks of the government's policy on private medicine. It cheekily suggested that "there was not a complete appreciation of the nature or complexity of this inter-dependence [between the public and private health care systems] in all national policy-making circles".

Three potential policy approaches by government "to meeting frustrated demand in the public system" could prove costly to the exchequer, "if aggressively pursued", the report argued. The promotion of new private hospital developments, the restriction of private patients' access to public hospitals or the competitive purchase by the public sector of care for public patients in private hospitals could each in turn lead to cost increases and premium hikes in the private sector, which would drive more patients back onto the public sector, the report argued. It further provoked the Department by suggesting that the private sector offered superior care and the government was unlikely to fund the health strategy.

Michael Kelly, secretary general of the Department, observed of the PWC report, in a letter to Sheridan, that the Department found "some of the analysis surprising, many of the conclusions equally surprising and much of the language, particularly in its references to the public system, careless to say the least".[42]

Sheridan argued that the VHI's decision to discourage further private beds was consistent with government policy, as outlined in the health strategy. "The shortage of public beds will be addressed by significant investment in additional public beds and not by encouraging the creation of more private beds accompanied by an expansion of the private treatment fund."[43] Sheridan was in part reiterating to the Department of Health the arguments it had put to the Department of Finance in its failed rearguard action against the tax incentives. But Health was now forced to defend the new logic imposed upon it by the introduction of the tax incentives and by the desire of the government to use the private sector to treat public patients. Sheridan could perceive that unplanned expansion of private capacity might create an enormous drain on the VHI, as Blackrock and the Mater had done in the 1980s. On this, he doubtless had the Department's private agreement. He was, however, unlikely to win official sympathy for his attempts to preserve the *status quo* – that private patients might continue to receive preferential access to public hospitals, albeit much better-resourced. He argued against economic charging for private beds in public hospitals – "there should be no question of 'full cost' for private patients, who are already full subscribers for their public entitlement".[44]

Sheridan's refusal to accommodate the consequences of McCreevy's tax incentives was courageous. Although the government had been committed since the 1999 White Paper to giving the VHI full commercial freedom of operation, it had not yet taken any legislative steps in that direction. The Minister for Health continued to appoint all the members of Sheridan's board, who in turn had appointed him, subject to the Minister's consent. Although not a civil servant, Sheridan was operating in one of the dangerous grey areas in Irish public life. He was essentially presuming that the government would remain loyal to the spirit of the White Paper and permit him to pursue his own commercial logic. Against Jimmy Sheehan's gamble that the VHI would be forced to see his reason, Sheridan was venturing a gamble of his own.

Sheridan urged that the VHI and the Department of Health should reconcile their differences:

> The consequences of the public and private sectors advocating different solutions can only be to the detriment of the overall health system. It is with a sense of urgency therefore that I renew my call for a coordinated approach to the provision of bed capacity.[45]

For-profit insurance – privatisation of the VHI?

Having evinced little concern about the implications for the health system of fostering for-profit hospitals, the 1997–2002 government showed equally limited awareness of the dangers in developing a for-profit health insurance market. The 1999 White Paper never canvassed the possibility that it might be undesirable for decisions about health care to be taken by for-profit institutions. Nor did it show any concern that these institutions might be based outside the state. The government was quite content, it seemed, to foresee a future when a privatised VHI might be sold to the highest bidder. The emphasis of the White Paper was on giving the VHI commercial freedom "in the areas of product development and pricing". While judging that "an immediate full sale of VHI, at this time, would not be in the best interests of the VHI", the White Paper proposed that outside investment in the company should be pursued "as a matter of urgency" and that new legislation would "include provision for the eventual full sale of the State's interest in VHI if deemed desirable". The discussion of the future of the VHI was entirely from the viewpoint of the interests of the company, not of the health care system.[46] The VHI itself lobbied for privatisation. Employees of the VHI, in common with employees of other privatised state companies, could look forward to having share options in the new company.

The VHI retained AIB Corporate Finance as their advisers, the government retained Davy Corporate Finance and William Fry solicitors. These advisers were not hired for their knowledge of the intricacies of health care, nor of the impact of commercial insurance companies on the systems of other states. They were hired for their expertise in realising the highest possible value for the sale of state companies and in securing the future viability of the VHI as a commercial enterprise. The advisors concurred that the company should not be floated on the stock market but should be sold wholly or in part. Sources suggested that the view of the VHI's advisers, in particular, was that a partial sale could only be a first step, since a prospective purchaser would want to have an option to buy the company in full.[47] While the Department of Health declined to release the advice it had received under Freedom of Information, its very refusal made clear the thrust of the advice: a "blueprint for possible action by the State" which might "entail important financial negotiations".[48]

While the advisers worked on their reports during 2001 and 2002, the news that the VHI might be for sale was percolating through international insurance markets. US, European and Irish insurance firms paid courtesy calls on McCreevy to inform him of their interest.[49] The final Davy/Fry report of "Strategic Options for the VHI" was only submitted to the Departments of Health and Finance on May 8th 2002, ten days before the general election in which Labour had made clear that it opposed the privatisation of the VHI.[50] The Department of Health had planned to draft legislation to change the corporate status of the VHI later in the year, once the government decided what path it wished to take. The Department recognised in its annual business plan that this would be subject to the "continuation of Government policy in relation to VHI corporate change", an oblique reference to the possibility that the general election would return a government with a different view of the future of the VHI.[51] With the return of Fianna Fáil and a strengthened Progressive Democrats, committed to privatisation of state assets, it was now more likely then ever that the government would opt to sell the VHI. There was a very real danger that the immediate need to secure revenues for the state would take precedence over health policy considerations.

The tax incentives for private hospitals introduced in the Finance Acts of 2001 and 2002 were an ill-conceived departure in health policy. The state was now prepared to subsidise and invite for-profit hospitals to operate in Ireland. While private hospitals play a role in delivering care in many states' systems, how they do so is critical. Where private, non-profit hospitals sell care to an equitable, tax- or insurance-funded health care system, they are just one other provider, like Ireland's existing voluntary hospitals. Their presence may diversify and enrich care. However, for the state to encourage hospitals to operate for profit threatened the caring ethos in Irish health care and raised the possibility that public health funds would contribute to the profits of overseas health care corporations and domestic entrepreneurs. Equally, if the VHI were sold off to be run as a commercial concern, as the government appeared to contemplate, its members' treatments and coverage, and the terms on which it would remunerate doctors and hospitals, would be dictated by a for-profit and, in all probability, overseas company. Not only hospitals but also insurance companies would be feeding on the health care system for profit. These critical decisions for the future of Irish health care provoked virtually no debate.

The McCreevy tax concessions were further ill-conceived because they gifted state funds to private medicine at a time of constrained public provision, when private patients were already the beneficiaries of significant state subsidy. Given the nature of the consultants' contract, the new private hospitals would be staffed by consultants from public hospitals, which would further undermine the public health care system. Having been forced against its better judgement to accommodate these tax concessions and to embrace the Treatment

Purchase Fund, the Department of Health became committed not only to channelling private patient care into the private sector, but also to a programme of purchasing private care for public patients. Despite its fundamental belief and the central plank of its health strategy, that the answer to the crisis in the health service was to build public sector capacity, the Department was locked into a policy of fostering the private sector.

This state support for small, unplanned private hospitals, staffed from the public sector, was completely at odds with the overall direction of health policy, in particular the proposals for planned hospital networks and dedicated public hospital teams, recommended by the Hanly task force on medical staffing. With increasing pressures on the public finances, there was a serious risk that private beds in any form might be welcomed by government, whatever the consequences for staffing of public hospitals or for optimal regional planning of hospital services. The alternative that the private sector might tender to provide public hospitals for lease back and eventual sale to the state, a model pursued in the UK, remained open to the government as a more planned way of involving the private sector in supplying additional public beds.[52]

Politics not policy explained this new departure. It reflected the balance of power and ideology within the government and had nothing to do with logical planning for the health system. The response of the VHI provided a helpful space, in which Health might convince Finance to revoke its incentives, or at the very least insist that private hospitals should be staffed purely by private staff and that their size and location should be subject to the agreement of the new National Hospitals' Agency or Office. These new tax incentives were incompatible with the efforts of Health to plan the health service or the concern of Finance for efficacious health spending. A state-subsidised private sector, staffed by public consultants, would retard rather than advance the development of quality, public hospital care for the majority of the population.

15

CHANGING THE SYSTEM

"There will be no public/private distinction between patients and any discrimination will be impossible."
– Labour Party's 2001 health policy.

From 2000 to 2002, the opposition parties attempted to address the evident need for reform in the health care system by proposing a complete change in how the system was funded. The proposals for a European-style compulsory health insurance system, advanced by Labour and Fine Gael, offered a means of achieving equitable access to health care and a committed stream of funding for health. The implications of the change were radical and complex but the potential gains – equity and assured funding – were so great, and so manifestly lacking in the existing system and in the government's proposals for reform, that the opposition proposals deserved serious scrutiny. That they were not accorded this during the 2002 general election campaign was a missed opportunity, for the electorate had been offered a genuine choice. In this proposed historic shift to an insurance-based health system, Labour and Fine Gael would abandon the mix of public and private care in public hospitals, which Fianna Fáil and the Progressive Democrats proposed to preserve, even though the Progressive Democrats had earlier espoused just such an insurance-based system. There remained important differences between the opposition parties' approaches, however. The Labour Party's proposals were more comprehensive: they would end distinctions between public and private patients in both hospital and primary care. While Fine Gael claimed that its proposals would end two-tier hospital care, their detail was inconsistent with their aim – two-tier care might continue on public hospital campuses, if not in public hospital buildings.

Debate about the merits of an insurance-based approach may not have captured the imagination of the public during the election but had been engaging smaller circles of people, who had been actively thinking about health reform, over the preceding few years. Thinking had been evolving on the finer details of an insurance-based system, on issues like the role of insurance companies, the role of hospitals and the regulatory role of the EU. Wider dissemination of information about how other states organised their health care systems informed the debate. In addition, other, simpler proposals for achieving equity – such as merely changing how consultants were paid, or banning private practice in public hospitals, within the existing tax-based system – had been suggested as alternatives to the insurance-based approach.

Alternative models for funding a health care system

Within the three broad alternatives for health system financing – from general taxation like the UK, from compulsory social insurance like France and Germany or by private finance based on voluntary insurance like the US – there are refinements. In the US there is public insurance for the elderly and the poorest. In the UK, a private insurance sector is permitted to compete with the public system in providing care. In France, a growing proportion of health funding comes from taxation. At the most egalitarian extreme of the spectrum, Canada does not permit the use of private health insurance to purchase medical services which are available from publicly funded hospitals and physicians. No two systems are alike: like Ireland, each state has developed a system of health care which reflects its own history, culture and politics.[1]

The hybrid Irish system combines tax funding from the state and private insurance. The state funds the bulk of the health care budget from the central exchequer's general pool of taxation receipts: the needs of health must compete for priority with all other areas of government spending. Private health spending, either in the form of private insurance or as cash payments for drugs, doctors' visits or hospital charges, contributes about a quarter of health spending.

In European states with systems funded from social insurance, health care is primarily financed by payroll taxes levied on workers and employers in some proportion to income, like Pay Related Social Insurance (PRSI) in Ireland, which funds pay-related benefits. These payroll taxes are then channelled into the health care system via non-profit social insurance or sickness funds, in which membership is generally related to employment. The funds purchase health care for their members. Private, for-profit insurers play a subsidiary role.

The Irish tax-funded system is unusual in its degree of toleration for discrimination between categories of patient within the state system. Other states have achieved equitable access to health care in both tax-funded and insurance-funded systems. Equity is not a function of the system of funding. Nevertheless, the failure over many years to achieve equity in the Irish tax-funded system has, for varying reasons, encouraged reformers to seek inspiration in the compulsory insurance systems of other states.

The evolution of Labour's advocacy of compulsory health insurance

From the launch of her discussion document on health in April 2000 to the publication of a revised version in the autumn of 2001, Liz McManus of the Labour Party travelled around Ireland to discuss her evolving policy with health professionals and party members. The party hosted meetings and invited doctors, nurses and others to come and discuss health reform. "Sometimes, they didn't bother turning up. In Wexford, we had a really good debate. In Dublin West, where quite a number of doctors and patients turned up, there developed an almighty row. It was clear that they had never heard each other saying these things before." McManus's odyssey developed her views and was catalytic for others':

> I had invited these doctors to come to our house one evening and share their views on how the health system should be reformed. We broke up our meeting at the agreed hour and said our goodbyes. Some time later I went out – to put out the bins, I think – and there they all were, on the pavement, outside our house, still talking. "You have no idea", they told me, "how great it is to have an opportunity to get together and talk about the system. We never do this in our normal lives."[2]

McManus knew from her previous experience as a Minister of State that, if she were ever appointed Minister for Health, she would achieve little unless she had already drafted her plans for reform. "Once you are in government, clarity and time to work things out is lost because a lot of issues hit you and you are working with the civil servants, who are slow to change. A lot of the detail has to be clear in your head from day one."

Her policy reflected many influences. She cited the earlier work of her husband, the GP John McManus, a consistent advocate of equal access to state-funded care. Consultants, nurses, academics and others attended private Labour Party round table discussions to debate the policy's details. Since 1989, Pat Rabbitte, then McManus's Workers' Party colleague in the Dáil, had been willing to contemplate funding health care through insurance. As a member of Democratic Left, McManus had published a discussion document in 1998 which suggested that access to care might be funded by either universal insurance or taxation.[3] Two years later, she and the Labour Party were committed to the former option.

For Labour, this adoption of an insurance-funded route to equity was a return to its antecedents. In 1969, the party had supported a comprehensive health service funded from social insurance. In the early 1980s, Barry Desmond had advocated a national health insurance system incorporating the VHI. Subsequently, the party had appeared to favour the introduction of an NHS-style tax-funded health system, but had then endorsed Brendan Howlin's 1994 health strategy, with its commitment to maintaining the position of private practice.

After Labour's disappointing performance in the 2002 election, McManus nonetheless perceived progress. "The whole idea of an insurance-based system was nowhere four years ago. It is now part of the debate. That in itself is at least setting up the possibility of real reform."[4] In 2002, McManus was elected deputy leader of the party and remained spokesperson on health. Rabbitte was elected leader. The party now had a leadership with a record of advocacy for health system reform.

Labour's approach to compulsory health insurance

In its 2001 policy, a refinement of its 2000 discussion document, Labour promised that, in government, it would "introduce an insurance-based system for everyone, to cover health care including GP services and hospital treatment, with substantial state funding and strict supervision, all underpinned by a statutory Health Care Guarantee".[5]

All patients would be permitted to choose their insurer, their hospital and their specialist. The state would pay insurance premiums for, approximately, the 50 per cent of the population on lower incomes, and a further 10 per cent would be partly assisted on a sliding scale. The remaining 40 per cent of the population would continue to pay their own premiums, on which they would receive income tax relief. This was to be a compulsory insurance system. The state would pay the premium for any higher earner who neglected to do so, and it would recover the cost through income tax. Since the insurance system would now cover GP care, premiums could be expected to rise to cover that additional cost.

Patients would not have to make any top-up payments to doctors or hospitals but the top 60 per cent of earners would have to pay for medication, unless it exceeded a monthly threshold (a continuation of the existing system). Insurers would be required to cover a range of services governed by a statutory Health Care Guarantee. Hospitals would not be permitted to discriminate between patients and there would be a statutory requirement that they provide a single standard of care for all. The state would continue to fund A & E services, ambulance services and GPs' preventive care directly and would contribute to investment in GPs' practices. Labour argued:

> The outstanding benefit of this new system is that as far as hospitals and GPs are concerned, there will be no difference between rich, middling or poor patients. No matter how the insurance premium is paid, hospitals and practitioners will charge the same fees for everybody; there will be no public/private distinction between patients, and any discrimination will be impossible ... EU countries with good health outcomes tend to have mandatory insurance, a mix of public, private and voluntary hospitals and a strong supervisory role for the state. That's the balance that will be applied here.[6]

Once Labour started campaigning, this detailed document was cryptically summarised in an election pledge as: "Free GP care for all – As Labour delivers a fair, high quality health service, not continued health apartheid." Labour had undoubtedly deliberately chosen to emphasise what the middle classes stood to gain from the new system – free GP care – rather than what they stood to lose – preferential access to hospital care. Had they been targeting a working class electorate, they might have placed greater emphasis on achieving hospital treatment prioritised by need not income.

The evolution of Fine Gael's advocacy of compulsory health insurance

The Fine Gael leader, John Bruton, phoned his Foreign Affairs spokesman, Gay Mitchell, in the summer of 2000 to tell him that health was going to be "the major issue" and he wanted him to take the brief. Representing the working class constituency of Dublin South-Central, where he had been reared by a widowed mother in a family of nine and had gone to work at the age of 16, Mitchell knew how the health system affected the poor of Dublin: the disaster of failing to qualify for a medical card, the cancelled appointments, the long waits. An ambitious career politician, former Lord Mayor of Dublin, and member of the Dáil for nearly 20 years who had never held full ministerial office, Mitchell vigorously attacked his new brief: he visited hospitals, met professionals, administrators, trade unionists. He developed and wrote the party's new policy with the help of a small group: a chartered accountant, a hospital administrator and a general practitioner, Declan Murphy, former president of the ICGP.

Fine Gael's advocacy of a health insurance system was not without precedent. In 1961, former Minister for Health Tom O'Higgins had argued for a comprehensive health service "based on the principle of insurance". Fine Gael had retained its commitment to an insurance system in its 1965 "Just Society" document. Whereas O'Higgins had proposed that everyone should pay an equal "health stamp", Mitchell proposed that his insurance system should be funded from taxation, so its costs would fall more heavily on higher earners, anathema to O'Higgins, who would have considered this "state paternalism".

The party had forgotten this history. Mitchell started with a blank sheet and his advisers had considerable influence. Declan Murphy was an enthusiast for managed care, which was central to the policy. Front-bench members initially balked at Mitchell's radicalism and met four times before endorsing his policy. Later Mitchell proved to be a less than convincing proponent of compulsory health insurance: he would advocate a Health Ombudsman, rather than explain his complex proposals for reform. Fianna Fáil policy analysts didn't even dignify his policy by critiquing it during the 2002 election campaign. Labour, they correctly discerned, was the party that had given more thought to its position, against which they needed to find counter-arguments.[7]

Mitchell later admitted that he found it hard to sell his complex policy during the election. "It was a bit like telling people, when their house is on fire, that you are building a fire station." However, he became progressively more outspoken about the need for equity and was prepared to state that private patients would no longer receive priority in public hospitals, under the Fine Gael reforms.[8]

Fine Gael's approach to "state funded, insurance based" care

Fine Gael's policy, published in November 2000, proposed a universal health insurance system to cover hospital care but not primary care. Access to free GP care would be greatly expanded but by an extension of the existing medical card scheme. Unlike Labour, who proposed that most of the existing insured would continue to pay their own insurance premiums, Fine Gael proposed that all premiums should be paid by the state and funded through taxation. Because Fine Gael subsequently went to the electorate offering lower taxes, its policy offered a windfall gain to the existing insured.

Fine Gael described its system as "state funded but insurance based".[9] Insurance companies would receive state funds, on the nomination of individual taxpayers, for which they would provide core essential services. Private insurance would continue to cover non-medical benefits in hospitals (such as private rooms) and admission to private hospitals. Fine Gael applied the language of the market to health care. Insurance companies would be "the patients' purchasing agents". Patients would select the insurer, "whose product best meets their needs".[10]

> The reason for involving insurance companies in the process is to separate the function of providing health services from that of purchasing health services. Furthermore, there are likely to be a number of insurance companies actively seeking business. In this way competition can be created in health care which will bring about greater equity and cost effectiveness. This might be called managed competition.[11]

This language and thinking bore evidence of the influence of developments in health care in the NHS in the UK during the Conservative era, which were also exported to New Zealand, and had mixed success in both states. Fine Gael presented its policy to the electorate in 2002 in stripped-down form. The language of managed competition had disappeared. The emphasis now was on ending "apartheid in our two-tier health service". The essential proposals in regard to primary and secondary care had survived.[12]

Labour and Fine Gael compared

Superficially similar, there were important differences between the Labour and Fine Gael approaches to an insurance-based system. Each would involve insurance companies as the conduit for funding health care. But Labour would keep the middle class paying its own premiums; Fine Gael would pay all from taxation and did not pursue the consequent implication of increased taxation. The parties' motivations for going the route of a universal insurance system subtly differed. Labour said its advocacy of reform was "for the sake of efficiency and above all for the sake of justice";[13] Fine Gael's emphasis was on "creating competition ... for greater equity and cost effectiveness".[14]

Both Labour and Fine Gael were motivated by the desire to remove distinctions between public and private patients, but for Labour this critically meant removing distinctions throughout the health system; Fine Gael would merely remove the distinction in public hospitals. Both saw benefits in a system in which insurers competed for the custom of patients, and hospitals and doctors competed to treat those patients. The difference in emphasis between the two parties, however, was that Labour was proposing that, by insuring all patients, all patients would now receive their care as service, rather than largesse; Fine Gael was enamoured of the idea of managed competition as a means of making the health service more efficient and would continue to have two categories of patient – the public and the private. These differences became more obvious in how the two parties regarded the role of insurance companies and hospitals and in their approach to GP care.

Explaining why she had opted for proposing compulsory insurance, rather than an NHS-style tax-funded service, Liz McManus said "with up to 45 per cent of the population now covered by private insurance, they would appear to like what they get. It does create a different relationship between the patient and the health services."[15] For McManus "the really important thing" was "empowering the patient and having the money follow the patient". An insurance-based system, with a number of insurers, gave the "benefit of competition".[16]

Labour explicitly addressed the issue of "why wouldn't an NHS-type system work?" The UK's NHS shared with Ireland problems of waiting lists and crisis management, Labour argued. And

> even a reformed NHS type model would be extremely difficult to adapt to this country given our tradition of supported private health insurance. Socially, politically and economically, it would be almost impossible to transfer all but a very small proportion of the current 42 per cent of private policyholders onto the public system ... we need to progress beyond the current system, not by eliminating the advantages given by health insurance but by ensuring that those advantages are extended to all.[17]

The Labour and Fine Gael philosophies most obviously diverged in their approaches to GP care. Labour would include GP care in the insurance-funded system; Fine Gael would exclude it, so that GPs would retain two classes of patient and two forms of payment.

This exclusion was apparently driven by Mitchell's often-stated concern that covering all patients for free GP care would make GPs civil servants. His insistence on retaining private-fee income for GPs was driven by his belief that salaried GPs would be less productive.[18] He did not, apparently, consider the possibility that rewards for productivity could be built into a universal system. This retention of private-fee income for GPs was inconsistent with the party's stated philosophical stance that health care was "a social responsibility ... not a commodity for individual consumers who can or cannot afford it"[19] and was at odds with the personal view of Mitchell's adviser, the general practitioner Declan Murphy, that "we should remove all financial barriers to consulting GPs".[20]

Fine Gael remained, therefore, only a partial convert to the principle of social solidarity, which informs European insurance-based systems and is established on "the premise that health care is not a normally traded good and access to it is a fundamental right".[21] Mitchell had not been persuaded that individuals, whatever their level of income, might wish to insure against ill-health and that the doctor-patient relationship might benefit from the absence of a direct cash payment. Labour's stated underlying principle was that health care should be "delivered to all citizens as a right".[22]

The philosophical differences between Labour, Fine Gael and the government parties

For their part, the government parties – Fianna Fáil and the Progressive Democrats – remained philosophically wedded to the view of health care as a traded good, expressed so clearly by Rory O'Hanlon: "I believe in Ireland that if people want to pay for their own medical treatment out of their own disposable income, that is their right." Patients, it followed, must remain divided between the fee-paying and the clients of the state.

The Progressive Democrats advocated continued distinctions between patients in their 2002 election manifesto, which stated that "the solution [to the different treatment of public and private patients] is not to try to make one size fits all or to bring in a new PRSI tax under the guise of universal private health insurance". Instead, they proposed to focus on results and service levels, "where unacceptable differences in treatment between public and private health matter".[23] Committed as an outgoing government party to the implementation of the 2001 health strategy, they shared with Fianna Fáil the heroic assumption that increased capacity would remove equity as an issue. A more effective opposition might have exploited to better effect the Progressive Democrats' former advocacy of an insurance-based system.

Both the Progressive Democrats and Fianna Fáil implicitly viewed access to health care as a commodity to be purchased, most markedly in their limited proposals to extend access to free GP services. Fianna Fáil would extend medical cards to "over 200,000" extra people at an unspecified time, which would increase the proportion of the population with medical cards from 31 to 35 per cent.[24] The PDs stated that they would ensure medical card eligibility at least kept pace with income growth, implying that the proportion of the population covered might remain unchanged.[25]

Questions about universal insurance systems

The role of hospitals

Fine Gael and Labour, with greater refinements, proposed that an advantage of an insurance-based system would be to give hospitals greater autonomy. In the language of health economics, this is referred to as the purchaser-provider split. Under the traditional Irish health system, where the state funds most health care from taxation and, through the health boards, also runs the hospitals, effectively including the voluntary hospitals, the state, therefore, both purchases and provides most health care.[26] In the opposition parties' proposals for insurance-based systems, insurance companies would become the purchasers of health care on behalf of their patients and hospitals – private, public or voluntary – would compete to supply them.

Purchaser-provider splits have been tried in states which do not have insurance-based systems. In the UK, this system of managed competition led to some hospital closures under Conservative governments. In New Zealand, it was tried and abandoned in the 1990s. The New Zealanders discovered that providers of care had ceased to cooperate and share information, and hospitals were pursuing efficiency at the expense of care.

In its 2000 discussion document, Labour initially proposed that hospitals would be given "greater autonomy" in day-to-day operation and recruitment of staff and would be "required to cover their costs through income from health insurers and patient co-payments where applicable". The state would still fund capital projects. Health insurers would not be obliged to contract with all providers, unless the government considered this necessary "to ensure access to and choice of hospital services".[27]

Fianna Fáil, in the person of Micheál Martin, was quick to spot the political Achilles' heel in the proposal:

> Where one of the smaller regional hospitals is unable to win a service contract from a private insurer it may be forced to restrict services or close altogether ... to expose our local hospitals and the population who rely on these hospitals to such a perilous and uncertain future would be folly indeed. The Labour Party too often forgets that there is an Ireland beyond the cities.[28]

While commending Labour's discussion document as "extraordinarily far-seeing", the US economist Dale Tussing also cautioned about the consequences of introducing "budget-responsible autonomous hospitals". He pointed out that they were not a necessary corollary of universal health insurance, which he separately described as "a change which is very much in harmony with recent thinking and innovations in both Europe and North America".[29] Tussing later elaborated that, while there were some powerful arguments for autonomous or, in effect, privatised hospitals – resources would automatically go to areas of greatest need, hospitals would economise, the role of politics would be reduced – there remained reasons for state subvention to hospitals to continue, "perhaps indefinitely".

> Some hospitals may thrive under such a system; others, raised and nurtured under a wholly different environment may fail. When hospitals fail, either the population served will be denied hospital service, or the government will have to bail out the endangered institutions, a practice which would undermine the integrity of the entire system.

Tussing proposed a transitional period of increasing autonomy for hospitals, when the state would continue to support them:

> The state might consider it appropriate to continue some hospital subventions indefinitely. This is a concession that the market can't recognise and deal with all instances of societal need ... The public will want and deserve assurance that hospital decisions are not mainly or even largely budget driven.

Investor-driven hospitals were rare because the public was reassured by the "not-for-profit method of organisation that the hospital's first objective is patient care".[30]

In its refined policy, Labour recognised these concerns and now proposed that hospitals' income from insurers' fees would be matched by payments from the state. Public hospitals owned by health boards would continue to be an "important pillar" of the service. Addressing Micheál Martin's specific attack, Labour proposed that when "the operation of patient choice" caused "unsustainable decline in revenue" for a hospital, a new Health Services Authority would "help the institution refocus its activities and specialisations in a way that responds to the actual needs of the local community".[31]

Having refined the mechanism of hospital autonomy, Labour had also found a means to address the issue of hospital location. Patient choice would soon make clear if a local hospital's standards were inadequate or, if local people truly considered local care an overriding need, would facilitate raising standards because revenues would follow patients. It was too much to expect, however, that Fianna Fáil would acknowledge that there was some merit in this proposal. Labour's policy "would potentially shut local hospitals", Fianna Fáil continued to claim.[32]

Labour's motivation for giving hospitals greater freedom was now more clearly and persuasively stated:

> Hospitals must be freed from bureaucratic control from above by multiple centres of power (Department of Health and Health Boards). The absurdity of budget capping must be replaced by a payment system where "the money follows the patient" and hospitals that treat more patients will earn more revenue.[33]

To prevent conflict between insurers' desire to reduce costs and patients' needs, Labour proposed that insurers would not be permitted to own or operate hospitals. This would prevent the emergence of US-style health maintenance organisations (HMOs).[34] An advocate of universal health insurance from well to the right of Labour, UCD economist Moore McDowell took the precisely opposite stance: that the development of insurer-owned HMOs should be a mechanism to control health care costs.[35]

Fine Gael proposed that hospitals should be autonomous, non-profit and self-governing. They should have significant voluntary input and their management should be put out to tender at regular intervals. Fine Gael suggested that wasteful spending within hospitals could be as high as 20 per cent.[36] There were real echoes here of New Zealand's experimental period, when it was believed that up to 32 per cent of expenditure on hospitals could be saved by shorter stays, better management and recruiting hospital managers from outside the public service.

The future of private medicine

In a system which no longer distinguished between public and private patients, would there be any future for private medicine? If all patients were to be insured for "all necessary health care", statutorily defined in a Health Care Guarantee and which all insurers must offer, as Labour proposed, would there be any reason for them to seek top-up insurance? Would they be permitted to purchase it? Labour proposed to allow insurers to offer additional services "like luxury hospital suites or elective cosmetic surgery", which would not attract any state subsidy. Fine Gael, like Labour, proposed to permit additional private insurance for "non-medical benefits", such as private rooms, in public hospitals but, critically, would also allow additional insurance cover for treatment in private hospitals.[37]

Here was an important difference in the parties' thinking. Labour essentially foresaw a system in which all hospitals, public and private, would opt to supply services to all patients on an equal footing, since all would be equally covered by the compulsory insurance system. Fine Gael foresaw compulsory insurance achieving equality of access and care in public hospitals but, by permitting insurers to offer separate cover for medical care in private hospitals, was apparently prepared to permit continued fast-track access to essential care by this route. Fine Gael continued to speak of "private patients" as a separate category.

In its first discussion document, Labour had also envisaged that private medicine might continue, provided it did not operate within "the framework of state supported facilities". Consultants and hospitals might opt to work in a "super-private" system, without any state subvention, provided they did not also work in the "universal hospital system". A private hospital, which opted to sell care to the state system, would not be permitted simultaneously to sell preferential care to patients who paid more.[38] Labour's more refined policy no longer mentioned the possibility of a "super-private" system, now apparently taking the view that, as top-up insurance would only be permitted for non-medical benefits or inessential treatments, all hospitals could be expected to opt to sell their services to the state-regulated compulsory insurance system.[39]

Although Fine Gael's policy was intended to end the two-tier system in public hospitals, the party's policy document showed an openness to the continuation of private practice, which, if put into effect, would undermine that objective. Fine Gael envisaged that "private patients could continue to use privately funded health insurance at private hospitals", without stipulating whether or not those hospitals might simultaneously transact into the public system. Although the policy document did not explicitly address the issue of the consultants' contract, it emerged that the party proposed to continue to permit consultants on public salaries to undertake private practice off the site of their public commitment.[40] This logic then trapped Fine Gael into a continuation of two-tier care on public hospital campuses. To prevent undue absences by consultants, the party suggested that "separate, privately funded private hospital facilities on the same campus as public hospitals could be considered and might contribute to easing pressure on public hospitals' lists." Private hospitals for "private patients", staffed by consultants with public commitments, would leave the door wide open to the continuation of two rates of payment to doctors, for two classes of patient, in a recognisably two-tier system.[41]

Fine Gael also proposed the creation of a new "specialist" grade in hospitals "to take the pressure of routine work off consultants".[42] Mitchell had envisaged that such specialists would be salaried and undertake no private practice, a suggestion which did not go down well with Finbarr Fitzpatrick, secretary-general of the IHCA, who remained a party activist and was Fine Gael director of elections in 2002. Mitchell's salaried, public-only specialists were not included in the policy document.[43]

Labour kept an open mind on the question of how doctors would be paid. Provided contracts established "the principle of equality of patients", doctors might be paid by salary and/or fee per capita or service.[44] Labour later clarified that there would be the "same fee payment system for all patients"[45] and "a new contract based on universal health insurance will be offered to consultants and family doctors", its detail to be "subject to negotiation".[46]

The role of insurance companies

The fundamental question about universal insurance systems is whether it is desirable for health care to be run by insurance companies. Critics point to the experience of the US system, where managed care is increasingly run as a business by for-profit corporations, and where health care costs a great deal and is often less than humane. On the other hand, the much-admired health systems of France and Germany are also insurance-based and rate highly in patient satisfaction. These are profoundly different systems. The most important distinction is that in the US, health care is funded by private, voluntary insurance, whereas in France and Germany, the insurance system is compulsory and universal. In the US, many people are uninsured. In France and Germany, everyone must be insured and workers and employers pay for health care through social insurance contributions. The US system is driven by profit: it has been estimated that the profits of insurance companies and medical care organisations account for 1 to 2 per cent of the entire income of the United States.[47] In France and Germany, most insurance cover is channelled through non-profit social insurance or sickness funds, in which membership is generally related to employment. Private, for-profit insurers play a subsidiary role. In the US, insurers dictate what they will and will not cover. In Germany, the Federal Ministry of Health sets rules to ensure that all citizens have equal access to care and are covered for the same benefit package, a formula which the Labour Party proposed to emulate with its statutory Health Care Guarantee. In the US, health care is a marketable commodity. The state retains control of health care in the European model.

In some confused debate about the Labour and Fine Gael proposals, they were perceived as arguing for a US-style system, because they intended to fund health care through private insurance companies. In reality, their proposals were much closer to the European model. However, given the structure of the Irish insurance market, which is dominated by one large state company, their proposed insurance-based systems did not share the starting points of France and Germany, where the systems' roots go back to forms of worker cooperation. Whereas in France and Germany the insurance system is funded through payroll taxes, Labour proposed the Irish system should be part-funded by individuals' payment of premiums and partly by the state; Fine Gael proposed that the exchequer would fund the insurance system. That these funds would then go to private insurance companies raised the spectre for some critics that, as in the US, the health care system might become driven by the profit motive. If the VHI were to be privatised, then introduction of an insurance-based system could indeed make this spectre a flesh-and-blood reality.

To guard against this, the Labour Party proposed that while the VHI should be separated from direct state ownership to comply with EU competition requirements, it should not be privatised.[48] Labour also supported the enforcement of risk equalisation, in which insurers who cherry-pick low risks, such as the younger and healthier, must compensate those insurers, like the VHI, with more high-risk members. Because for-profit competitors would therefore be forced to compete on a level playing field with the not-for-profit VHI, Labour seemed content that these measures would be sufficient to prevent the emergence of a for-profit motivated health insurance industry in Ireland. Fine Gael did not state its view on the future of the VHI.

How constrained are Irish reformers by EU law?

There are other models that the Irish proponents of compulsory health insurance might have explored. In Canada, not-for-profit provincial health insurance plans, accountable to provincial government, purchase health care from independently run, not-for-profit hospitals. The plans operate either from within the Ministry of Health or through a separate agency closely linked to the Ministry. There is a split between purchasers and providers, but it is the providers (the hospitals) not the purchasers (the insurance plans) that are private.

In its policy formulation, Labour apparently shared the commonly held belief that, since Ireland is required under EU law to permit open competition in the *voluntary* health insurance market, this would make it impossible to restrict *compulsory* health insurance to not-for-profit or state companies, such as the VHI. However, EU law has limited application to statutory health care provisions. In EU treaties, member states have explicitly stated that the organisation and delivery of health services and medical care remains a matter of national competence. The EU accepts the principle that, when a state is determining its form of social provision, competition law must take second place. When health insurance forms part of a statutory system of social security, it is explicitly excluded from the EU insurance directives. Thus, where French *mutuelles* or German insurance funds provide services in line with public policy goals, in a manner regulated to meet those goals, they are not judged to be engaged in traded services and are therefore not subject to single market rules. Where, however, *mutuelles* use their client bases and their sheltered positions to offer services over and above statutory provisions, they are subject to competition rules.

There has, however, been scope for confusion, since different definitions of social security exist. In one judgment, the European Court of Justice specified that this exclusion from the insurance directives only applied to public social security institutions. If private, for-profit insurance firms administered a compulsory statutory scheme of social security, the directives would apply. This judgment related to insurance for accidents at work, not health insurance. The question whether a compulsory health insurance scheme administered through private companies, as Labour and Fine Gael proposed, would also be subject to the directives and forced to permit the participation of for-profit companies, has not come before the court. However, the Dutch decided to choose a public framework of health insurance because they feared a private model would entail application of the EU insurance directives.

An international study of the influence of EU law on health care systems, which was commissioned by the Belgian Presidency of the EU, advised in 2001:

> Member states decide the goals they wish to pursue, such as equity and more effective care, and must then find mechanisms by which to do this that are consistent with European law ... health policy makers are confronted with a mass of contradictory advice from those who take either a restricted or expansive view of the scope of European law in health care ... While many of the transactions within statutory systems may be exempt on social grounds, health authorities must be aware of the possibility of removing this protection through deregulation and privatisation ... poorly considered health care reforms, especially where they introduce market mechanisms and decentralisation, might render organisations unexpectedly subject to competition law.[49]

This caution might have been written for Labour and Fine Gael. Yet they might also find encouragement in knowing that they are by no means alone in Europe in seeking to devise a system of health insurance that preserves the values of social solidarity while employing the mechanisms of the market. If an Irish government were elected with a mandate to design a compulsory health insurance system from scratch, this would be an unprecedented undertaking for any EU member state. Other states became members with the principles of their systems already in place. Ireland would be on untested ground. It appears that a system of compulsory health insurance, which was explicitly not-for-profit and channelled through the state-owned VHI, would indeed be exempt from EU competition directives and could not be forced to admit private for-profit insurers. However, a system channelled through private insurance companies would need to be carefully crafted if it were not to trigger competition requirements and provide a beach-head for the profit motive in health care. The clearer and more coherent the social policy goals of the new system, the more secure it is likely to be from the enforcement of EU competition law. Reformers who wish to design a unique Irish system, taking the best from the experience of other states, may have wider and more creative options than the backroom thinkers of Labour envisaged. It should be possible to design a system of compulsory insurance-purchased care which is in the European tradition of social solidarity and in which health care is not run by private insurance companies.

Arguments against compulsory health insurance

Why not just change how consultants are paid?

Why not achieve equity by a simpler route than changing the entire system of health funding, some critics have asked. In his early response to the Labour policy, Dale Tussing suggested that equity might instead be achieved by simply paying consultants in the same way for every patient. The economic incentive for doctors to maintain class distinctions in hospital care would end, by simply slicing through the complex knot of the public/private mix. This liberation would presumably please those doctors who had expressed their abhorrence of the two-tier system and their desire to work in another way. Tussing wrote:

> The Labour Party has proposed rectifying this problem by buying insurance for public patients. Paying specialists by FFS [fee-for-service] for all patients is a simpler, more obvious, and more immediate reform which could achieve the same results. The same amounts of money currently used to pay salaries could be instead used to pay physicians according to fee-for-service.[50]

He later expanded:

> If all patients, and not only private patients, are paid for by fee-for-service, that will remove the incentive to create two separate waiting lists. It won't get rid of the waiting list; that requires an inflow of resources. But it should get rid of the inequitable distribution of the list.[51]

The medical profession sought payment by fee-for-service in 1974, when they reached their impasse with Brendan Corish over free hospitalisation. When Corish's official, Dermot Condon, went to Canada to investigate fee-for-service, he concluded "to introduce it here would have been a license to print money". Tussing's counter-argument in 2001 was that, while no method of payment was perfect, where there was "evidence of inadequate provision of care, one might want to try FFS".[52] In effect, he was arguing not just for a different system but, in opposition to Condon's views, that the consequence that this would lead to increased investment in Irish health care was no bad thing. However, in systems with evidence of excessive utilisation of health care, Tussing has argued that doctors should instead be paid by salary or capitation.

He later amended his view of the superiority of his approach to the Labour Party's. If doctors were paid by FFS for all patients, and there was consequently a common waiting list, this would remove a major motive for buying private insurance, which would be a windfall gain for purchasers of insurance who ceased to do so, and a corresponding windfall loss for the state, which would pay the fees for these people. A compulsory health insurance system, as advocated by the Labour Party, in which higher earners would continue to fund their own insurance payments and people on lower incomes would have their premiums paid by the state, would limit windfall gains. Tussing nonetheless suggested that "if it is true that people of modest means today buy private insurance cover because they fear that they won't get timely care, any reform which addresses this problem will shift some premium costs from those patients to the Government."[53]

It costs too much

Some analysts of the health care system have expressed concern about a compulsory insurance system on the grounds that it would cost too much. ESRI economics professor Brian Nolan argued that reliance on funding health care via competing private insurers "can be a recipe for (even greater) cost inflation". He suggested that universal coverage could instead be achieved through social insurance or direct state funding. The complete split proposed by Labour in its original discussion document between the public and private sectors, with consultants in public hospitals no longer working in private hospitals, could be achieved without changing the system of funding, he implied.[54]

Ruth Barrington, chief executive of the Health Research Board, objected that, while people liked insurance-based systems because they were "very responsive", giving patients "what they want – quick access to a doctor and to hospital", they were also the most expensive systems in the world because they created "a climate, in which doctors want to please patients and patients can take advantage of doctors", who will provide whatever they think the insurance system will cover, a risk described as "moral hazard":

> From the point of view of the public good it doesn't make much sense to move from a system, where you encourage people to be more responsible about their health and their use of the health services to one which encourages people to be less responsible.[55]

It costs too much and it means ceding power to insurers

The government parties' opposition to compulsory health insurance was bolstered by Deloitte and Touche's study of the health system. At the

Ballymascanlon cabinet meeting in 2001, officials of the Department of Health told Ministers that the study pointed to "administrative and logistical problems of shifting to an insurance based system" with little obvious benefit to health outcomes. While such a system might make services and new technology more accessible to patients and would provide more incentives for providers, it could lead to excess capacity in hospital beds and personnel, high labour costs and lack of service integration and planning. It would mean "a significant degree of future planning of health services is given to private insurers". They said most of these objections also applied to the alternative of a French- or German-style social insurance fund covering the entire population. The strengths of the existing central-taxation-funded system, the Department reported, were "good service planning, integration of services helped by present arrangements and strict budgetary control" – claims for the system, as applied in Ireland, which the subsequent Prospectus and Brennan studies disputed. The Department acknowledged that weaknesses of the tax-funded system were "lack of incentives for providers"; it was "slower in patient responsiveness"; and "full multi-annual budgeting" was "not in place".[56]

When the Deloitte and Touche study was published, it became apparent that this had been a Department of Health interpretation, presumably to support its own predispositions. The consultants, who drew on the expertise of the York Health Economics Consortium, actually stopped short of making a recommendation. "Changing a nation's health financing system requires serious consideration and is beyond the remit of this study," they wrote. While they did point out that the risk of excess capacity was greater where services were "purchased through individual fees and by multiple insurers", on the other hand, they elaborated that waiting lists and rationing were more likely in tax-funded systems, where health spending would be affected by issues like the wider state of the economy.[57]

The objection that an insurance-based system might give undue power to private insurers was a real one, which the Labour Party addressed by stipulating that the state would enforce a Health Care Guarantee and that a statutory state agency, the Health Services Authority, would be responsible for approving proposals for new hospitals. Although it is a legitimate position to object to giving a role to insurance companies in determining medical cover and planning services, some Irish proponents of this view may be vulnerable to the accusation of intellectual dishonesty. They conveniently choose to disregard that if, as tends to be the case, they are themselves insured with the VHI or another company, they have opted to place the determination of the nature and quality of their care in the hands of the same companies.

Arguments in support of compulsory health insurance

A secure source of funding for health care

The strongest argument for compulsory insurance as a route to health care funding is the precise converse of the most frequently adduced argument against it. If the weakness of insurance systems is that they lead to more spending on health, that is also their strength. Since each citizen is covered by a premium for a defined set of benefits, the system raises the funds necessary to deliver those benefits and can then commission them. Health care has a ring-fenced fund, an earmarked tax, to use the jargon, which will increase in response to rises in population and will remain independent of fluctuations in the state of the economy.

Against the backdrop of Ireland's experience of stop-start health care funding, this is a persuasive argument in favour of compulsory insurance. In 1989, the Commission on Health Funding rejected it, although Cormac MacNamara put the minority dissenting case that earmarked taxation or insurance contributions would raise public consciousness of the cost of health care. A further dissenter has been Kevin Murphy, the Ombudsman, who argued, in his 2001 report on nursing home subventions, that the time had come to revisit this issue of a "secure source of funding for health care".[58]

One of the reasons insurance-based systems cost more is that they provide more care. UCD economist Joe Durkan observed in a discussion of the arguments for compulsory health insurance: "I am not saying it will be cheap. Costs will rise because additional people will be treated who aren't being treated now."[59] He suggested that among the reasons why such a system was unlikely was that governments would be reluctant to commit the resources needed to deliver equity.

Durkan attempted to cost the system. An annual premium of £1,500 (€1,900) per adult would be required to replace the existing system, he calculated in 2001. However, since citizens would now be funding care through premiums which had formerly been funded directly by the exchequer, the exchequer would have substantial savings which could be used to reduce taxes. Durkan addressed with clarity an issue which Fianna Fáil did its best to confuse. Fianna Fáil persistently demanded costings for the new system, as though its entire cost would be in addition to funding the existing system. In reality, the new system would involve a rerouting through insurance companies, instead of through the state, of the existing contributions provided by society to the running of the health care system. That equity would mean greater demand, as Durkan pointed out, was in effect impossible to cost, an "open-ended commitment". As Aneurin Bevan reportedly told the Chancellor of the Exchequer prior to the establishment of the NHS, the cost of a free health service would depend on the behaviour of the public and the only way to discover it was to permit the public to behave.

It achieves equity without antagonising doctors or the middle class

That a compulsory insurance system would remove inequities in access and treatment is a compelling argument in its favour, but it is not a sufficient argument, since this could also be achieved in a tax-funded system which simply banned private practice in public hospitals and paid doctors equally for each patient they treated. To support the case for going the further distance to reorganising the Irish system of funding health care requires additional arguments. Labour's Liz McManus has repeatedly emphasised that insurance changes the nature of the relationship between doctor and patient. Reading between the lines, it also appears that Labour's advocacy of compulsory health insurance has been driven by the political judgement that simply to banish private practice from public hospitals would provoke the ire of the insured middle classes and the medical profession.

Some doctors prefer insurance companies to the state

The medical profession has episodically proposed an insurance-based system. Jimmy Sheehan, the private hospital promoter, described as "ideal" a compulsory insurance system, purchasing care from a network of independent hospitals neither constructed nor run by the state. He objected to the rationing of health care by either the state or insurers, which ultimately led him into a conceptual cul-de-sac in which medical professionals alone might decide how health care resources should be spent. "It must become the prerogative of the medical profession to decide what is relevant for the individual. There has to be some form of accountability. I think you have to trust your professionals."[60] Nowhere would government or insurers countenance this blank cheque for medicine.

Other doctors see particular merit in insurance systems because they can deliver equity and universal coverage without making doctors employees of the state. For the "single payer" state, the system substitutes multiple payers: the insurance companies. Critics of insurance systems might suspect that these professionals anticipate that insurance companies will prove easier and more generous taskmasters than the state. This is not necessarily the case, as doctors discovered in the US, where HMOs have been aggressive in controlling their activity and income. If an Irish insurance-based system were to protect the quality of patient care from the business imperatives of the insurance companies, it would only do so by state regulation. Doctors would need the state as their ally.

One of the most vocal medical proponents of compulsory insurance has been the Dublin oncologist John Crown, director of the Cancer Chemotherapy Research Unit at St Vincent's Hospital, whose support for an insurance-based system has appeared driven as much by his distaste for the state as an employer, as by his disavowal of the "offensive" two-tier system.[61] Crown harbours deep suspicions of the role of the state in health care: "all of the non-publicly answerable quangos, which run Irish medicine, wish us to concentrate power in the hands of an unelected, unanswerable, ideologically-driven, administrative élite".[62] He has argued for a German-style system of "mandatory, occupationally based insurance, with a social security net for the unwaged", regulated by government and "financed principally by not-for-profit, non-governmental agencies". "The way forward is not to bureaucratise the private system but rather to democratise it, by making access to it equitable."[63] Some GPs are also better disposed to a free GP scheme which is insurance rather than tax-based because they believe their freedom as patient advocates would be compromised in a "single payer" state system.

Finbarr Fitzpatrick, who was implicated in the election argument for compulsory insurance as Fine Gael's director of elections, nonetheless subsequently adopted a stance of indifference to the proposal, as did the IHCA.[64] The amount of funding was more important than the method, he observed. He did not share Crown's enthusiasm for an insurance-based system as a means of ensuring that consultants would have multiple payers. "I don't think the manner in which consultants are remunerated necessarily affects their clinical independence or their advocacy role." Fitzpatrick foresaw "eternal friction" between "the advocacy role, clinical independence and the resource provider and salary payer, be that the state or a major health insurer".[65]

In 2002, the opposition proponents of compulsory health insurance were competing with assurances from Fianna Fáil that they would abolish waiting lists and deliver excellent public patient care by massively investing in health care, even though the two-tier system would survive. The immediate post-election realisation that this best of all worlds was a spindoctors' illusion strengthened arguments for a system which would deliver a secure source of funding for health care, end inequity and offer incentives to hospitals and doctors to treat more patients. If the health strategy's calculation of the investment needs of the health service, or even a scaled-down version of it, were to be accepted, how might it be funded? Introducing a compulsory insurance system would offer the electorate assurances that their extra contributions would go directly to health care.

But why go this route to equity and assured funding? Why not merely ban private practice in public hospitals and fund equitable public health care through taxation or social insurance, without the intermediary role of the insurance companies? To ignore the warnings about the potential cost of such a system required a compelling motivation. For the Labour reformers, the overriding attraction of compulsory health insurance was that it offered a politically achievable route to dismantling two-tier care. If instead the public and the private were merely separated in the existing system, there would remain a thriving private health insurance industry funding care in a potentially growing private hospital sector, particularly if the public sector were underfunded, as had historically been the case. To avoid the risk of deepening the schism in Irish health care might require going the further distance to nationalising private hospitals, as Bevan did in the UK in the 1940s, a politically unlikely departure in Ireland with its constitutionally enshrined and culturally engrained respect for the rights of private property. On the other hand, if the entire population were enlisted in a compulsory health insurance system, which incorporated the VHI, and to which private hospitals would sell their care on an equal basis for all patients, such a schism would never arise. Private hospitals need not be nationalised to ensure their participation in the system.

No reform quite like this has been attempted anywhere else, but then no other state has developed a system quite like Ireland's and no states' health care reforms or systems have been identical. In evolving their policies, Labour and Fine Gael were feeling their way, with Labour having teased out the implications to a much greater degree. The strength of a universal system, as ultimately proposed by Labour, was that it enforced the participation of all citizens and this in itself was the best assurance that standards of care would not suffer. To avoid levelling down, the middle class and the articulate would ensure that the system was better resourced.

Insurance systems differ greatly. They can be a route to equity but how they are implemented is critical. There were important differences in the Labour and Fine Gael proposals. The Fine Gael policy fell at the first hurdle: it would not have delivered the equity it aimed to achieve. Labour's system was unnecessarily market-led, reflecting Labour's apparent belief that EU law would require that its system should involve for-profit, private insurers. Provided it chose to administer its system through a public body like the VHI, this need not necessarily be the case. EU competition law need not apply. With the EU's blessing, or at least without its objection, Ireland could develop a publicly accountable system of health insurance as an intrinsic part of its social security system. Ireland could legitimately reject any attempts under EU competition law to enforce the participation of for-profit companies in its system.

There existed the option, therefore, unexplored by either party, of an insurance system administered by a public insurance body, the original Canadian system.[66] This would not have the absolute arm's length distance between the purchasers and providers of care – the managed competition element, which particularly appealed to Fine Gael – unless all hospitals were privatised. What it would achieve, in addition to the critical removal of discrimination between patients, would be the application of insurance principles to health care – that defined payments would purchase defined benefits – in place of the rationed and capriciously funded tax-based system. It could still foster competition between hospitals without requiring their privatisation. Public hospitals could be required to compete with private hospitals to provide services to the insurance system.

Although the status of hospitals has been linked with debate on the merits of compulsory insurance, these are two separate issues. Labour advanced a strong case for freeing hospitals from bureaucratic control, ending budget capping and allowing the money to follow the patient. While this Labour approach appeared in conflict with the vision of a rationally ordered hospital network, subsequently proposed by the Hanly task force on medical staffing, it was not irreconcilable with it. Labour envisaged that a new Health Services Authority would assist local hospitals in determining their place in the scheme of things. Were a brave new dawn of rational hospital organisation to arrive, there would still be merits in letting revenue flows follow patients, so that, for instance, if regional hospitals failed to deliver acceptable care and patients continued to travel to Dublin, Dublin hospitals would receive correspondingly larger budgets. If, on the other hand, more patients opted for regional care, then the insurance plan would channel funds to their regional centre. There would have to be a role for government in ensuring the continued viability of each level of the planned network.

Labour and Fine Gael's proposal that multiple insurance companies should purchase care – a model of competitive health care purchase as well as competitive supply – could not, however, be reconciled with the centralised, *dirigiste* proposals of the Department-of-Health-sponsored Prospectus group for a national health services executive (HSE), with responsibility for planning, commissioning and funding services. While Labour proposed a Health Services Authority, this state agency would plan and deliver but not purchase care, a role consigned to the competing, albeit state-regulated, insurers. In the alternative model with a single state-controlled insurance body, compulsory health insurance could be reconciled with proposals for a centralised system of health administration and funding. In this case, the new HSE would also act as the public insurance body, mandated to administer and purchase care.

An insurance-funded HSE could have the security of a reliable, earmarked stream of funding, whereas the Department of Health's proposed HSE would depend for funding on the Department's ability to fulfil one of its remaining roles – "acquisition of resources from Government"[67] – and would therefore ration care, depending on the prevailing political and economic climate. Funding would never be unlimited, nor should it be. If health costs became too great, the electorate would doubtless object to the level of their insurance contributions, but at least they would be able to make an explicit connection between their payments and their care and, in this centralised system, could hold one body accountable for the efficiency of health spending. The medical profession would not have achieved "multiple payers" in this model and might see the HSE – insurance-funded or not – as the new "non-publicly answerable quango", in John Crown's phrase, but this model would offer equity, earmarked funding and the prospect of promoting competition between suppliers of health care.

A compulsory insurance system could be funded through taxation (as generally in Canada and proposed by Fine Gael), by the payment of premiums (proposed by Labour) or through payroll taxes (as in France and Germany). There is a strong argument for the latter, which would achieve two desirable consequences: payment would be proportionate to income; and employers would contribute, as well as employees. Increases in UK health spending announced in 2002 were to be funded by this route. One of the chief reasons for poor social provision in Ireland is the low rate of taxation levied on companies, many of whom contribute to voluntary health insurance for their employees. All employers' enforced contribution to the health care system would increase the revenue from this sector and broaden the tax base, a desirable end in itself. In the tradition of social partnership, this might be negotiated between the partners, with wage moderation or productivity gains as the reward for companies paying their share of this new social pact and insuring their workers' health.

How would a citizen experience this new system? Each person would be insured for care, either by payment of a premium or by tax or social insurance. For that payment, the state would guarantee a package of care which providers – hospitals, primary care centres, individual doctors – would compete to supply. Any patient might be treated in the Blackrock Clinic or in the Mater Private Hospital, provided the hospitals had contracted to sell their services to the compulsory insurance system.

Would there be arguments about resources and quality of care? Unquestionably. No state is free of them. But a compulsory health insurance system would put equity and access at its centre and, with a defined contribution of funding for each citizen to purchase this equitable care, the delivery of sustained investment over decades to meet the changing health care needs of the population would become a feasible project. A compulsory insurance system offers one route to addressing the funding needs and the inequity of the Irish health care system. There are others. Before examining the political feasibility of the alternative pathways to reform and discussing the challenges which face reformers, it is illuminating to explore how other states have developed and manage their health care systems.

16

LESSONS FROM ABROAD

"Most Canadians would not stand idly by and accept changes that would destroy this symbol of national identity."
– *The 2002 Romanow Commission comments on the egalitarian Canada Health Act.*[1]

No state believes its health care system to be perfect. All states face the challenge that health care is expensive. Technology, medicine and people's expectations change. Since better health may cheat mortality, demand for care is potentially infinite.

But some states do better than others – measurably so. Life expectancy, the ultimate measure of health outcome, differs. Citizens' access to care and their consequent quality of life differs. The relationship between investment and outcome differs. The priority accorded to prevention and primary care differs. Wider aspects of a society than health care systems – such as income inequality, quality of housing and of education – contribute to differing experiences of health.

This chapter examines health care systems internationally to review how and why they differ from Ireland's and what Ireland might learn from their experiences – both good and bad. It reviews the experience of seven states: the UK, which despite great differences in its history and system, continues to influence health care in Ireland; Canada, which has built a strongly egalitarian system; Germany and France, where health is funded by the European model of compulsory health insurance; Denmark and New Zealand, where health care is funded from taxation, but with widely differing results; and the United States, where the mixed system of voluntary insurance and taxation has bred great inequity.

These states' experiences reveal that it is possible to have no or negligible waiting lists, equitable access to care and a higher life expectancy than in Ireland. Canada, France and Germany have achieved all three. In Denmark, life expectancy is disappointing. In the UK, waiting lists are greater than in continental Europe, reflecting lower health spending. In New Zealand and the US, fees are a barrier to care. Most European states offer free or reimbursed GP care and equitable access to hospital services.

States generally develop health care systems which reflect their values. In the US, the provision of health care is not seen as society's obligation but as a voluntary consumer purchase. In Germany, the system of compulsory health insurance was established in the 19th century as an expression of the belief that social welfare for the poor was essential for national survival in a hostile world, so that the better-off had a shared interest in securing the health of the entire society. From those roots has grown the powerful European support for the value of social solidarity: that all citizens should contribute in proportion to their means to ensure that everyone experiences equal access to health care (and other necessary social services), independent of means or social class. When a society believes in social solidarity, as the UK did after the unifying experience of the Second World War, it sees the logic for an equitable health care system, like the original National Health Service (NHS). Ireland's two-tier health care system manifests values that are closer to Boston than Berlin (or Paris or Copenhagen or Ottawa or London).

In other states, as in Ireland, the development of health care has been a political story. Political reformers have met reversal in the US. The UK and Canada achieved equitable systems only after immense battles with the medical profession. How doctors work and how they are paid has remained an issue of contention in many states. The issue of who owns the health care system – the professional, who delivers care, or the citizen, who funds it – is often still disputed territory.

The UK – the underfunded, embattled NHS

Older people in Ireland recall when the NHS was the flagship of the UK's welfare state. Many Irish people have been employees or patients of the NHS. Since before independence, there have been close links in professional associations and work practices between the two states. Yet defenders of Ireland's two-tier system cite the failures of the NHS as evidence that comprehensive, equitable systems don't work. Such comparisons ignore the successes of the NHS, its underfunding by European standards and the success of other equitable systems.

Founded in 1948, the NHS will remain forever associated with the radical and combative Aneurin (Nye) Bevan, Labour Minister for Health, who famously confronted the militant opposition of the medical profession to achieve its genesis. He won the support of hospital consultants by the generosity of their terms of employment. As he remarked to a friend, "I stuffed their mouths with gold."[2] By curious coincidence, Bevan resigned over the issue of patient charges in the same month, April 1951, that Noel Browne resigned as Minister for Health in Ireland when his relatively modest reform efforts were defeated.

The son of a Welsh miner, Bevan had worked in the mines for 9 years from the age of 13. As a militant trade unionist and socialist campaigner in an era of great unemployment and poverty, he was deeply sceptical of the vested interests of middle class groups such as the medical profession.[3] A formidable orator with a lifelong stammer, as Minister of Health from 1945 to 1951 he compromised to achieve his goal – a comprehensive, universal and free health service. Its delivery was a secondary issue, so he was prepared to make concessions to doctors on how they were paid and employed and on private practice.[4]

The ground work had been laid for a national health service in the Beveridge Report (1942), which proposed a universal health service, funded not from social insurance, as health care had been since 1911, but from taxation. Medical need not insurance status should dictate treatment. Bevan's Conservative predecessor had tried to introduce a form of national health service but so diluted his proposed legislation in response to medical opposition that it was eventually abandoned.[5] When Bevan came into office, the British Medical Association (BMA) had already adopted an entrenched position. He insisted that he would consult but not negotiate with a body outside parliament. The BMA's chief objection to his proposals was that they would ultimately lead to civil service status for salaried general practitioners.

The British Medical Journal, the association's mouthpiece, wrote that their conflict centred on one fundamental principle: "The National Health Insurance Act … leads unmistakably to the eventual establishment of a wholetime State medical service." In a forthcoming plebiscite, the profession would be voting about "their continued existence as a body of free men". Capable of both charm and invective, Bevan accused the leaders of the BMA of "a squalid political conspiracy"[6] to oppose the will of parliament, describing them as a "small body of politically poisoned people".[7] The doctors were not notable for their restraint either. Bevan was described as a "would-be

Fuehrer" pointing a pistol at the doctor's heads.[8] Roland Cockshut, a BMA spokesman, suggested after one negotiating triumph, "Some people say that we must not kick a man when he is down. Why not? He's still breathing, isn't he?"[9]

Charles Hill, the BMA's secretary, claimed doctors would become salaried officers of the state. "Break into that [the doctor-patient relationship], make the doctor not your doctor but the State's doctor; no longer your friend,your advocate and you will have done something to medicine that it will be impossible to repair." As one of Bevan's biographer's pointed out, "coming from the spokesman of a profession which was still insisting on its freedom to buy and sell practices, this was rich".[10] Bevan removed this right, compensating the profession for it.

Bevan found some allies in the medical profession. The *Lancet* editorialised: "the doctor-patient relationship ... can never be wholly satisfactory while the doctor is not only a friend in need but also a friend in need of his patient's money".[11] Bevan told parliament that "nothing should please a good doctor more than to realise that, in future, neither he nor his patient will have any financial anxiety arising out of illness".[12]

In the NHS Act of 1946 and the National Health Service, which came into being on July 5th 1948, Bevan achieved a service in which all citizens could receive free health care from nationalised state-owned hospitals and from general practitioners, who were now paid by the state in a combination of salary and capitation. They could also receive free drugs, dental and other benefits. The service was funded by the exchequer from general taxation. Both general practitioners and hospital consultants retained the right to private practice. Consultants were allowed to retain "pay beds" in NHS hospitals and were given substantial representation on the new management structures.[13]

Bevan was aware that, if the concessions on private practice were not "properly controlled, we can have a two-tier system in which it will be thought that members of the general public will be having worse treatment than those who are able to pay". This was an argument, he said, for full participation in the NHS. He deplored a letter to *The Times* "from a distinguished orthopaedist, who talked about private practice as though it should be the glory of the profession. What should be the glory of the profession is that a doctor should be able to meet his patients with no financial anxiety."[14]

The BMA eventually acquiesced to the NHS, as its support eroded, when Bevan did not insist on a salaried GP service. The government gave a legislative guarantee that there would be no full-time, salaried GP service except under fresh legislation.[15] Within months of its foundation,

97 per cent of the population had enrolled in the NHS and 90 per cent of GPs participated from its inception.[16] There was one fly in the ointment. Bevan and his Ministry had never fully costed the service. The true provision for a free health service must depend on the behaviour of the public and the only way to discover it must be to permit the public to behave, he reportedly told the Chancellor of the Exchequer.[17] Early funding crises led to Bevan's reluctant acceptance of a one shilling charge on prescriptions and his resignation in 1951 over dental and optical charges.[18] The overwhelming majority of services would remain free at the point of use, and these charges were not applied to children, the poor or the elderly.

Opinion polls have continued to show a strong attachment to the NHS as a national institution. Despite frequent funding crises, resulting from tight finance limits set by successive governments, there has been no serious attempt to move away from a system of general tax-based funding.[19] Although a five-year investment plan announced by the Blair Labour government in 2002 was to be funded from increases in employees' and employers' social insurance contributions, this did not signify a shift to a system designed on insurance principles. The government planned to increase health spending from below the EU average at 7.7 per cent of national income to above the average at 9.4 per cent by 2008.[20] A review of the health service commissioned by the Treasury in 2001 conceived that health spending might need to rise to as much as 12.5 per cent of national income by 2022 to respond to the needs of an ageing population.[21] This would be comparable to US health spending as a proportion of national income and to the level of spending envisaged for Ireland, were the 2001 health strategy to be implemented. It was hoped, however, that a better health service with improved preventive care and health promotion might so improve health that its cost would not exceed 10.6 per cent of national income.

This planned investment reflected a realisation that the NHS had been underfunded for decades, which was manifest in long waiting lists, poor quality hospital buildings and in life expectancy, which was below the EU average for women and barely exceeded the average for men.[22] UK public spending on health had been less than the EU per capita average since 1970. Health spending fell in real terms in 1996, the final year of Conservative Party government before the election of Labour under Blair.[23] Irish per capita public health spending has exceeded the UK's since 1999.[24]

The five-year plan envisaged an increase of 10,000 general and acute beds, at least 15,000 more GPs and consultants, 35,000 more nurses and thousands of other health professionals. It promised a drop in waiting times to a maximum of three months by 2008. The government showed an acute awareness of the need to pace its investment, which was lacking in the electorally driven increases in Irish spending over the five years from 1997 to 2002. "Too slow, and we miss the opportunuity to improve the nation's health care, with the risk that people simply give up on the NHS. Too fast, and investment might produce input price inflation, rather than improved output and responsiveness," explained Health Secretary, Alan Milburn. Although it was decided that 7.5 per cent was the optimal annual level of real NHS growth,[25] 9 per cent real growth was expected in 2002.[26]

While waiting lists have been controversial in the UK, they compare favourably with Ireland's. In September 2002, in England, only 6 patients in total had waited longer than 18 months for either inpatient or day treatment. Only 3 patients in every 10,000 people had waited for over a year. This compared to 21 adult patients in every 10,000 people who had waited for over a year in Ireland. In Northern Ireland, however, waiting lists have been worse than in the Republic. In September 2002, Northern Ireland had 9,158 "excess waiters" – people waiting over 18 months, or over 12 months in the case of cardiac surgery – a ratio of 54 patients in every 10,000 people.[27] Northern Ireland suffered badly from cutbacks under the Conservatives and has not had spending increases comparable to England's. In 2002, the UK had fewer acute beds (3.3 per 1,000 people) than the EU average, but marginally more than the Republic.[28]

NHS hospitals are owned by the state and hospital doctors are salaried.[29] In 2002, consultants' salaries ranged from €80,808 to €138,873 (£52,640 to £90,465) with maximum allowances. A few might earn up to €205,071 (£133,585) through a complex system of merit awards.[30] Although pay beds for private patients survived Labour efforts to remove them in the 1970s, in 1998 they constituted just 1 per cent of all beds and, in 2001, private patients were 1 per cent of total NHS admissions. While there is evidence that private patients can gain faster admission to NHS hospitals, the scale of this two-tier access is negligible compared to Ireland's.[31] The vast majority of NHS consultants' private practice takes place in private hospitals.[32] These are predominantly for-profit, offer straightforward elective procedures, of which abortion is the most numerous, and supply fewer than 5 per cent of all beds.[33] Approximately 11 per cent of the population has some form of private insurance cover.

Traditionally, full-time NHS consultants (58 per cent) were not permitted to earn more than 10 per cent of their gross income in private practice. Maximum part-time consultants (25 per cent) received ten-elevenths of their salary for giving up one NHS session per week and were allowed unlimited private practice. Part-time consultants (11 per cent) had a smaller weekly commitment to the NHS.[34]

Debates have been ongoing about the possibility that private earnings might reduce commitment to NHS work. However, a survey in 1992 by the Mergers and Monopolies Commission reported that full-time consultants spent a mean of 53 weekly hours on NHS work and 6 hours on private work.[35] In 2000, the government threatened to ban private practice for consultants for their first seven years, requiring them to work exclusively for the NHS, unless a new contract could be achieved which made private practice rights contingent on meeting NHS service requirements.[36] The influence of these developments was apparent in the 2001 Irish health strategy proposal that new consultant appointees should have a full-time commitment to public patients. In England, the BMA rejected the reformed contract in 2002, although consultants in Northern Ireland and Scotland, who traditionally had fewer private practice opportunities, voted for it. While lengthening their working week, the contract would increase their salary.[37] Health Secretary Alan Milburn responded to the BMA's resistance by proposing to introduce a sub-consultant grade for new appointees.

General practitioners work for the NHS on contract as independent, self-employed professionals and, in 2002, earned an average of €94,590 (£61,618) after expenses.[38] The state is their primary employer, with only an estimated 3 per cent of GP consultations paid for privately.[39] They may not see NHS patients privately. Their contract is negotiated between the BMA and the Department of Health and payment is by a mixture of capitation, allowances and fees. The UK and the Republic have the same proportion of GPs to population – 6 to 10,000 – well below the EU average.[40] While Irish GPs pride themselves on offering a same-day service, waits of seven to ten days are not unusual for routine appointments in the UK, which gives some indication of the unmet demand which a free GP service could reveal in Ireland. But it may also reflect the mode of paying GPs, which might benefit from the incentive effect of a greater element of fee-for-service.

The NHS has undergone a series of administrative reforms. The Conservatives attempted to make health care market-driven, with local health authorities and GP practices being funded as "purchasers" to buy services for patients from hospitals and other community health "providers". Resources and contracts flowed away from some hospitals to others, leading to closures.[41] Providers faced uncertainty and competitive bargaining increased administration costs. Since some GPs were funded to purchase services (fundholders) and others not, inequities in access emerged and the Labour Party pledged to abolish GP fundholding, which they did on entering office.[42]

In power, Labour devolved health policy to the administrations of Scotland, Wales and Northern Ireland, where it became increasingly divergent. The abolition of GP fundholding in Northern Ireland did not take place until 2002. The Labour government rejected the Conservatives' "market ethos", which it said had undermined teamwork and hampered planning, leading to cuts in nurse training and stalled hospital building.[43] In England, Labour retained a split between the commissioning of care and its provision but ended the competitive bargaining process. Scotland abandoned the split altogether in early 2003 and reverted to the more old-fashioned NHS, with health boards both planning and providing services.[44] Northern Ireland had yet to decide its approach.

GPs in England have been required to become members of primary care groups with local nurses and managers – sometimes under the leadership of a nurse – which are expected to evolve from advising on local health needs to taking responsibility for the commissioning of care, when they become Primary Care Trusts (PCTs). The PCTs are intended to control 75 per cent of the NHS budget by 2004 and to commission care from hospitals – public, private or voluntary – run community services and oversee the performance of family doctors.[45]

This English reform represents a complete change in the way in which health care is funded and controlled. It ends the NHS role as a largely monopoly provider of care through state-owned, nationalised hospitals. These will now be given greater freedom of operation and more financial incentives to perform. The government had already encouraged private provision of hospitals for leaseback to the NHS and permitted the building of private hospitals on NHS sites. Health authorities have been much reduced in number and have lost their power to purchase care.

Milburn's reforms have been driven by his belief in the need to remove layers of administration and to let power flow from the bottom up rather than the top down, but he also shares common ground with the Conservatives in valuing market competition in health care. While retaining care free at the point of delivery and based on need not income, the reforms are intended to ensure that "who provides the service becomes less important than the service that is provided".[46]

Milburn could yet be remembered "as the man who destroyed the NHS," one commentator cautioned, when he unveiled his plans.[47] The Scottish chairman of the BMA welcomed Scotland's divergent approach because he believed it would not lead the NHS "into the same abyss" as Milburn had in England.[48]

In the greater freedom of operation which these reforms give to hospitals, they are akin to the reforms proposed by Labour and Fine Gael. In their emphasis on devolved power, they run completely contrary to the current Irish government-sponsored proposals for a centralised and top-down Health Services Executive, which appears to be modelled on the old-style NHS executive.

Canada – where equitable access is a symbol of national identity

Canada has a strongly egalitarian, one-tier system of health care, which delivers results: life expectancy in Canada exceeds the EU average by over a year for women and nearly two years for men.[49] Canadians believe so strongly in equal access to health care that Canada prohibits private insurance for benefits which are already covered by the public health care system. In Canada, as in Ireland, politicians and doctors have engaged in intense battles about access to and control of health care, with the difference that, in Canada, the politicians have prevailed.

While the UK's system is tax-funded and was traditionally publicly delivered, Canada's system, while mainly funded from taxation, is administered through provincial insurance programmes and is privately delivered. The state does not own hospitals and most doctors are self-employed. Canada's system offers universal coverage for medically necessary care. Some provinces offer additional services, such as physiotherapy, as part of their package of benefits.

The system developed as a compromise in battles between the medical profession and the state. Since 1972, every Canadian has been covered by national health insurance for medical and hospital care. The province of Saskatchewan provided a model for the rest of Canada when it was first to introduce public insurance for hospital services in 1947 and first to extend cover to all medical care from 1962, despite a three-week physicians' strike.[50] The doctors sought to reverse legislation which introduced province-wide medical care covered by insurance at a time when one-third of Saskatchewan's population was uninsured. The compulsory insurance scheme was to be supported by taxation and administered by a government commission.

This government control was the sticking point for doctors. That the health service, however funded, should be run by government was anathema to the profession. Under the existing system, insurance prepayment plans, some run by doctors themselves, covered a majority of the population, and nearly half of physicians' incomes came from direct cash payments by patients. Doctors wanted to preserve their independent schemes and, like some doctors in contemporary Ireland, objected to the state being their "sole payer". According to Lord Taylor, a British socialist peer who eventually mediated an end to the strike:

> What they [the doctors] objected to was a universal scheme which would abolish their independent schemes and provide them with only a single pay-master. It was this belief – that they were to be forcibly enrolled as civil servants – rather than any real anxiety about finance which caused them to refuse their co-operation.[51]

A doctor and early supporter of the NHS, he observed that the Saskatchewan government was

> quite ignorant of the pattern of thought of the ordinary medical practitioner. Its members could not conceive of people who did not believe in collective action, who were resolutely opposed to public control, and who believed that even the most benign of civil services would all too soon turn into a dangerous tyranny.

The doctors of Saskatchewan described their fellow-citizens as "recipients of physicians' services" in a declaration issued in response to the announcement of the government's plan. As a Canadian historian of this saga later observed:

> Citizens might object that they are not simply "recipients": not only do they finance the services, they are the sole reason for the services to exist. They might also object ... that they are not permitted to choose, as one of their democratic rights, to make their payments through their elected government.[52]

Since 1944, Saskatchewan had been governed by the Co-operative Commonwealth Federation Party (CCF), "a farmer-dominated party of socialist reformers" – a novel concept in Ireland. Tommy Douglas, CCF premier and Minister for Health, who successfully introduced Canada's first health insurance plan to cover hospital treatment in 1946, believed that people should "be able to get health services just as they are able to get educational services, as an inalienable right of being a citizen of a Christian country."

Taylor succeeded in mediating between government and doctors because he decided that, since they spoke different languages, they should not meet. He engaged in shuttle diplomacy between the two sides until compromise was reached. The strike lasted for twenty-three days and became an international *cause célèbre*. To break the strike, the government recruited 110 doctors from other parts of Canada, the UK and the US. English doctors were airlifted to Saskatchewan. The Saskatchewan premier, Woodrow Lloyd, said the issue in dispute had become "whether the people of Saskatchewan shall be governed by a democratically elected legislature or by a small, highly organised group".

Domestic Saskatchewan newspapers were critical of Lloyd's government but, nationally and internationally, the action of the doctors was condemned. The strike was "a mutiny" (*The Observer*); "wrong" (*Lancet*); "desecrates the Hippocratic oath" (*The Washington Post*). The doctors' action in disobeying "a law duly enacted by a duly elected government of the people" could not be condoned in a law-abiding community (*The Toronto Globe and Mail*).

The strike was eventually settled when it had become clear to the doctors that their support was eroding. They did not achieve their objective although the government made some compromises. Doctors' prepayment plans survived as agencies for paying doctors but were not permitted to continue acting as insurance plans raising premiums from the public. Many doctors left the province but many more remained who had come during the strike or afterwards. In an echo of Bevan's compromise, the government stated that it had no intention of establishing a full-time, salaried government medical service.

A further landmark in the development of the Canadian health service, again achieved despite strenuous opposition from organised medicine, was the passage of the Canada Health Act by the Federal Parliament in 1984. The Act provided for financial penalties for provinces which permitted hospital user charges or physician extra-billing, indicating how seriously Canadians viewed equal access to health care. It strengthened the application of the five principles that govern Canadian health care: universal coverage – 100 per cent of the insured population must receive the same services on the same terms and conditions; comprehensive coverage – the plan must cover all insured health services; reasonable access – there should be no barriers such as user charges or extra billing; portability of coverage – when Canadians moved within Canada and sometimes abroad; and public administration of the insurance plans on a non-profit basis.[53]

Despite ongoing debate about the nature of the Canadian health care system, an accord between the Prime Minister and provincial governors reaffirmed these principles in February 2003, apart from limiting coverage to within Canada.[54] They took their lead from the influential government-appointed Romanow Commission that, in 2002, described the 1984 Act as a "symbol of Canadian identity".[55] The Canadian system continues to provide universal coverage, free at the point of delivery, for all "medically necessary services". Canadians who take out private health insurance may do so only to cover what are regarded as non-medically necessary services such as dental care, physiotherapy and prescription drugs. It is not legally permissible to use private health insurance to obtain medical services that are available from publicly funded hospitals and physicians. The Romanow Commission recommended that the Act should be revised to extend the definition of "medically necessary services" to include diagnostic services, such as MRI and CT scans, now on offer from specialised private clinics, to prevent the privately insured from gaining more rapid access to these forms of diagnosis and, therefore, to treatment.[56]

While Saskatchewan's pioneering medicare programme was insurance based, with payment of insurance premiums securing coverage for a package of benefits, most Canadians now pay for their health care primarily through their federal government tax, which is channelled to the provinces. Two provinces raise funds through individual health care premiums, which are considered an alternative form of taxation.[57] Since most funding now comes through taxation, rather than social insurance payments or insurance premiums, some analysts define Canada's system as a tax- rather than insurance-based system.[58] The administration and purchase of health care is managed by a provincial health insurance plan accountable to provincial government.[59] These plans are not-for-profit and in each province act as the single purchaser of health care either from not-for-profit hospitals, which are generally owned by charitable bodies, religious orders or municipalities, or from physicians, who are mostly self-employed.[60] The plans operate either from within the Ministry of Health or through a separate agency closely linked to the Ministry. The Romanow Commission asserted that "a single-payer system will continue to be a cornerstone of the Canadian system" because it achieved better cost control and more equitable access than a multi-payer, private insurance system.[61]

The Commission was answering growing debate about extending the role for private health insurance in Canada. In a study of this debate, which compared Canada's experience to Ireland's, Thomas Rathwell, a Canadian professor of health administration, argued in 2001 against the extension of private insurance because it "would create a two-tier system whereby those with private insurance would get preferential treatment". He recommended that, if Canada were to extend opportunities for private insurance, "drawing on the Irish experience, the conditions to avoid are the designation of private beds in public hospitals and permitting specialists to have both a public and private practice".[62]

Arguments for private insurance have been driven in part by concern about the level of state investment in health. Historically, Canada has spent very much more on health care than Ireland. Total health spending exceeded 9 per cent of national income from 1989, peaking at 10.1 per cent in 1992. Its share of national income fell as a consequence of cutbacks in the mid-1990s and it was 9.3 per cent in 2001.[63] In 2000, 80 per cent of Canadians believed their system to be in crisis.[64] The Romanow Commission criticised national and provincial governments for "corrosive and divisive debates" about the relative financial responsibilities of federal and provincial governments and called for a "truly national approach to medicare". The 2003 First Ministers' Accord responded with a federal commitment to a five-year Health Reform Fund, which would transfer federal resources to the provinces and provide investment for home care, primary care and better public diagnostic services.

Waiting lists for care remain an issue of concern to Canadians, yet waiting times are in another universe from Ireland's. While a Canada-wide waiting list has yet to be developed, one study reported that, between seeing a specialist and undergoing surgery, Canadians waited on average nine weeks for treatment in 2000. Since Irish public patients who see a specialist and are recommended for surgery must wait three months before they qualify for inclusion on a waiting list, the average Canadian (and this means all Canadians, since there are no public and private patients) would not be considered to have "waited" at all in Ireland. Patients waited on average 16.2 weeks in 2000–2001 between their general practitioner's referral and eventual surgical treatment.[65] In Ireland, the length of time between a GP's referral and seeing a specialist is not counted as waiting.

Doctors in Canada are paid primarily on a fee-for-service basis. Their payments are defined in detailed lists of fees based on negotiations between provincial governments and medical associations. Family doctors' gross incomes averaged €132,958 ($188,601), medical specialists' €162,401 ($230,366) and surgical specialists' €213,872 ($303,377) in 2000/2001.[66] These gross incomes also cover practice expenses, which the Canadian Medical Association estimates range from 26 to 42 per cent of income.[67] Some provinces have sought to limit doctors' earnings by capping them, clawing back earnings above a specified threshold and auditing high earners. Others are looking at changing the model of payment from fee-for-service. Alternative payment plans, such as forms of capitation payment, accounted for 11 per cent of physician remuneration in 2000/2001.[68]

Health care is a highly political issue in Canada, yet, although they may not realise it, Canadians have an enviable system: equitable, accessible, with relatively short waits and good health outcomes. Hostile commentary suggests that Canadians escape to the US for care but, in fact, few Canadians opt for US over Canadian care.[69] Canadians share many Irish concerns – for more accountable administration of the health care system, better evaluation of spending, a better-developed primary care system – but they get it right more often than they appear to appreciate.

Germany – no waiting lists, equal access to care

With many more hospital beds and doctors than Ireland, Germans take their ready access to quality health care for granted. They are accustomed to receiving most of their care without payment. The continental system of compulsory health insurance that was developed in Germany subsequently became the main mechanism for financing health care in France, Belgium and the Netherlands and influenced early attempts at comprehensive systems in other states, including the UK and Canada, which later developed their own models.

Among the member states of the OECD, only the US and Switzerland spend a higher proportion of national income on health care than Germany. Germany has spent close to or above 9 per cent of national income on health care since 1980 and above 10 per cent since 1995. It has spent well above the EU per capita average on health care since the 1960s.[70] Ireland's per capita public spending on health care fell below 40 per cent of the German level in the late 1980s and in 1998 remained at only 65 per cent of the German level. Although Irish per capita health spending has since exceeded the EU average, in 2002 it had still not attained the German level.[71] Many years of higher spending would be required for Irish health care to rival the system Germany established during the Irish decades of neglect.

The German system of compulsory health insurance is described as Bismarckian, after the Chancellor of the Prussian-dominated German Empire who introduced the first national system of social security and compulsory health insurance in 1883.[72] Germany's system has its roots in medieval guilds, which provided mutual aid to their members. Germans are insured by sickness funds, which may be regional but can be company- or employment-based, such as farmers' or miners' funds. The funds receive their income from payroll taxes, levied on employees and employers.[73] Membership of a sickness fund is mandatory up to a certain level of income: in 2000, 74 per cent of the population were mandatory members, 14 per cent voluntary, 9 per cent bought private health insurance and the remainder were state employees, like soldiers, who received free government care. In 1999, there were 453 sickness funds, all non-profit, and 52 private health insurance companies, 25 of which were traded on the stock market.[74]

The German constitution states that living conditions should be of equal standard in the 16 states of the federal republic, so the Federal Ministry of Health sets rules to ensure that all citizens have equal access to care and are covered for the same benefit package. It also sets the terms for the financing and provision of health care.[75] The sickness funds then purchase health care for their members either from hospitals or from physicians' associations. Hospitals can be publicly owned (55 per cent of all beds), private not-for-profit (38 per cent) or private for-profit (7 per cent).[76] All hospital staff are salaried. The physicians' associations pay doctors according to an agreed scale of fees, federally regulated since a threatened doctors' strike in 1913.[77] The associations are legally obliged to provide care, including emergency services, which is evenly distributed both socially and geographically. In 1996, the average doctor's income was between three and five times as much as blue-collar workers and between two and three times as much as white-collar workers.[78]

Unlike in Ireland, general practitioners do not act as the "gatekeepers" to the health care system, through whom patients must be referred for specialist visits. To this and the practice of "doctor-hopping" – shopping around for second opinions at the expense of the insurance company – is attributed some of the high cost of the German health care system. To encourage more integrated provision of services, the German government has proposed to give GPs a greater gatekeeping role.[79]

Germans pay few fees directly, contributing a fraction of prescription charges, some small hospital charges and some dental charges. Many categories of patient, including children and those on low incomes, are exempt from charges. Additional patient payments, which were introduced as cost-cutting measures in the mid-1990s, were subsequently reversed in 1998. A proposal in 2000 to set global limits for spending by sickness funds provoked such fierce opposition from physicians – who threatened to put patients on waiting lists, hitherto unknown except for transplants – that it was dropped.[80]

Since reunification, German health care has had to provide equal services to the poorer East, which, coupled with lower health insurance contributions due to higher unemployment, provoked a financing crisis.[81] Whereas in France the social insurance system has been increasingly supported by general taxation, in Germany taxes have contributed a declining share to health spending – 10 per cent in 1995, representing government payment for care for state employees and welfare recipients and capital investment in hospitals. Statutory insurance contributes nearly 70 per cent of funding and private insurance and out of pocket payments the remainder.[82] Statutory health insurance again recorded deficits in 2001 and the first half of 2002, provoking the government to raise the income threshold for mandatory insurance (thereby preventing some higher earners from opting for private insurance); to freeze hospital and doctors' remuneration; and to act to control drug costs.[83]

Germany has a very well-endowed system: 10 general practitioners for every 10,000 people compared to 6 in Ireland; nearly twice as many practising doctors overall in proportion to population; 6.4 acute care beds for every 1,000 people compared to Ireland's 3; an average bed occupancy rate of 80 per cent. German life expectancy for both men and women is marginally above the EU average.[84]

France – ranked number one for health system performance

When the World Health Organisation ranked health care systems' performances in 1997, France came in number one.[85] There are no waiting lists for treatment in France. Women live longer than in any other OECD state except Japan. With a life expectancy at birth of 82.5 years, they live over three years longer than Irish women.[86] The French system, while complex, achieves equity or close to it, and has many similarities to the German system.

But no system is perfect. The French remain concerned about how to control health spending, which consumes 9.5 per cent of national income, only exceeded by the US, Switzerland and Germany, and rivalled by Ireland in 2002.[87] Hospitals face a nursing shortage.[88] And the life expectancy for men (75 years) ranks 11th in the OECD – the same as in the UK, although over a year higher than in Ireland. One study attributed this mortality rate to factors outside the health care system, such as a high incidence of AIDS and violent deaths from suicide and road accidents, although tobacco and alcohol consumption also played a role.[89]

In a study of waiting lists, Liz McManus of the Labour Party attributed the French success to the number of beds in hospitals – 4.2 per 1,000 population in 2000 compared to under 3 in Ireland. Paris has nearly 10 acute beds per 1,000 population, way above the French average, in contrast to Dublin, which has below the Irish average.[90] The French have concentrated their beds in their national centre of expertise, whereas Ireland has dispersed beds throughout the state and starved its national centre. With bed occupancy rates at around 75 per cent, McManus concluded the French had "over capacity built into their system".[91] All planned surgery is arranged under a booking system in which the patient is given a date for surgery immediately when it is prescribed, although this may involve a few months' wait.

In France as in Germany, health care is funded by social insurance through workers' and employers' contributions. The social security system was established in 1945, building on occupational health insurance schemes introduced in the 1920s. The powerful French left in the post-war years preferred this system, which gave the trade unions a role, to a tax-funded and state-controlled system like the NHS.[92] Compulsory social insurance covers 99.5 per cent of the population.[93] Marginalised groups such as asylum seekers have their costs met by the state. Social insurance contributions are channelled into 18 social insurance funds (the largest of which covers four-fifths of the population).[94] The funds have traditionally been governed by union and employer representatives and administer benefits.

Patients pay general practitioners and specialists outside hospitals directly, for which they are reimbursed by social security for some but not all of the cost – the remainder is met by supplementary insurance offered by private insurers or non-profit *mutuelles*. In practice, virtually all health care is covered by insurance. On average, working households spend 20 per cent of their gross income on health.[95] Under a universal health insurance scheme introduced in 2000, the poorest households do not have to pay fees up front.

The social security system is bureaucratic, with administration costs accounting for over 10 per cent of the funds' out-goings, mostly due to "the refund of endless small sums paid directly to doctors by their patients". Opponents of continental-style social insurance cite these administrative costs as a reason for avoiding such a health care funding system. However, this is not a prerequisite of the system, contrasting "with the system applying in some Canadian provinces where doctors are paid directly by the public insurance scheme, which permits substantial savings"[96] – generally, this is also how voluntary insurance operates in Ireland.

French hospitals can be publicly or privately run. Private hospitals account for a third of all beds[97] and may be for profit or not-for-profit. Hospitals (public or private) that participate in the public service are financed by overall global budgets, which are paid by the insurance funds, while those that do not participate charge daily rates and fees.[98] Public hospital staff have the status of civil servants.[99] Private patients may be treated in public hospitals.

A hybrid system has evolved in which approximately one-third of France's doctors are both self-employed and work for the government; another third work for the government only; and the last third are solely self-employed. Pay varies widely, with radiologists, cardiologists and gastroenterologists on earnings comparable to those of company directors,[100] salaried public hospital doctors earning from €45,000 to €83,000 in 2002 and doctors in university hospitals earning some 50 per cent more. While doctors in university hospitals seldom conduct private practice, salaried doctors in public hospitals may do so provided it is strictly limited to two half days a week or treatment of patients in up to four beds.[101] Patients may therefore pay privately for treatment but, given the absence of waiting lists, there is no apparent concern in France that this causes two-tier access. As in Ireland, public hospitals have a virtual monopoly of emergency treatment, do most major operations, most research and treat the elderly and poor, while private hospitals "cream off" profitable areas of minor surgery and frequently transfer patients with complications or life-threatening conditions to public hospitals.[102] The sickness funds agree payments for doctors in private practice in negotiation with their unions.

General practitioners do not play a gatekeeper role to the health care system. A minority of GPs are paid by capitation, the majority are paid on a fee-for-service basis, according to a schedule determined by the Ministry of Health. Since the French can choose their doctors and there is competition for income between abundant doctors, half of whom are specialists, the volume of procedures offered and of medicines prescribed is high. France vies with Japan and the US for the world's highest per capita consumption of pharmaceuticals.[103] France had 30 practising physicians for every 10,000 people in 1998 compared to 20 in Ireland.[104] Doctors prescribe more "in response to implicit pressure from their patients", one study commented, which "makes it very difficult to control expenditure".[105] Patients may reclaim the cost of drugs. One assessment found that nearly 15 per cent of drugs examined were of "insufficient medical benefit". Other states have attempted to control drug costs by insisting on the use of generic drugs, which accounted for only 8 per cent of drug sales in France in 1999, compared to nearly 70 per cent in the UK,[106] but the French have since begun to encourage their greater use.

During the 30 years of economic growth after the Second World War, rising wages and employment provided an increasing fund to finance medical expenditure. However, in the economic downturn of the 1970s, expenditures continued to rise without increases in income to fund them, resulting in steadily worsening finances for the health insurance funds during the 1980s and early 1990s.[107] Following three consecutive years in which income from social security failed to match expenditure, causing health care to require greater funding from general taxation, the French government decided to reform the social security system.[108] The 1996 Juppé reform required amendments to the Constitution so that parliament could set targets for spending and reimbursements by the insurance funds, a significant shift of power from the funds to the state.[109] The setting of a ceiling for doctors' fees antagonised the profession and the main medical union refused to agree fees with the funds.[110] Growth in health spending slowed but picked up again from 1998, leading the OECD to comment that doctors and patients might be reverting to "their previous habits of over-prescribing and over-consuming".[111] A new tax, the RDS (reimbursement of social debt), was introduced to bridge the gap between the insurance funds' income and expenditure – the *trou de la Sécu* or "social security hole". The CSG (general social contribution) levied on all income, not just salaries, replaced most of the employee component of social insurance contributions and came to account for one-third of insurance funds' revenues. Although the growing contribution of taxation to funding health care leads some commentators to say that France is moving from a Bismarckian system, the important distinction remains that the new taxes have been earmarked for health.[112] Parliament's targets were overrun following the Juppé reforms, so the government further required the largest health insurance fund to report regularly on meeting targets and propose remedial measures where necessary. In

2001 the employers' federation, Medef, ended its role in managing the social insurance system, arguing that it was not the role of a modern entrepreneur to be involved in public health management, especially as it had no say over how contributions were used.

While the politics of health in France remain complex and controversial, the French like their health care system. A Eurobarometer survey in 1997 showed that two-thirds of the French population were fairly satisfied with their health care compared to 40 per cent in the UK and 20 per cent in Italy.[113]

Denmark – a traditionally public system which is turning to the private sector

Strategists in the Irish Department of Health like to look to the Danish health care model.[114] Denmark is like Ireland and the UK in funding health from general taxation – in contrast to other European states with compulsory health insurance systems, which the Department does not favour. Denmark shares other characteristics with Ireland: a shortage of nurses, chiefly due to low pay and poor working conditions; and a failure of life expectancy to keep pace with the increase in the European average.[115] Because Denmark has consistently invested above the EU per capita average in health and yet achieved poor increases in life expectancy, the World Health Organisation ranked its health system performance as worst in the EU in 1997.[116]

This assessment is disputed by Danes – and with good cause. The WHO ranked Ireland's under-resourced and inaccessible system well above the much better endowed and accessible Danish system, apparently reflecting a WHO view that Ireland was doing well considering how little it had invested in care. Although waiting lists have recently become a political issue in Denmark, Danes have generally been very content with their care. A 1998 Eurobarometer survey showed them to be the most satisfied Europeans, while, in 1999, 76 per cent of Danes were satisfied with their health care, fourth among the EU states.[117]

Defenders of the Danish system point out that it offers a high degree of equity, has expanded services in many areas, such as cataract surgery or care for the dying, that offer improved quality of life rather than prolonged life, and provides care for the elderly which is superior to many other European states'. They argue that mortality is a poor measure of a health system's performance.[118] However, Denmark has responded to its disappointing life expectancy performance with a

345

national programme aimed at improving public health and reducing social inequality in health. GPs are paid for preventive consultations in which they discuss patients' diet and lifestyle.[119]

Denmark, like the UK, delivers equitable access to care within a tax-funded system. It has a deep-seated culture of egalitarianism and support for state solutions to social needs. The roots of the welfare state date to the 18th century, when this constitutional monarchy began to employ doctors with responsibility for public health and the care of the poor, believing a large, healthy and industrious population to be crucial to the nation's wealth. Since the Second World War, in a political system which values consensus, Danish political parties on all sides have supported access to health care independent of ability to pay.[120] Although other states which have achieved equitable access to care permit its delivery by private hospitals or self-employed doctors, and the UK is now encouraging diverse providers of care to the state-funded system, Denmark has up to very recently regarded the growth of private medicine as a potential threat to the public system's delivery of equitable care. Even the Danish Medical Association has not supported calls for greater privatisation.[121]

For the individual patient, most health care is free. There are some payments for drugs, dentists (free to the age of 18) and other therapies. A small voluntary health insurance scheme dominated by one large not-for-profit company exists to cover these. While private hospitals provide less than 1 per cent of beds, voluntary insurance has begun to cover treatment in these hospitals for those who want to avoid public waiting lists.[122] There are, however, no private beds in public hospitals.[123]

Most doctors (60 per cent) are salaried hospital employees with salaries including allowances in 2002 which ranged from €40,389 (300,000 Danish krone) for a junior doctor starting out to €87,996 (653,612 Danish krone) for a consultant and €99,626 (740,000 Danish krone) for a "managing consultant".[124] General practitioners are paid by a combination of capitation and fee-for-service, from which they must meet their practice costs because they are not state employees. Before costs, they earn an income comparable to that of a consultant.[125]

Denmark has a highly decentralised system of government with many powers devolved to the counties, which both finance and deliver health care – the model that Ruth Barrington proposed for Ireland. Health care is financed from state, county and municipal taxes and accounts for 70 per cent of councils' spending. Councils own and run hospitals and pay doctors and other health professionals. One disadvantage of this decentralisation is that there have been uneven standards of care around the country, an effect which central government is attempting to ameliorate by offering waiting time guarantees and free choice of hospitals.[126] Waiting times, however, compare favourably with those of Ireland. In 2000, only 7 per cent of patients had to wait more than three months for treatment.[127]

After waiting times became an issue in the 2001 general election, the new centre-right coalition government guaranteed that patients who were not treated within two months in the public sector would have the right to treatment in private facilities or abroad.[128] This has led to growth in small clinics contracting to sell treatments to the publicly funded system and to growing opportunities for publicly salaried doctors to supplement their salaries with these additional earnings.[129] Hitherto, only a very limited number of public hospital doctors chose to avail of their unrestricted right to treat the privately insured in their spare time.[130] The new government's willingness to channel public funds into a private sector, staffed by public hospital consultants, has echoes of developments in Ireland and could potentially undermine standards of public sector care, which has been at the heart of the Danish system. However, the government's rhetoric has remained committed to the welfare state ideals of a tax-based and universal health care system.[131]

New Zealand – the cautionary tale of disappointing market reforms

New Zealand's story has acquired the status of a cautionary tale of health care reform. New Zealand, like Ireland, has two-tier access to hospital care – albeit not in public hospitals – and charges the majority of patients for GP visits. It spends less than Ireland on health. Another former British colony, it too has retained attributes of the British health system prior to the foundation of the NHS. Attempts to introduce market efficiencies in the provision of care in the 1990s caused deteriorating standards, were hugely unpopular and were reversed at the end of the decade. Life expectancy is longer than in Ireland, however, a year and a half longer for both men and women. New Zealand's system shares many of the shortcomings of Ireland's system and its more recent efforts to reform primary care have been influential in the development of the Irish primary care strategy.

New Zealand achieved full constitutional independence in 1947, before the foundation of the NHS, and never sought to establish a comprehensive NHS-style system, free at the point of use for all services. It has a predominantly tax-funded health care system, in which hospital inpatient treatment has been free since 1938, but waiting lists for public care have encouraged the growth of private health insurance to purchase care in private hospitals. While GP care is subsidised for lower income patients and children under six, GPs may set their own fees.[132] Just as in Ireland, primary care is dominated by private, general medical practice and "charges are seen as a significant barrier to accessing primary medical care".[133] Prescription drugs are subsidised so that the maximum a patient must pay is NZ$15 (€7). There are no official figures on GPs' earnings but, because around 60 per cent of their income comes from direct patient payments, which affords GPs great independence from the state, the New Zealand government has shared Ireland's difficulties in developing a comprehensive, population-based approach to primary care.

New Zealand, like Ireland, must recover from past underinvestment in health care. In 1987, New Zealand spent only 5.7 per cent of national income on health and, while this has since grown to around 8 per cent, New Zealand's per capita health spending remains below the EU average and has been exceeded by Ireland's since 1993.[134] Irish per capita national income overtook New Zealand's in the late 1990s.

In 1991, the National Party government initiated radical health care reform in a political climate that promoted market solutions to social problems. In a purchaser/provider split, then also in vogue in UK Conservative politics, a national health funding authority purchased care from competing hospitals and community services, which were expected to perform as businesses. A report by management consultants Arthur Andersen had suggested that up to 32 per cent of expenditure on hospitals could be saved by shorter stays and better management.[135] Managers were recruited from outside the public service. It was not a happy experiment. Childhood immunisations fell by 10 per cent between 1996 and 1998 and the number of women requiring readmission to hospitals after childbirth increased from 6 to 10 per cent between 1996 and 1999.[136] Competing for their funding, providers of care ceased to cooperate and share information.[137] In 1998, 90 per cent of New Zealanders thought their system needed fundamental change.[138]

The Labour-Alliance coalition government, elected in 1999 under Prime Minister Helen Clark, ended the purchaser/provider split in the hospital sector, while retaining it in primary care, and devolved responsibility for health care to district health boards, with a majority of elected members, going in the diametrically opposite direction to the proponents of the abolition of health boards in Ireland. The 2000 health strategy stated that "the commercial focus of health care in recent years" with competition "for the largest share of the health dollar" was undermining public trust in the health system.[139]

The district health boards own and operate hospitals and are responsible for purchasing primary care for their local population from primary health organisations (PHOs), which provide general practice, nursing and community services in a model similar to the primary care teams envisaged for Ireland. While the Irish strategy has not proposed a system for payment of GPs, in New Zealand it is proposed that these PHOs will be paid a capitation fee per enrolled patient.[140] The level of the capitation fee and the level of payment required from the patient vary with the patient's income. However, it is envisaged that capitation payments will rise, as resources permit, so that every patient eventually has low-cost access to care.[141]

The New Zealand government has been targeting public hospital waiting lists, growth in which provoked 51 per cent of New Zealanders to take out private health insurance in 1990. The proportion of privately insured has since fallen to 33–37 per cent, as waiting times have improved. Despite a government goal that no one should wait more than six months for either their first specialist assessment or an elective procedure, the number of people waiting and the length of waits grew rather than reduced in 2002. While there is no private practice in public hospitals, private insurance purchases care in private hospitals. The majority of public hospital doctors are salaried but may significantly supplement their income by private practice in private hospitals. In 2002, public salaries ranged from €50,000 ($100,000) to €79,700 ($159,578),[142] while in 2001 incomes in excess of €125,000 ($250,000) were not uncommon for specialists with substantial or exclusively private practices.[143]

New Zealand's appetite for health system reform has not been matched by a sense of urgency about removing financial barriers to access – another attribute which it shares with contemporary Ireland.

The United States – where health care is a marketable commodity

The United States is distinguished by having the most expensive and technologically advanced health care system in the world and yet failing to provide adequate care for a sizeable minority of its population. An estimated 43 million people including 10 million children – nearly 16 per cent of the population – were uninsured in 2000. These were mainly the working poor, who must either pay for their care or go to public hospitals' emergency departments, which may not legally refuse treatment. They received less and lower quality medical care.

The wealthiest state in the OECD apart from Luxembourg, the US consistently spends about 13 per cent of its national income on health, compared to an EU average of 8 per cent. Total per capita health spending is over twice the EU average. Yet life expectancy for men and women is lower than the European average. Canada, in contrast, spends just over 9 per cent of national income on health care, delivers equitable access and has a life expectancy that comfortably exceeds the European average.[144]

Whereas European states have opted for systems funded by general taxation or compulsory social insurance, the US, like Ireland, has a hybrid system that combines tax funding with private voluntary insurance. The state pays for less than half of US health care. Individuals and companies pay for the rest in private fees or by private voluntary insurance. Government schemes covering the elderly and disabled (Medicare) and the poor (Medicaid) finance care for 25 per cent of the population and constitute 40 per cent of health spending. Medicaid covers only 40 per cent of those below the poverty line and coverage varies with state of residence, so that very poor people are denied coverage in some states. The rest of the population is either covered by employer-provided medical benefit schemes, which not all employers offer, by hugely expensive private insurance or remains uninsured. The annual cost of employment-based schemes in 2001 ranged between €2,245 and €4,490 ($2,000 and $4,000), including employer and employee contributions.[145]

How Americans regard their health care system depends on who they are. The many tiers of care go beyond the four of Medicaid, Medicare, uninsured and insured. With competing profit-motivated insurance companies, access to care differs from insurer to insurer, state to state and year to year.[146] Medicare patients are not fully covered for all treatments and for prescription drugs, which are costly. Medicaid is also often inadequate and, since its rates of payment are very low, doctors who agree to accept Medicaid patients may be less qualified. The minority of the population who vote generally have good health care. Politicians receive campaign funds from political action committees linked to lobby groups, an estimated 500 of which represent health care interests.[147]

This inadequate system has persisted despite generations of efforts to effect change, culminating in the 1990s with President Clinton's ill-fated reforms. Efforts to introduce compulsory social insurance began as early as 1910, when they failed as they had in Ireland. At that time, the rich paid for care provided by self-employed physicians and voluntary, not-for-profit hospitals. The poor received care as charity from public hospitals, staffed by medical students, and the middle class struggled in between. Voluntary health insurance, provided by employers and untaxed by the state, emerged to fill the gap. Unions preferred to bargain for health benefits as part of employees' remuneration rather than to lobby for a state scheme.[148] President Truman sought to introduce compulsory health insurance in the late 1940s but was defeated by massive opposition from health insurers and the American Medical Association (AMA), who labelled the proposal "government controlled socialised medicine". Medicare and Medicaid were introduced in the 1960s. Senator Ted Kennedy espoused the cause of national health insurance in the 1970s and also failed.[149]

From the 1970s, employers and insurance companies sought to control costs through so-called "managed care" by bodies such as health maintenance organisations (HMOs), which generally paid doctors a salary or a fixed sum for each patient, rather than on a fee-for-service basis, and offered restricted patient care. By 1997, 92 per cent of physicians had managed care contracts, generally accounting for some half of their incomes.[150] In the 1980s, many employers began to pay their employees' medical costs directly rather than by buying insurance for them. Community rating collapsed, so insurers no longer charged uniform rates by cross-subsidising from the young and healthy to the old and sick. Insurance became so expensive that more employers opted out of providing medical benefit. This and reduced eligibility for Medicaid led to growing numbers of uninsured people.[151] This was the backdrop in the 1990s to President Clinton's reform proposals, which sought to combine German-style compulsory workplace insurance with managed care, retaining for-profit health insurers, HMOs and physician practices.

President Clinton's immensely complex package alienated a broad spectrum of interests and failed to win the support of Congress.[152] Some doctors and the middle class insured feared that the scheme would force them into managed care organisations. The health insurance industry sponsored television advertisements that played on these fears. The AMA vigorously opposed the reform, although other medical associations supported it. Small and medium businesses opposed the scheme, because it required employers to provide insurance for their employees. Big business feared that the savings they had made by managed care would be used to subsidise the uninsured. Conservatives attacked it as another example of "socialised medicine".[153] Ironically, after President Clinton's defeat, managed care grew to dominance.

Some of the more liberal states, such as Hawaii, Massachusetts, Oregon and Minnesota, subsequently sought with mixed success to address the problem of the growing numbers of uninsured by measures like expanding Medicaid or offering affordable insurance.[154] States are, however, barred by federal law from regulating or insisting on employee health benefits. Conservative states, on the other hand, have set eligibility levels so low that many of the poor do not qualify for Medicaid. Since 1997, a new federal programme known as CHIPS (Children's Health Insurance Programme) assists states to provide for uninsured children but has reached only three million of the ten million uninsured.[155]

Of the 13 per cent of national income that goes to health care, it has been estimated that the profits of insurance companies and medical care organisations account for 1 to 2 percentage points – 1 to 2 per cent, that is, of the entire income of the United States.[156] While only 13 per cent of US hospitals are run for-profit, with the remainder being voluntary non-profit (55 per cent), public (27 per cent) or federal (5 per cent), for-profit managed care organisations now dominate American health care.[157] They have, however, become less rigid. Preferred Provider Organisations (PPOs), which restrict patients to specific providers but do not generally otherwise manage their care, now exceed HMOs.

In a culture in love with high technology and which pays higher physician fees for higher tech medicine, competition to offer high tech care drives up costs. In the mid-1990s one county in California with a population of 2.5 million had more MRI scanners than all of Canada, with the consequence that MRI units advertised for business.[158] Doctors have traditionally been self-employed and the highest paid professionals in the US, with an average income in the mid-1990s that was ten times that of the average production worker.[159] In 2001 specialists earned from €225,000 to €1,123,000 ($200,000 to $1 million) with cardio-vascular surgeons earning a median income of €515,000 (US$459,000) and oncologists and anaesthetists approximately €314,000 (US$280,000). Doctors in primary care earned a median of €162,800 (US$145,000).[160]

Although Ireland and the US both have hybrid tax and insurance systems, the US discriminates between patients on a far more exotic scale. Yet citizens who cannot afford care have the option of free public hospital emergency room treatment, while Irish people who cannot afford care have no free option, unless they need acute hospital treatment. Supporters of Boston in the "Boston versus Berlin" debate may envy the US its low taxes but no one seriously advocates that

Ireland should emulate its health care system. The dominance of the profit motive and the huge profit margin in US health care should give pause for thought to Irish government supporters of the privatisation of the VHI and the introduction of for-profit hospitals, run by US and other international health care corporations.

It comes down to values in the end. "Cherish your commitment to solidarity and equity. Cherish your universal coverage and relatively low costs. You may not realise how good your systems really are": so one US author advised Europeans at the end of a gloomy review of the failings of his own health system.[161] But Ireland is not committed to solidarity, equity or universal coverage. Five of the seven states whose systems are reviewed in this chapter – Canada, France, Germany, the UK and Denmark – can claim that commitment. The remaining two – New Zealand and the US – have inequities, which are comparable to our own in the case of New Zealand and on an altogether different scale in the US.

Ireland shares with many states concerns about shortages of nurses, expensive medical technology and drugs, ageing population and pressure on hospital services. Where Ireland differs is in its two-tier system of access and care, its long hospital waiting lists for the bottom tier, its financial barriers to accessing primary care, its medical hierarchy and staffing system that compound a shortage of doctors, its virtual absence of preventive medicine and its high levels of cancer and heart disease, resulting in a lower than average life expectancy. While states with better health care have invested at above average rates for decades, Ireland is grappling with the after-effects of decades of underinvestment. Although some states, such as Canada and Denmark, consider they have waiting list problems, Ireland's are in another league.

The level of health spending matters. Good quality health care does not come cheap. But high health spending does not ensure good quality, accessible care and good health outcomes, as illustrated by the experience of the US. The manner in which health systems are organised and accessed remains critical.

Citizens of some states have shown a greater willingness to spend on health care, which may be related to how they contribute to it. Insurance-based systems are generally more responsive to patients' needs than tax-based systems, which are more likely to ration care. Thus, health spending has been consistently high in France and Germany and tightly controlled in the UK. Private or social insurance explicitly defines the basket of health care benefits that it covers. The tax-funded NHS does not specify an explicit list of guaranteed services, a shortcoming also of the Irish public health care system.[162] Yet Denmark, which does not define benefits either, has delivered relatively high health spending.

Some states have publicly funded health care systems, which deliver care through publicly funded institutions where doctors are salaried. Some states' public systems purchase care from private hospitals and self-employed doctors. Some do both. Some states fund through insurance, some through tax. All these arrangements can deliver equitable care. Outside Ireland, very few developed states permit private practice in public hospitals. In the UK and France, it is extremely limited and subject to considerable control in an effort to avoid preferential access.[163] Ireland's institutionalised two-tier public hospital system, in which private practice is provided for in consultants' public contracts and private patients gain preferential access to designated private beds, whatever their relative need, is quite exceptional and leads to quite exceptional inequity.

The US experience discloses that the dominance of the profit motive in insurance and managed care makes for expensive health care systems, in which patient care may suffer. At the other extreme, all Canada's hospitals are not-for-profit. In Germany, the for-profit sector is very small indeed. Private not-for-profit hospitals play a role in providing care in many states.

It would appear that no system of health administration is ideal. In France, the state is taking more centralised control. In England, power is being devolved to primary care organisations. In New Zealand, district health boards dominated by locally elected representatives have reappeared. Experiments with markets continue in England and have largely been abandoned in New Zealand and Scotland. Irish reformers will ultimately have to have the courage of their convictions about what suits this small state. There is no universally acknowledged template for a superior system of administration.

Who owns health care? The citizen, the state or the doctors? It was the issue of state control and employment, the fear of civil service status, which provoked doctors to strike in Canada in 1962 and to confront Bevan in the UK in the 1940s. Yet many doctors in many states appear to derive professional satisfaction as salaried state employees. The self-employed GPs of the UK in effect work for state contracts.

There was a time when health care was primarily a private enterprise, which doctors could control. The rising cost of care and the rising expectations of patients have left that era behind. Since doctors do not fund health care, they cannot hope to control it. In the US, they came under the control of for-profit managed care organisations, by no means a preferred destiny to control by the state, albeit somewhat less rigid from the late 1990s. In Germany, the state has frozen their remuneration. The French have put a ceiling on it. Canadian provinces have variously capped, clawed back and audited doctors' earnings. Like any trade union or professional group, doctors will inevitably find themselves fighting for improved conditions of employment. That is quite another matter from dictating to the state or their fellow citizens about how they should access care, which doctors attempted and failed to do in Canada and the UK and succeeded in doing in Ireland in the 1950s and the 1970s.

There are many international options for reform: in how the health system is funded and administered, how care is purchased and delivered. But the central anomalies in Irish care remain two-tier hospital care and financial barriers to primary care. Designing an accessible, equitable Irish system will require change in how doctors relate to the health care system and in how they are paid and employed. There is more than one model to achieve that. But there remains the question of what values we Irish espouse as a society. Do we perceive health care as a consumer purchase or do we believe in social solidarity – that as a community we will no longer stand by while our neighbours suffer needless ill-health and premature death?

PART FIVE
A HEALTHIER STATE

17

A HEALTHIER STATE

"No society can legitimately call itself civilised if a sick person is denied medical aid because of lack of means."
— Aneurin Bevan.[1]

"It is inevitable that people will demand that health care should be available as a human right, and that care be provided on a basis of need rather than on an ability to pay."
— James Deeny, former chief medical officer of the Department of Health, reflecting when in his eighties.[2]

This book began with the enquiry "why not reform?" Why has it been that, despite the obvious need for accessible health care, despite the plans of men like James Deeny in the 1940s, despite the great successes elsewhere of reformers like Aneurin Bevan, Ireland has retained a shameful system in which access to care is determined by means not need?

The barriers to reform were readily apparent in the early decades of the state: the Catholic Church with its antagonism to state control of health care and its obsession with controlling sexual morality; the medical profession with its fear of state employment and its desire to retain private fees. But the Church supported reform attempts in the 1970s and put the case for a universal health care system from the 1980s.

The same cannot be said of the medical profession. There have been exceptions, doctors such as James Deeny, Noel Browne and James Ryan who championed reform in the 1940s and 1950s, the GP and political activist John McManus who has campaigned for reform since the 1970s and UCD's dean of medicine, Muiris FitzGerald, who has argued for change in how hospital doctors work. But organised medicine, the official voice of the profession as represented by the IMO and by the IHCA in particular, has been a continuing obstacle to reform. In 2002, Finbarr Fitzpatrick, the IHCA's singularly effective frontman, could still state with seeming confidence that if the Minister for Health insisted on a public-only contract for new consultant appointees, "we will use all our influence to make sure nobody takes it and it doesn't become a reality. We might fail but I am confident that we won't."

As with its politicians, a society gets the doctors it deserves. Doctors work in the system that society condones. They are not its creators. When the government of Saskatchewan won its battle to introduce compulsory medical insurance, some doctors emigrated, more came to stay. It is striking how the experience of working in Canada has influenced many Irish medical advocates for reform, such as John Barton, the cardiologist from Ballinasloe, who described its system as "beautiful" and Sean Conroy, regional manager with the Western Health Board, who has compared the Irish public/private divide to a "caste system".

James Deeny pointed out that would-be reformers are stuck with the existing cadre of trained medical personnel – "You cannot take them out and shoot them"[3] – but that does not mean that medical politics should determine national politics. Politicians intent on reform have prevailed over medical opposition in other countries – and in Ireland. With the 1953 Health Act, a Fianna Fáil government introduced free hospital care for the majority of the population despite the opposition of organised medicine. It was in the evolution of national politics in the years that followed that reform became derailed. Seán Lemass may have promised Noel Browne "we'll try to give you a good health service" in 1951 but in the 1960s, under Lemass's leadership, Fianna Fáil adopted the comfortable and comforting philosophy that "a rising tide lifts all the boats" and became beholden to the new rich. It would pursue incremental reforms demanded by the higher paid, such as the extension of eligibility for free hospital care, but no longer would it risk confrontation with the medical profession or disturbing the interests of its wealthy backers. So universal free hospital maintenance offered by Charles Haughey in 1979 was rapidly followed in 1981 by his government's agreement to unlimited private practice for consultants on public salaries, which undermined the purported universality of the system. Universal eligibility for free consultant care, introduced in 1991, was equally undermined by the new system of bed designation which ring-fenced at least 20 per cent of the beds in public hospitals for the use of private patients, whatever their condition or the length of public waiting lists.

The political system was a barrier to reform, "if not the major one", concluded Miriam Hederman O'Brien, chairwoman of the Commission on Health Funding, after she watched the shelving of the Commission's 1989 report, which had recommended the introduction of a common waiting list for public and private patients. Reform would take time and the attention span of politics was too short, she feared. Barry Desmond, Labour's most controversial incumbent in Health, observed that for reform to happen "you really have to come into government in the first month with the bill almost drafted". Bevan had that advantage when he became Minister of Health in the UK in 1945 – a blueprint for reform from the Beveridge Report, an earlier attempt by a Conservative Minister, even a medical opposition which had shown its hand, so that he began his reforming efforts with the battle lines already drawn.

Not since the 1950s has an Irish government started out with a comprehensive blueprint for health care reform. In its attempts to please every category of voter, Fianna Fáil has preferred short-term winning strategies – keeping county hospitals open, extending medical cards to over-70-year-olds, targeting waiting lists – to the electorally riskier course of embarking on genuine reform. Fine Gael, a lesser version of a catch-all party and grappling with an apparently terminal identity crisis, appears equally incapable of developing a consistent health care policy. Its strategy to end two-tier care in 2002 would have preserved the distinction between public and private patients and continued to permit public hospital consultants to conduct private practice off-site. Labour has espoused reform in opposition, but, in government in conservative coalitions, Labour Ministers have not been distinguished by their espousal of reform – not since Brendan Corish met defeat at the hands of the hospital consultants in 1974. Outside the Dáil, although ICTU has traditionally supported a comprehensive national health service, in the mid-1990s social partnership institutions became a voice for organised and higher paid employees who were members of the VHI, rather than for the low paid on the margins who could not afford GP care. Not until the voluntary sector gained a voice in social partnership did access to medical cards become a priority issue.

How is it that the need for health care as a right, which was apparent to James Deeny in the 1940s and still apparent to him in his eighties, 40 years later, could so fail to engage the majority of Irish politicians and the Irish political system? What does this say about Irish society? Political scientists speak of Ireland's "exceptional" politics: the very large percentage of voters who support parties of the right and centre; the very small percentage support for the left; how on closer examination Irish political parties do not fit the standard European left-right definitions; that Fianna Fáil's radical populist past is not shared by other European conservative parties. From the perspective of health care reform, the analogy with the US is compelling. In both Ireland and the US, the political party system has its roots in a civil war, the major parties are catch-all coalitions of interests and in neither country has there been political space for the emergence of a major social democratic party that would champion rights such as equitable access to health care.[4]

Is this sufficient explanation for the complacency of Irish society in the face of the neglect of medical need? The US has a society which believes in individualism, in private provision, in untrammelled capitalism. What does Irish society believe in? The Boston versus Berlin debate has crystallised the sense that Ireland is now at a crossroads and must decide if it will take the European road of higher taxes to fund better social provision or the American road of lower taxes and continued inadequate social provision. The stalling of the boom since 2001 has reawakened atavistic fears, deep-seated insecurities that paralyse this society in indecision about its future. What if the sense of choice is an illusion? What if the multinationals go, the jobs evaporate and emigration begins again? Can we afford to think like a civilised society and provide health care for the next generation of emigrants? It is at this level of the Irish subconscious, this level of defeatism that social solidarity is undermined. If the citizens of a society do not believe deep down in the viability of that society, then they are inclined to pursue self-interest rather than to build for a future in which the good of one affects the good of all. Not until that defeatism is confronted, not until the Irish subconscious catches up with the Irish reality – that this is a state with higher than EU average income, with above average inequality, where self-interest has been pursued at the expense of the good, the health and the education of all – will the electorate and its representatives wake up to the realisation that the time has long since come to build an equitable and accessible health care system within a more egalitarian society.

Rory O'Hanlon, that most gentlemanly of doctor politicians, has expressed the reigning political philosophy of Irish health care: "If people want to pay for their own medical treatment out of their own disposable income, that is their right." Jimmy Sheehan, the medical entrepreneur, considers that health is like housing: "People are entitled to different levels". That the health of one affects the health of all and that it is uncivilised to have tiers of access depending on means are not accepted propositions in Ireland. If such propositions were accepted, Ireland would not have its extraordinary health care system.

And it *is* an extraordinary system. Consuming 10 per cent of national income yet denying care to many families. Consuming nearly one-quarter of government spending yet fostering two-tier access to hospitals. Channelling state funds into private for-profit hospitals. Channelling them into preferential care for private patients through tax relief for insurance, subsidised charges for private accommodation in public hospitals and the payment of public salaries to hospital consultants while they earn private fees.

The ill-considered use of state funds to subsidise and promote private care contrasts with the resistance of government to improving access to primary care for those who cannot afford it. If improving health rather than placating the more vocal political constituencies were the objective of health spending, improved access to primary care would be the first priority of government and universal access its next objective. But to deliver either would require an acceptance of the need to increase taxes for some in order to fund better access to care for others, not a short-term winning strategy. It would require a philosophical conversion to the proposition that health care should be seen as a right rather than a marketable commodity and that its universal provision is in the interests of all.

The agenda for reform is self-evident. Primary care needs to be taken seriously. It needs investment in people and facilities. And it needs to be accessible. No one should face financial barriers to seeing their family doctor, not even the relatively well-off. Society should collectively insure the individual against ill-health, either through taxation or through an insurance system. Everyone with the means to do so should contribute to a system which ensures that no one must worry about money when they are ill. If it is a genuine fear that free access would swamp the existing primary care system, then access could be gradually extended as resources are developed. But the counter-argument is that giving free access to all immediately, while simultaneously requiring that all contribute to the provision of resources through tax or insurance, the "big bang" approach, would inject the sense of urgency to the development of primary care which has been so lacking.

In hospitals, the two-tier system of access and care must end. The route to that is also evident: a common waiting list "at a minimum", as the NESF recommended; the same method of payment for consultants, whoever their patient, which implies an end to private practice in public hospitals because distinction between patients would become redundant; and an end to off-site private practice for publicly salaried consultants. As the Canadian academic Thomas Rathwell observed when advising Canadians about the risk that their greater use of private insurance would create a two-tier system: "drawing on the Irish experience, the conditions to avoid are the designation of private beds in public hospitals and permitting specialists to\ have both public and private practice".

Not only two-tier care but also care by unsupervised junior doctors must end – and the sooner the better. The standard of care which the Irish health system has tolerated and continues to tolerate is indefensible. It has persisted because of the failure of politicians and officials to take on the consultant establishment, to insist on the dismantling of the medical hierarchy and on reform of how hospital consultants work, and because of the unwillingness of politicians to face down local interests and rationalise small rural hospitals. The work of the Hanly task force on medical staffing promises to provide the political system with a blueprint for change in how hospitals are organised and in how hospital doctors work. Regional centres of excellence with satellite hospitals offering elective rather than acute care, a doubling of consultant numbers to provide a cadre of fully trained doctors, who deliver care in person, work as teams and earn less than the former gods at the apex of the hierarchy, changing the consultants' contract to ensure their full-time commitment to the public hospital system – these are the implications of its recommendations.

These changes are not primarily about the working conditions of doctors. They are about safer care for patients. In place of behind-doors negotiations between intimidated health officials and the medical organisations, these reforms should therefore be announced in the Dáil by a Minister who makes it clear that he has a democratic mandate which will not be denied. Reorganising local hospitals will require administrative reform. There are essentially two options: either to give power to the centre, which means removing the health boards' veto and requiring the Minister to take political responsibility for decisions on the location of hospital services, acting perhaps through a new Health Services Executive; or to give responsibility as well as power to the regions and require health boards to fund hospital services locally. Since the Irish political culture has been averse to developing local democracy in this Scandinavian manner, the former reform appears better suited to the needs of the moment: centralised decision-making, because the time for decision is long overdue.

These are the essentials of a reform agenda in what is popularly understood as health care: accessible primary care, an end to two-tier hospital care, consultant-delivered care in a reorganised hospital network. For the patient, the present system would end. He would no longer face the possibility of being sent, if he can afford it, by his expensive and ill-equipped GP to wait to be seen by a young graduate doctor or an immigrant doctor outside a formal training programme in a hospital which is not adequately equipped to treat him if he is seriously ill. Instead he would first be seen without charge in a well-equipped primary care centre, staffed by a team of professionals, who might even have asked him to come for a health check. He might be advised on lifestyle changes which would improve his health. If he is ill, his condition might be investigated and treated there. If in need of hospital investigation or specialist treatment, he would be referred to an appropriately equipped and staffed hospital, where, depending on the severity of his condition, he would be seen as an outpatient immediately or within a few days by a consultant or, at least, a fully trained doctor. If he required surgery or a further procedure, he would be given a date for treatment immediately, if necessary, or within three months at the longest.

This transformation is achievable – but for a price. Health in all its aspects requires sustained investment. That requires a collective commitment to funding it either in the form of tax or insurance. The legacy of underfunding will not be erased because in one year or two Irish health spending has exceeded the EU average. We will be deluding ourselves if we ignore the investment needs identified in the health strategy, collectively decide that health does not need more investment and choose to subscribe to the mandarins' view that "shortage of funding may no longer be the key issue in the health service". Quite apart from the investment required to develop what is popularly understood as health care – in beds, staff, equipment – Irish society also needs more facilities for the disabled, the mentally ill, the elderly, the convalescent, the homeless, children at risk and more people to staff these facilities. Investment must be paced, planned, committed in advance. The UK has looked into the future and faced the fact that health spending may need to rise to 12 per cent of national income to cope with an ageing population. Wealthier states with enviable systems have consistently spent between 9 and 10 per cent of national income. Ireland's spending has just approached 10 per cent of national income. Since this investment has been made in an unreformed, inequitable system at an inflationary time, when state funds still subsidise preferential access for private patients, hospital consultants receive public and private incomes in excess of those of many of their international colleagues and junior doctors are paid huge sums in overtime to staff a system that offers inappropriate care in too many acute hospitals, reform should eventually deliver better value for money. But it will not obviate the need for sustained investment if Ireland is to build a service which compares with those of states like France and Germany. There is no right level of health spending. How much Irish society spends is a collective decision, a function of the standards of care which this society wants and of our ability to design a system which will deliver acceptable care at an acceptable price. While every state grapples with health care costs, it appears to be the case that as states get wealthier, they generally choose to spend a higher proportion of income on health care.

How to fund this investment? By tax or by introducing a compulsory insurance system? Either route could achieve an equitable system of care. In the existing tax-funded system, this could be achieved by introducing free primary care in which the state would pay GPs by salary, capitation, fees or a mixture of methods, and by banning private practice in public hospitals and investing in public care so that the majority would opt to be treated in one-tier public hospitals by salaried consultants. This would not be such a radical departure. It would be similar to the system in the UK or Denmark, much more mainstream internationally than the existing Irish system. The VHI would revert to insuring a much smaller proportion of the population for elective care in the small number of private hospitals. Provided the state invested sufficiently in the public system, the nascent private hospital industry would lose its appeal. But if the state did not invest sufficiently in the public system, there would exist a risk that patients and doctors would take flight into the private system and the schism in Irish care would deepen.

Reformers have turned to the alternative compulsory insurance system because it avoids some of these risks. It creates a system in which all must participate. The distinction between public and private patients ends. Private hospitals contract to treat patients within the state system. The VHI becomes part of the new system. The payment of an insurance premium for each individual for a defined package of benefits provides an earmarked fund for health care. Consultants might be paid by fees rather than by salary, politically easier to achieve although bringing with it problems of spiralling cost. States who pay doctors by fees have been forced to take measures to control costs, such as capping their incomes or freezing their rates of pay. No system is perfect and no system will end the battle between states and doctors over who owns and controls health care.

But it is clear what reform must achieve and what must be avoided. Reform must achieve equitable access. It must avoid permitting the mutation of Irish health care into a private, for-profit industry. The Labour proponents of compulsory insurance have, by and large, thought through how to avoid this and would receive support from the EU in designing an insurance system that is not driven by profit. It is the government parties who are sleepwalking their way towards a for-profit health industry with their apparent willingness to privatise the VHI and allow its sale to the highest bidder, their support for for-profit hospitals and their use of state funds for the treatment of public patients in the private sector while they cut back on treatments in public hospitals. In its draft report, the Department-of-Finance-sponsored Brennan Commission identified a managerial vacuum in Irish health care. Far more important has been the political vacuum: the avoidance of difficult decisions in areas such as hospital reorganisation, the unwillingness to confront hospital consultants, the glaring contradictions in health policy caused by the interventions of the Minister for Finance, the inconsistencies in the health strategy, the absence of explicit values and of vision. To reform Irish health care, incrementalism will not suffice. That got us into this fine mess. Getting out of it requires political leadership. Canada developed its egalitarian health service because Tommy Douglas in Saskatchewan believed that people should "be able to get health services just as they are able to get educational services, as an inalienable right of being a citizen in a Christian country". There is no substitute for political leadership.

If reform is driven merely by a preoccupation with administrative structures and value for money, we will be rearranging the deck chairs on the Titanic. This is the perspective of the Department of Finance which, having seen no objection to state subsidy for for-profit private hospitals, has lost any claim to credibility as an arbiter of health policy. Reform must take access to care as its starting point, its lodestone.

The state of health care is a metaphor for the condition of this society, this Unhealthy State. Directionless during the boom, Irish society is at risk of rediscovering its former fatalism, of accepting passively that the boats will remain beached until the tide turns: that children must remain awaiting tonsillectomies, old people awaiting the drug therapy which could alleviate their arthritis, the intellectually disabled awaiting the community care which would remove them from psychiatric wards. Since an election fought on the promise of massive investment in health, there has been a concerted effort to throw dust in the eyes of the public and imply that wasteful spending is the central problem in the health service. This has been part of a political agenda to distract from the service's investment needs and defend the low-tax regime achieved during the boom. The proponents of this point of view are motivated by their rearguard defence of lower taxes. To every speaker who talks about value for money, the response should be "what about access?"

The Berliners among us, those who aspire to building a civilised society and a healthier state, should not be distracted from the essential questions. Why not reform? Why not universal access? Why not social solidarity? If this book has contributed to answering those questions, it has served its purpose.

APPENDIX

Table A.1 Chronology

Minister for Health[a]	Period in office	Government	Elected in	Significant events
James Ryan[b]	Jan. '47–Feb. '48	FF	1944	1947 Health Act provides for free treatment for children during school years and mothers before and after birth. Never implemented.
Noel Browne	Feb. '48–Apr. '51	Inter-party	1948	1950 Mother and Child scheme proposes free care for mothers before and after birth and children to the age of 16. Browne loses government support.
John A. Costello	Apr. '51–Jun. '51	FF	1951	1953 Health Act provides free hospital care for majority, free care for mothers before and after birth and for infants to six weeks, subject to income limit.
James Ryan[b]	Jun. '51–Jun. '54			1957 Establishment of VHI, offering private insurance to cover hospital care.
T. F. O'Higgins	Jun. '54–Mar. '57	Inter-party	1954	
Seán MacEntee[b]	Mar. '57–Oct. '61	FF	1957	
Seán MacEntee[b]	Oct. '61–Apr. '65	FF	1961	1962 Irish Medical Union (IMU) established.
Donogh O'Malley	Apr. '65–Jul. '66	FF	1965	1966 White Paper: Fianna Fáil abandons support for free care for all.
Seán Flanagan	Jul. '66–Jul. '69			1968 FitzGerald Report advocates reducing number of acute hospitals.
Erskine Childers	Jul. '69–Mar. '73	FF	1969	1970 Health Act establishes health boards, choice of doctor in GMS.
Brendan Corish[b]	Mar. '73–Jul. '77	FG/Lab	1973	1974 Corish fails in attempt to extend free hospital care to all. Bill to legalise import of contraceptives defeated.
C. J. Haughey[b]	Jul. '77–Dec. '79	FF	1977	1979 Regulations extend free hospital maintenance to all. Legalisation of limited sale of contraceptives.
Michael Woods[b]	Dec. '79–Jul. '81			1981 Consultants combine public salaries with unlimited private practice in their new common contract.
Eileen Desmond[b]	Jul. '81–Mar. '82	FG/Lab	1981	
Michael Woods[b]	Mar. '82–Dec. '82	FF	Feb. '82	
Barry Desmond[b]	Dec. '82–Jan. '87	FG/Lab	Nov. '82	1983 Constitutional ban on abortion. 1984 IMA and IMU merge to form Irish Medical Organisation (IMO). Supreme Court says the Minister has no power to order hospital to discontinue services. 1985 Liberalisation of sale of contraceptives. 1986 Public hospital closures. Blackrock Clinic and Mater Private Hospital open.
John Boland	Jan. '87–Mar. '87			
Rory O'Hanlon	Mar. '87–Jul. '89	FF	1987	1987 Massive spending cuts. 1989 Irish Hospital Consultants' Association founded. Government defeat over compensation for haemophiliacs infected with HIV from contaminated blood products provokes election.

Minister for Health[a]	Period in office	Government	Elected in	Significant events
Rory O'Hanlon	Jul. '89–Nov. '91	FF/PD	1989	Sept 1989 Commission on Health Funding recommends common waiting list, national Health Services Executive Authority and abolition of health boards. 1991 Health (Amendment) Act extends free consultant care to all and introduces system of designated public and private beds in hospitals. 1991 revision of consultants' common contract attempts to introduce monitoring of consultants' private practice.
Mary O'Rourke	Nov. '91–Feb. '92			1992 "X" case. Constitutional amendments to protect freedom of information and right to travel passed, amendment to remove threat of suicide as grounds for abortion defeated.
John O'Connell	Feb. '92–Jan. '93			
Brendan Howlin	Jan. '93–Nov. '94	FF/Lab	1992	1993 Purchase of condoms allowed at any age. 1994 Health Strategy *Shaping a Healthier Future* accepts public/private mix. Over 1,000 women test positive for hepatitis C following infection by contaminated blood products.
Michael Woods	Nov. '94–Dec. '94	FG/Lab/DL	1994c	1995 Legislation to permit doctors to counsel women on abortion. 1996 Death of Brigid McCole. 1997 Report of Finlay Tribunal.
Michael Noonan	Dec. '94–Jun. '97			
Brian Cowen[d]	Jun. '97–Jan. 2000	FF/PD	1997	1997 Revision of consultants' common contract removes the option of a public-only contract. 1999 White Paper on Private Health Insurance restates support for public/private mix.
Micheál Martin	Jan. 2000–May '02			2001 Health Strategy retains the public/private mix but advocates massive investment in public health care and public-only contract for consultants in early years. 2002 Defeat of constitutional amendment to remove threat of suicide as grounds for abortion. Report of Lindsay Tribunal.
Micheál Martin	May '02–	FF/PD	2002	2003 Budget provides no funding for implementing strategy or extending medical card eligibility.

[a]Department of Health established 1947.
[b]Also Minister for Social Welfare.
[c]Change of government without election.
[d]Remit broadened to become Department of Health and Children.

Table A.2 The history of Irish health spending 1980–2002: current spending and EU comparison

Year and govt. in power at time of Budget	Gross non-capital health spending^a €'m	Increase on previous year %	Non-capital spending in 1995 prices^b €'m	Increase in real terms^c %	Spending on general hospital programme^f €'m	Increase on previous year %	Spending on general hospital programme in 1995 prices^b €'m	Increase in real terms^c %	Irish per capita public health spending as % of EU averaged^d %
1980 FF	929.4		2,561.1		500.3		1,378.4		82
1981 FF; FG/Lab^e	1,089.4	17.2	2,478.7	-3.2	581.5	16.2	1,323.1	-4.0	74
1982 FF	1,268.1	16.4	2,544.4	2.7	645.0	10.9	1,294.2	-2.2	72
1983 FG/Lab	1,384.6	9.2	2,563.6	0.8	708.5	9.8	1,311.8	1.4	70
1984 FG/Lab	1,466.5	5.9	2,512.3	-2.0	753.0	6.3	1,289.9	-1.7	68
1985 FG/Lab	1,580.8	7.8	2,561.7	2.0	808.8	7.4	1,310.6	1.6	67
1986 FG/Lab	1,649.4	4.3	2,556.2	-0.2	822.8	1.7	1,275.2	-2.7	64
1987 FF	1,676.0	1.6	2,448.9	-4.2	832.9	1.2	1,217.0	-4.6	62
1988 FF	1,699.5	1.1	2,383.2	-2.7	841.8	1.1	1,180.5	-3.0	58
1989 FF	1,809.4	6.5	2,415.3	1.4	886.3	5.3	1,183.1	0.2	57
1990 FF/PD	2,001.0	10.6	2,541.5	5.2	1,017.1	14.8	1,291.8	9.2	61
1991 FF/PD	2,224.6	11.2	2,638.9	3.8	1,139.0	12.0	1,351.1	4.6	66
1992 FF/PD	2,484.0	11.7	2,791.1	5.8	1,262.1	10.8	1,418.2	5.0	72
1993 FF/Lab	2,743.4	10.4	2,879.6	3.2	1,392.9	10.4	1,462.1	3.1	74
1994 FF/Lab	2,908.5	6.0	2,992.1	3.9	1,455.1	4.5	1,497.0	2.4	78
1995 FG/Lab/DL	3,105.4	6.8	3,105.4	3.8	1,558.0	7.1	1,558.0	4.1	78
1996 FG/Lab/DL	3,183.1	2.5	3,120.4	0.5	1,621.5	4.1	1,589.5	2.0	76
1997 FG/Lab/DL	3,648.3	14.6	3,380.3	8.3	1,861.4	14.8	1,724.7	8.5	87
1998 FF/PD	4,040.1	10.7	3,614.6	6.9	2,043.0	9.8	1,827.9	6.0	87
1999 FF/PD	4,807.4	19.0	4,111.7	13.8	2,380.8	16.5	2,036.3	11.4	92
2000 FF/PD	5,610.3	16.7	4,542.7	10.5	2,679.6	12.6	2,169.7	6.6	97
2001 FF/PD	7,010.1	25.0	5,297.8	16.6	3,384.5	26.3	2,557.8	17.9	> 100
2002 FF/PD	8,166.7	16.5	6,001.8	13.3	3,922.8	15.9	2,882.9	12.7	> 100

^aCurrent spending measured on a programme basis, one of a number of differing measures used in the national accounts. Source: *Revised Estimates for Public Services*.

^bAdjusted for inflation in public authorities' spending on goods and services. Source: Central Statistics Office.

^cMeasures change in inflation-adjusted spending.

^dSource: Unweighted average calculated from *OECD Health Data 2002*, and including Irish spending. Includes current and capital spending. Full comparable EU data only available to 1998. 1999 and 2000 EU averages calculated using trends in spending in three states.

^eIn 1981, there were two Budgets, the second following a change of government.

^fIncludes contributions to patients in private nursing homes.

Table A.2.1 The history of Irish health spending 1980–2002: capital spending

Year and govt. in power at time of Budget	Capital Spending[a] €'m	Increase on previous year %	Capital spending in 1995 prices[b] €'m	Increase in real terms[c] %
1980 FF	44.4		92.1	
1981 FF; FG/Lab[d]	56.5	27.3	102.7	11.5
1982 FF	62.5	10.6	103.0	0.2
1983 FG/Lab	67.3	7.7	104.8	1.8
1984 FG/Lab	70.5	4.8	102.6	-2.1
1985 FG/Lab	72.4	2.7	100.4	-2.1
1986 FG/Lab	74.5	2.9	98.8	-1.6
1987 FF	73.1	-1.9	94.0	-4.9
1988 FF	56.2	-23.1	69.8	-25.7
1989 FF	61.0	8.5	72.4	3.6
1990 FF/PD	58.7	-3.8	66.8	-7.7
1991 FF/PD	54.0	-8.0	59.9	-10.4
1992 FF/PD	55.9	3.5	60.7	1.4
1993 FF/Lab	55.9	0.0	59.2	-2.5
1994 FF/Lab	83.2	48.9	86.0	45.5
1995 FG/Lab/DL	121.9	46.6	121.9	41.7
1996 FG/Lab/DL	152.1	24.8	143.5	17.7
1997 FG/Lab/DL	167.0	9.7	143.2	-0.2
1998 FF/PD	187.0	12.0	148.6	3.7
1999 FF/PD	230.7	23.4	166.6	12.2
2000 FF/PD	293.9	27.4	189.6	13.8
2001 FF/PD	373.6	27.1	220.9	16.6
2002 FF/PD	507.1	35.7	289.8	31.1

[a]Total public capital expenditure. Source: Department of Health *Health Statistics* volumes. Table L6.
[b]Adjusted for inflation in new construction in the health sector. Source: Department of the Environment, *Construction Industry Review and Outlook*.
[c]Measures change in inflation-adjusted spending.
[d]In 1981, there were two Budgets, the second following a change of government.

Table A.3 Health services in the 1990s: employment, nurse training and waiting lists

	Numbers employed in:					Total health service employment	Nurse-training places	Public waiting lists[c]
	Management administration[a]	Medical/Dental	Nursing	Paramedical	Support services[b]			
1990	6,607	3,994	24,574	4,180	19,383	58,738	1,237	–
1991	6,763	4,100	25,118	4,299	19,217	59,497	1,274	–
1992	6,930	4,155	25,771	4,395	19,211	60,462	1,255	–
1993	7,243	4,310	26,220	4,628	19,414	61,815	1,268	40,130
1994	7,607	4,417	26,839	5,024	20,051	63,938	1,179	24,778
1995	7,885	4,581	27,267	5,345	20,092	65,170	1,109	27,696
1996	8,151	4,684	27,170	5,576	20,174	65,755	1,099	30,447
1997	8,794	4,976	27,346	5,969	20,825	67,910	982	30,453
1998	9,474	5,153	26,611	6,422	22,066	69,726	968	34,331
1999	12,525	5,385	27,044	6,831	23,073	74,858	1,215	33,924
2000	12,366	5,698	29,177	7,613	26,658	81,512	1,500	31,851
2001	14,714	6,285	31,429	9,228	31,340	92,996	1,648	26,659
2002	–	–	–	–	–	–	–	29,174

[a]Includes staff directly serving the public, such as consultants' secretaries, telephonists and personnel in A & E, medical records and computers. All numbers are whole-time equivalents rather than numbers employed.

[b]Includes maintenance and technical staff.

[c]Comparable figures only available from the beginning of the 1993 Waiting Lists Initiative. Figures for June each year, except in 2002, when the growing category of patients waiting for day surgery were included for the first time in the September total.

Sources: Final Report of the Nursing and Midwifery Resource Steering Group, July 2002, and Department of Health personnel census and waiting list figures.

Table A.4 The 25-year roller-coaster (1977–2002): fluctuations in medical card holders, privately insured, acute beds, patients treated and jobs in public health care

Year and govt. in power at time of Budget	Patients treated in public hospitals as inpatients or day cases[a]	Percentage of the population with medical cards[b]	Percentage of the population with private health insurance[c]	Numbers of acute hospital beds[d]	Numbers employed in the public health service[e]
1977 FF	–	38.6	18.2	–	50,611
1978 FF	–	37.9	19.5	–	–
1979 FF	–	36.4	21.8	–	–
1980 FF	552,075	35.6	26.1	17,665	–
1981 FF; FG/Lab	571,429	35.6	28.6	17,668	66,060
1982 FF	582,622	37.1	30.2	17,582	–
1983 FG/Lab	–	38.3	30.9	17,633	–
1984 FG/Lab	581,455	37.0	31.2	17,636	63,077
1985 FG/Lab	–	36.8	31.2	17,223	–
1986 FG/Lab	616,241	37.4	31.3	16,878	62,464
1987 FF	597,171	37.9	31.4	15,225	58,091
1988 FF	598,826	37.4	32.7	13,632	56,357
1989 FF	626,179	35.8	33.8	13,634	–
1990 FF/PD	647,612	34.9	34.4	13,753	58,738
1991 FF/PD	662,965	35.1	35.3	13,806	59,497
1992 FF/PD	666,912	35.6	35.9	12,136	60,462
1993 FF/Lab	709,763	35.8	36.5	11,809	61,815
1994 FF/Lab	715,821	36.0	37.3	11,853	63,938
1995 FG/Lab/DL	736,701	35.8	37.9	11,953	65,170
1996 FG/Lab/DL	771,465	35.8	38.4	11,937	65,755
1997 FG/Lab/DL	785,708	34.6	39.2	11,861	67,910
1998 FF/PD	808,081	33.6	40.5	11,788	69,726
1999 FF/PD	827,989	31.9	41.8	11,781	74,858
2000 FF/PD	876,338	31.4	43.8	11,832	81,512
2001 FF/PD	919,268	31.2	46.2	11,985	92,996
2002 FF/PD	963,283	–	–	12,191	–

Note: Gaps in series occur where consistent figures are not available.
[a]Source: *Acute Hospital Bed Capacity Review*, Department of Health, 2002. Figures for 2000–2002 updated by Department of Health.
[b]Source: Reports of the General Medical Services Payments Board.
[c]Sources: Department of Health estimate in NESF, *Equity of Access to Hospital Care*, 2002, p. 21, for years 1979–2001. For years 1977 and 1978, this is only the percentage of population with VHI membership published in Nolan, 1991, p. 148. Understates percentage with private health insurance, as it does not include members of small occupational schemes.
[d]Source: *Acute Hospital Bed Capacity Review*. Updated by Department of Health for 2001 and 2002. 2002 figure for November.
[e]Source: Department of Health personnel census. Pre-1990 as reported in the *Report of the Commission on Health Funding*, p. 53.

Table A.5 Growth in health spending by programme 1990–2002

Programme	1990 €'m	1990 % of total	2002 €'m	2002 % of total	Increase 1990–2002 %
Community protection[a]	30	1	275	3	803
Community health services[b]	295	15	1,526	19	418
Community welfare[c]	182	9	704	9	287
Mental health[d]	215	11	564	7	163
Disability[e]	193	10	963	12	399
General hospital[f]	996	50	3,801	46	282
General support[g]	90	4	334	4	270
Total current spending	2,001	100	8,167	100	418

[a]Health promotion, prevention of disease, food hygiene.
[b]GMS (GP treatment and medication for medical card holders), Drug Payment Scheme (refunds of drug costs above a certain threshold), home nursing, family planning and pregnancy counselling, dental, ophthalmic and aural services.
[c]Home helps, meals-on-wheels, foster and residential care for children, homes for the elderly, private nursing home subventions, allowances for carers of disabled children and other allowances for the disabled.
[d]Diagnosis, care and prevention of mental illness.
[e]Residential and day care for the intellectually disabled, assessment and care of people with physical disabilities, rehabilitation.
[f]Hospital and ambulance services. Excludes private nursing home subventions, which had been included up to 1998.
[g]Administration, research, science and technology. Source: *Revised Estimates for Public Services.*

Appendix

Table A.6 International comparison of health and health care resources

Country	Life expectancy at birth[a]		Acute beds per 1,000 pop.[b]	Doctors per 1,000 pop.[c]	GPs per 1,000 pop.[d]	Spending on drugs as % EU per capita average[e]	Public health exp. as % EU per capita average[f]	Public health exp. as % national income[g]	Total health exp. as % national income[g]	National income per capita in 2000 US$[h]
	F	M								
United States	79.4	73.9	3.0	2.8	0.8	149	135	5.8	13.0	35,657
Canada	81.7	76.3	3.3	2.1	0.9	122	118	6.8	9.3	27,963
Germany	80.7	74.7	6.4	3.6	1.0	113	135	7.8	10.3	25,936
France	82.5	75.0	4.2	3.0	1.5	140	116	7.2	9.5	24,847
Denmark	79.0	74.2	3.3	3.4	0.6	73	133	6.8	8.3	29,050
New Zealand	80.8	75.7	n.a.	2.2	0.8	75	81	6.2	8.0	20,262
UK	79.8	75.0	3.3	1.8	0.6	91	89	5.9	7.7	24,323
EU average	80.4	74.4	4.1	3.3	0.9	100	100	5.8	8.0	26,052
Ireland	79.1	73.9	3.0	2.0	0.6	60	>100	7.2	9.6	24,709

[a]Data for 1999 except for EU average: last full comparison for 1997. Source: *OECD Health Data 2002*.

[b]International data for latest year available, ranging from 1998 to 2000. Source: *OECD Health Data 2002*. Irish bed count for 2001 from Department of Health and population count from 2002 Census of Population.

[c]International data for 1999 and 2000. Source: *OECD Health Data 2002*. Irish figure calculated for 2002 from published totals for GPs, consultants, NCHDs and doctors in public health.

[d]International data for 1998 to 2000. Source: *OECD Health Data 2002*. Irish figure for 2001: Department of Health presentation, Ballymascanlon. OECD only counts Irish GPs in the GMS.

[e]Source: *OECD Health Data 2002*. Data for spending on pharmaceuticals and other medical nondurables in 1997, the latest year for which it is available for all states. In 2000, among those states for which data was available, the US remained the highest spender and Ireland the lowest.

[f]International data for 1998, the last year for which full EU data is available. Among states whose comparable spending is available for the years to 2000, the relationship of their spending to the average has remained fairly constant. Source: *OECD Health Data 2002*. However, Ireland's spending exceeded EU average in 2001 and 2002 – see Table A.2, p. 372.

[g]International data for 1998 to 2000, and sourced from *OECD Health Data 2002*, apart from UK total spending, which is for 2002. Ireland's figures for 2002. Total health spending is public plus private spending. National income refers to GDP in all cases except Ireland's, where it refers to GNP. Irish GDP is an overstated measure of national income because it includes the repatriated profits of multinationals.

[h]Figures for 2000 in US$ adjusted for purchasing power parity. Source: *OECD Health Data 2002*. Ireland's national income is expressed as per capita GNP. Irish per capita GNP exceeded the EU average in 2001.

Figure A.1 International comparison of public health spending per capita 1980–2000

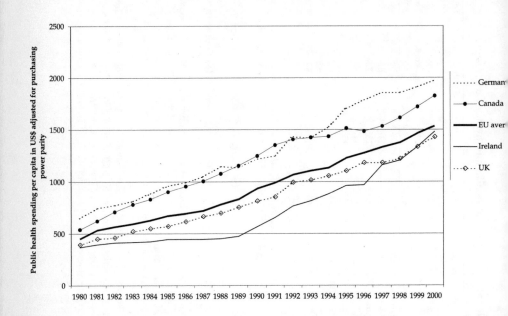

Source: *OECD Health Data 2002.* Post-1998 German and EU average spending extrapolated from past trer

GLOSSARY

Ard Fheis – Party conference.

Comhairle na nOspidéal – Hospitals' Council

Church – Refers to the Catholic Church, unless otherwise stated.

Dáil – Parliament.

Department – Department of Health.

FOI – Papers released under the 1997 Freedom of Information Act.

Ireland – Irish Free State from 1922; Republic of Ireland from 1949.

National income – GNP is used as the best measure of Irish national income, whereas GDP is used to measure other states'. Since Irish GDP includes the repatriated profits of multinationals, it is considered that GNP is a better measure of income.

Northern Ireland – Six counties which are part of the United Kingdom.

Seanad – Upper house of the Dáil.

Taoiseach – Prime Minister.

Tánaiste – Deputy Prime Minister.

NOTES

1. Health in an unhealthy state

[1] *Inequalities in Health in Ireland – hard facts*, Department of Community Health and General Practice, Trinity College Dublin, September 2001, p. 5. Data for 1996.

[2] National Economic and Social Forum, *Equity of Access to Hospital Care*, Forum Report No. 25, Government Publication Sales Office, 2002, p. 40.

[3] Irish GNP per capita exceeded the EU average in 2001. Department of Finance.

[4] Brian Nolan, "Income Inequality during Ireland's Boom", unpublished article to appear in *Studies*, summer 2003.

[5] In September 2002, 676 children had waited 6 months or more for an operation on their ears, nose or throat. No information was available on how much longer than 6 months they had waited. Department of Health waiting list data, December 3rd 2002.

[6] *The National Health and Lifestyle Surveys*, Centre for Health Promotion Studies, National University of Ireland Galway, 2003. Survey conducted in 2002.

[7] *Strategic Task Force on Alcohol Interim Report May 2002*, Department of Health and Children, 2002.

[8] 1999 ESPAD Report on health behaviour in children in all 26 European countries, quoted in *Quality and Fairness – a health system for you*, Department of Health and Children, Stationery Office Dublin, 2001.

[9] *The National Health and Lifestyle Surveys*, 2003 and 1999. Earlier evidence from the 1985 and 1990 Kilkenny Health Project, reported in Claire Collins and Emer Shelley, "Social Class Differences in Some Lifestyle and Health Characteristics in Ireland" in Cleary and Treacy (eds), *The Sociology of Health and Illness in Ireland*, University College Dublin Press, 1997.

[10] Tanya M. Cassidy, "Alcoholism in Ireland" in Cleary and Treacy. *OECD Health Data 2002* reported that Ireland had a mortality rate from liver disease and cirrhosis in 1998 of 4.4 per 100,000 people, compared to an EU average of 11 and rates in Germany of 16.2 and France of 13.5.

[11] RTÉ's *Prime Time*, November 28th 2002.

[12] *Quality and Fairness*, pp. 23–24. *Inequalities in Mortality 1989–1998: a report on all-Ireland mortality data*, The Institute of Public Health in Ireland, 2001, pp. 12, 38. The first quotes Eurostat data for 1997; the second uses an age-standardised measure averaged over the period of the study.

[13] Life expectancy at birth, 1999, *OECD Health Data 2002*.

[14] Ireland had 5.9 deaths per 1,000 live births in 2000 compared to an EU average of 5. Sweden had 3.4 deaths per 1,000; Finland had 3.8. *OECD Health Data 2002*.

[15] *Quality and Fairness*, pp. 26, 27.

[16] The mortality rate for women from cancer was 181 per 100,000 compared to 148 per 100,000 in the EU on average. *Inequalities in Mortality 1989–1998*, p. 52. The mortality rate

from cancer was 5 per cent higher in the Republic than in Northern Ireland, where it was 170 per 100,000.

17*Building Healthier Hearts*, Cardiovascular Health Strategy Group, Stationery Office, Dublin, 1999, p. 30.

18 *Annual Report of the Chief Medical Officer 1999*, Department of Health and Children.

19 Ibid. Based on the report of the Cardiovascular Health Strategy Group, 1999.

20 In May 2002, the Irish Heart Foundation (IHF) criticised the government for failing to increase the number of consultant cardiologists in line with its own stated priorities and for delay in implementing secondary prevention programmes in primary care.

21 *Cancer in Ireland 1994–1998*, National Cancer Registry Board Cork, 2001, p. 98.

22 Ireland had 29.2 deaths per 100,000 in 1998 compared to an EU average of 24.9. *OECD Health Data 2002*.

23 Organised screening was still only offered to women in the midlands and the east. *The Irish Times*, October 17th 2002.

24 Patients in the west were less likely to receive radiotherapy than those in other health board areas, *Cancer in Ireland 1994–1998*, p. 116.

25 *Report of the Forum on Medical Manpower*, Department of Health and Children, January 2001, pp. 63–64.

26 Socio-economic group D has a mortality rate of 792.4 per 100,000 compared to 232 for socio-economic group A. *Inequalities in Mortality 1989–1998*, pp. 11, 39. Measure used described in note 12 above. Socio-economic group relates to occupation not income so, strictly speaking, these groups are not necessarily synonymous with the poor and the rich but, in broad terms, they do reflect endowment in power, influence and status as well as income.

27 Richard Layte and Brian Nolan, "The Health Strategy and Socio-Economic Inequalities in Health" in Miriam Wiley, *Critique of Shaping a Healthier Future*, ESRI, 2001, p. 20.

28 *Inequalities in Health in Ireland*, pp. 41–46.

29 Ibid., pp. 35–37.

30 Yoav Ben-Shlomo and George Davey Smith, "Inequalities in Health: reasons and possible solutions", *The Journal of Health Gain*, Vol. 1. Issue 2, June 1997.

31 Ibid.

32 In his opening address to a seminar on health inequalities, April 21st 1999. Proceedings published by the Health Promotion Department of the Eastern Health Board, as *Towards Health for All: reducing inequalities in Ireland*.

33 *"One Long Struggle"– A Study of Low Income Families*, by the Vincentian Partnership for Social Justice, based on surveys and interviews in 2000 and 2001.

34 Discussed by Layte and Nolan in Wiley, 2001.

35 Michael Marmot and Richard G. Wilkinson, "Psychosocial and Material Pathways in the Relation between Income and Health: a response to Lynch et al.", *BMJ*, May 19th 2001.

36 Brian Nolan et al., *Monitoring Poverty Trends in Ireland*. Results from the 2000 Living in Ireland Survey, ESRI, 2002.

37 In the boom years 1994–2000, the share of income going to the bottom 30 per cent of the population fell from 14.3 to 13.2 per cent. Nolan, 2003.

38 Analysis by the Combat Poverty Agency, *The Irish Times*, April 17th 2002.

39 Eurostat, 2001. Social situation in the European Union.

40 Ben-Shlomo and Davey Smith, *The Journal of Health Gain*.

41 The relationship between low income and ill-health is a much-disputed topic. For a recent defence of the view that inequality affects health primarily though psychosocial

mechanisms, and that in rich countries well-being is more closely related to relative income than absolute income, see Marmot and Wilkinson, *BMJ*.

[42] Jane Wilde in a letter to the Editor, *The Irish Times*, May 7th 2001.

[43] *Annual Report of the Chief Medical Officer 1999*.

[44] Foreword to *Inequalities in Health in Ireland*, Trinity College Dublin, 2001.

[45] *Economic Surveys 1996–1997: Ireland*, OECD, 1997, p. 116.

[46] The Voluntary Health Insurance Board (VHI) introduced a scheme to cover primary care costs in February 2002. It would repay €25 for each GP visit, typically then costing €40. The annual adult premium was €199. By year end, a minority of the VHI's subscribers had joined this scheme.

[47] In the west Dublin suburb of Tallaght in 2001, 35 per cent of households had neither medical card nor private health insurance. Trinity College Dublin, Department of Community Health and General Practice, *People Living in Tallaght and their Health*, Adelaide Hospital Society, March 2002.

[48] Veronica O'Keane, Anne Jeffers, Eamon Moloney and Siobhan Barry, *The Stark Facts – the need for a national mental health strategy*, Irish Psychiatric Association, 2003.

[49] Concluding observations of the Committee on Economic, Social and Cultural Rights, 28th session, April–May 2002, United Nations.

[50] From summaries of the proceedings at meetings between the international panel and the steering group and project team who worked on the 2001 health strategy, May 23rd 2001. Released by the Department of Health under FOI. The panel comprised: Professor Richard Alderslade, regional advisor, WHO Regional Office for Europe; Dr Judith Kurland, regional director, Department of Health and Human Services (USA); and Dr Charlotte Dargie, senior research associate, Judge Institute of Management Studies, University of Cambridge (UK).

[51] Report of the Working Group on Eligibility, June 8th 2001. FOI.

[52] See Table A.2, p. 372.

[53] J. J. Lee, *Ireland 1912–1985*, Cambridge University Press, 1989, pp. 374–390.

[51] John FitzGerald, *Understanding Ireland's Economic Success*, ESRI Working Paper No. 111, July 1999.

[55] As argued by the Tánaiste, Mary Harney, at a meeting of the American Bar Association in the Law Society of Ireland, July 21st 2000.

2. Defeat of the early reformers

[1] Noel Browne, *Against the Tide*, Gill and Macmillan, 1986, pp. 86–88.

[2] The Catholic population of the future Republic neared 90 per cent in 1911, was 95 per cent in 1961 and was under 92 per cent in 1991.

[3] Mary E. Daly, *Social and Economic History of Ireland*, The Educational Company, 1981, p. 114; J. H. Whyte, *Church and State in Modern Ireland 1923–1979*, 2nd edn, Gill and Macmillan, 1980, p. 12; Peter Mair, "Party competition and the changing party system" in Coakley and Gallagher (eds), *Politics in the Republic of Ireland*, 3rd edn, Routledge, 1999, pp. 128–131.

[4] Tom Inglis, *Moral Monopoly: the rise and fall of the Catholic Church in modern Ireland*, 2nd edn, University College Dublin Press, 1998, pp. 125–128.

[5] See Whyte, 1980, pp. 24–34.

[6] By 1911, little over one-third of Irish women between the ages of 15 and 45 were married. Daly, pp. 92–94.

[7] Argument persists as to whether the Church caused the repressive climate or merely reflected the society from which it came. Inglis, pp. 166–169

[8] Whyte, 1980, pp. 160, 262–264.

9 First promulgated in the 1931 Papal encyclical, *Quadragesimo Anno*, ibid., pp. 67, 158–160.

10 Daly, p. 173.

11 Éamon Ó Cuív, "Building Blocks for the Future" in Hannon and Gallagher (eds), *Taking the Long View: 70 years of Fianna Fáil*, Blackwater Press, 1996, p. 181.

12 Mair in Coakley and Gallagher, p. 131.

13 Ruth Barrington, *Health, Medicine and Politics in Ireland 1900–1970*, Institute of Public Administration, Dublin, 1987, pp. 34–38.

14 Ibid., p. 4.

15 Inglis, p. 119.

16 Barrington, p. 49.

17 Ibid., pp. 50, 54.

18 Ibid., pp. 58–66.

19 Ibid., pp. 119–122.

20 James Deeny, *To Cure and To Care – memoirs of a Chief Medical Officer*, The Glendale Press, 1989, p. 74.

21 Kieran Allen, *Fianna Fáil and Irish Labour: 1926 to the present*, Pluto Press, 1997, pp. 10–11.

22 Barrington, p. 115

23 Ibid., pp. 134–135.

24 Ibid., p. 165.

25 This was not true of New Zealand in 2003. See pp. 347–349.

26 Deeny, p. 111.

27 Maurice Manning, *James Dillon: a biography*, Wolfhound Press, 1999, pp. 204–208.

28 Browne, p. 102.

29 Barrington, p. 176.

30 Ibid., p. 182.

31 Deeny, pp. 115–117

32 Barrington, pp. 188–189.

33 Deeny, p.116.

34 Dáil Debates, Volume 105, May 1st 1947.

35 Whyte, 1980, pp. 150–153; Barrington, pp. 179–181.

36 Whyte, 1980, p. 143.

37 Barrington, pp. 186–187.

38 Whyte, 1980, pp. 149–150.

39 Ibid., pp. 153–155.

40 John Horgan, *Noel Browne – passionate outsider*, Gill and Macmillan, 2000, p. 73.

41 Deeny, p. 127.

42 Barrington, p. 164.

43 Browne, p. 123.

44 Deeny, p. 166.

45 Barrington, p. 163.

46 Ibid., p. 199.

47 *Quality and Fairness*, p. 102.

48 Barrington, p. 200.

49 Horgan, p. 82.

50 Ibid., p. 84.

51 Browne, p. 82.

52 Ibid.

53 Horgan, p. 33.

[54] Browne, pp. 86–87. Browne was writing prior to the introduction of a capitation system of payment for GPs for their GMS patients. See p. 79.

[55] Whyte, 1980, p. 235.

[56] Dáil Debates, April 12th 1951.

[57] John Cooney, *John Charles McQuaid – ruler of Catholic Ireland*, The O'Brien Press, 1999, Chapter 10.

[58] Although the 1937 Constitution introduced a prohibition on divorce and gave special recognition to the Catholic Church, de Valera resisted many of McQuaid's demands.

[59] Cooney, p. 71.

[60] Ibid., p.86.

[61] Barrington, p. 146.

[62] Ibid., pp. 161–162.

[63] Cooney, p. 167.

[64] Browne, pp. 146–147.

[65] Later there was an attempted takeover by the Knights of St Columbanus. See Whyte, p. 166 and Browne, pp. 147–148.

[66] Browne, p. 142.

[67] See p. 101.

[68] Details of the scheme were published in Whyte, 1971, Appendix A.

[69] Barrington, pp. 204–206.

[70] Quoted in Horgan, p. 89.

[71] Barrington, p. 205.

[72] Ibid., p. 213.

[73] Whyte, 1980, p. 206; Barrington, pp. 207–208.

[74] Horgan, p. 122.

[75] In a letter from the hierarchy to the Taoiseach, which was read to Browne when he met McQuaid in October 1950. Reproduced in full in Browne, pp. 158–159. Also full correspondence in appendices to Whyte, 1980.

[76] Barrington, p. 211.

[77] Deeny, p. 120.

[78] Horgan, p. 146.

[79] Ibid., p. 144.

[80] Whyte, pp. 252–259.

[81] Barrington, p. 214.

[82] Ibid., p. 215.

[83] Browne, pp. 163–164 does not reveal Cremin's identity, which is discussed in Horgan, p. 143.

[84] Horgan, p. 137.

[85] Browne, pp. 176–177. Browne had earlier been prepared to compromise on a means test. His biographer, John Horgan (pp. 147–148), later posited that his subsequent principled stand on this was motivated by a battle for control of Clann na Poblachta.

[86] Browne, p. 210.

[87] Deeny, p. 178.

[88] Barrington, p. 223.

[89] Ibid., p. 224–227.

[90] Ibid., p. 233.

[91] Whyte, 1980, p. 282.

[92] Lee, p. 187.

93 In a letter to the papal nuncio, the Vatican's ambassador to Ireland, quoted in Cooney, p. 301.

94 *Journal of the Irish Medical Association*, Vol. 32 No. 188, February 1953.

95 Whyte, 1980. Full text in Appendix C.

96 Barrington, p. 237.

97 Ibid., p. 243.

98 Ibid., p. 242.

99 Horgan, pp. 170–171.

100 As described by Joseph Robins (*Custom House People*, Institute of Public Administration, 1993, p. 142), a former assistant secretary in the Department of Health.

101 Barrington, p. 245.

102 Ibid., p. 246.

103 Ibid.

3. Consultants obstruct free hospital care

1 Daly, 1981, p. 174.

2 Ibid.

3 Dáil Debates, Volume 163, June 26th 1957.

4 Whyte, 1980, pp. 299–300. O'Malley as reported in the *Irish Press*, February 25th 1966.

5 *The Health Services and their Further Development*, laid by the government before each House of the Oireachtas, Stationery Office Dublin, January 1966, p. 16.

6 FitzGerald, 1999.

7 Whyte, 1980, p. 300. Flanagan as reported in *The Irish Times*, April 18th 1967.

8 Dáil Debates, Volume 192, November 23rd 1961.

9 John Horgan, *Seán Lemass – the enigmatic patriot*, Gill and Macmillan, 1997, p. 110.

10 Dáil Debates, Volume 208, April 15th 1964.

11 Dick Walsh, *The Party – inside Fianna Fáil*, Gill and Macmillan, 1986, p. 77.

12 Cormac MacNamara interview, March 2002.

13 Ibid.

14 The GMS was introduced in 1972.

15 Eight health boards were set up under the 1970 Health Act.

16 Translates as the Hospitals' Council.

17 Anecdotal evidence from a former civil servant with the Department of Health.

18 1970 Health Act Section 45.

19 *The Health Services and their Further Development*, p. 64.

20 Warned against by MacEntee in 1960. Ibid., pp. 62–63.

21 *Outline of the Future Hospital System*, Report of the Consultative Council on the General Hospital Services, Stationery Office Dublin, 1968, *passim*.

22 Robins, 1993, pp. 133–135.

23 Dáil Debates, Oral Answers, July 22nd 1971.

24 In a letter quoted in Appendix D, *First Report of Comhairle na nOspidéal*, September 1972–December 1975.

25 As noted by Barrington, p. 272.

26 Health Act 1970, Section 55.

27 Corish's character as assessed by Michael McInerney, *The Irish Times*, June 27th 1977.

28 *The Labour Party Outline Policy: Health, Social Welfare*, as adopted by the Labour Party annual conference, January 1969.

29 Brian Nolan, *The Utilisation and Financing of Health Services in Ireland*, Economic and Social Research Institute, Dublin, 1991, p. 16.

NOTES TO PAGES 51-60

[30] *The Irish Times*, February 26th and March 28th 1974.
[31] Dáil Debates, Volume 271, March 27th 1974.
[32] *The Irish Times*, April 22nd and July 12th 1974.
[33] Dáil Debates, Volume 271, March 27th 1974.
[34] Memorandum from Dermot Condon, secretary of the Department of Health, to the Minister, Barry Desmond, February 10th 1983, Desmond's private papers.
[35] The politics were explored by Bruce Arnold in the *Irish Medical Times*, January 21st 1977.
[36] Desmond O'Malley, Dáil Debates, Volume 271, March 27th 1974.
[37] Charles Haughey in a private members' Bill, Dáil Debates, Volume 280, April 22nd 1975.
[38] Lee, pp. 470–471.
[39] *The Irish Times*, February 18th, August 6th and October 16th 1976.
[40] Dáil Debates, Volume 271, March 27th 1974.
[41] In his 1961 encyclical *Mater et Magistra*, quoted in Whyte, 1980, p. 356.
[42] *Pacem in Terris: encyclical letter of Pope John XXIII*, Catholic Truth Society, 1963.
[43] See Desmond Fisher, "The Church and Change" in Kieran A. Kennedy (ed.), *Ireland in Transition*, Mercier Press, 1986; Peadar Kirby, *Is Irish Catholicism Dying?*, Mercier Press, 1984; and Seán Freyne's introduction to Hans Küng, *Church and Change*, Gill and Macmillan, 1986.
[44] In a lecture in 1966, quoted in Whyte, 1980, p. 335.
[45] Tony Fahey, "The Catholic Church and Social Policy" in Seán Healy and Brigid Reynolds (eds), *Social Policy in Ireland*, Oaktree Press, 1998.
[46] *A Statement on Social Policy*, the Council for Social Welfare, a committee of the Catholic Bishops' Conference, November 1972.
[47] *The Work of Justice*, Irish Bishops' Pastoral, Veritas Publications, 1977.
[48] Tony Farmar, *Holles Street 1894–1994: the National Maternity Hospital – a centenary history*, A & A Farmar, 1994, pp. 152–154.
[49] "A Short History of the Pill in Ireland", Mary Maher, *The Irish Times*, March 14th 1968.
[50] In his Lenten pastoral letter, March 28th 1971, quoted in Chrystel Hug, *The Politics of Sexual Morality in Ireland*, Macmillan, 1999, p. 92.
[51] Bishops' statement, November 1973, quoted in Whyte, 1980, p. 407.
[52] Whyte, 1980, pp. 408–409.

4. The unleashing of private medicine

[1] *Magill* magazine poll reported in *The Irish Times*, May 10th 1979.
[2] Nolan, 1991, p. 150. Deflator for public authorities' expenditure.
[3] Brendan Hensey, *The Health Services of Ireland*, Institute of Public Administration, 4th edn, 1988, p. 180.
[4] See Table A.2, p. 372.
[5] As reported by Michael Finlan, *The Irish Times*, October 3rd 1978. See also p. 183.
[6] No figures for eligibility were published in the later 1970s. Nolan, 1991, p. 16.
[7] Hospital Services (Limited Eligibility) Regulations, 1979. Charles Haughey, Dáil Debates, Volume 313, March 27th 1979.
[8] *The Irish Times*, July 28th 1978.
[9] *The Irish Times*, October 16th 1978.
[10] At a public meeting of the Royal College of Physicians in 2001.
[11] Profiled from interview with MacNamara and contemporaries.
[12] Profiled from the reminiscences of colleagues.
[13] Barrington, p. 269.

14 *Report No. 32 to the Minister for Finance on Hospital Consultants,* Review Body on Higher Remuneration in the Public Sector, Stationery Office Dublin, 1990, Appendix, p. 65.

15 *Outline of the Future Hospital System,* Report of the Consultative Council on the General Hospital Services, Stationery Office Dublin, 1968, p. 14.

16 *Common Contract for Consultant Medical Staff,* 1981.

17 While employed under contract by the voluntary hospitals, the consultants were now in receipt of state-funded salaries.

18 Memorandum from Dermot Condon, secretary of the Department of Health, to the Minister, Barry Desmond, February 10th 1983, Desmond's private papers.

19 *The Irish Times,* April 14th 1980.

20 *Interim Report of the Working Party on a Common Contract and a Common Selection Procedure for Consultants,* paragraph 5.22, incorporated in the *Common Contract for Consultant Medical Staff,* paragraph 12.

21 Memorandum from Condon to Desmond.

22 *Common Contract for Consultant Medical Staff.*

23 Briefing note on private practice in public hospitals supplied to the Minister for Health, August 24th 1984, Desmond's private papers.

24 *Report No. 32 to the Minister for Finance on Hospital Consultants,* p. 66.

25 Memorandum from Condon to Desmond.

26 *The Irish Times,* October 23rd 1980.

27 Memorandum from Condon to Desmond.

28 Clause inserted in St. Vincent's University Hospital contract.

29 As described by Phelim Donnelly, a Medical Union activist, "Contract riddled by sectarian pressures", *The Irish Medical Times,* February 4th 1983.

30 *Archdiocese of Dublin: ethical code for hospitals* reprinted in Maurice Reidy (ed.), *Ethical Issues in Reproductive Medicine,* Gill and Macmillan, 1982, p. 158.

31 At an Irish Nurses Organisation seminar in 1977. Described in Emily O'Reilly, *Masterminds of the Right,* Attic Press , 1988, p. 44.

32 This account derives entirely from Farmar, pp. 176–179.

33 *Love is for Life,* quoted in Hug, pp. 132–133.

34 Whyte, 1980, p. 387.

35 Hug, p. 110.

36 Ibid., p. 112.

37 1979 Health (Family Planning) Act.

38 *The Irish Times,* January 6th 1979.

39 See Table A.2, p. 372.

40 Barry Desmond, *Finally and in Conclusion: a political memoir,* New Island, 2000, p. 105.

41 See Table A.2, p. 372.

42 *The Irish Times,* January 18th 1983.

43 Ibid., January 19th 1983.

44 Barry Desmond interview, February 20th 2002.

45 *Draft Green Paper on the Health Services,* May and July 1984, Barry Desmond's private papers.

46 *Draft Green Paper on the Health Services,* Volume One, Chapter 2, p. 13.

47 Ibid., Chapter 11, pp. 14–15.

48 *Health – the wider dimensions,* Department of Health, December 1986.

49 *Draft Green Paper on the Health Services,* Chapter 11, p. 11.

50 Barry Desmond interview, February 2002.

[51] Garret FitzGerald, *All in a Life – an autobiography*, Gill and Macmillan, 1991, pp. 367, 636.

[52] See Table A.2, p. 372.

[53] Desmond, p. 220.

[54] Ibid., p. 222.

[55] Dáil Debates, Volume 363, January 30th 1986.

[56] *The Irish Times*, January 18th–20th 1983.

[57] *Proposals for Plan 1984–1987*, National Planning Board, 1984, p. 306.

[58] Described in the 2001 Deloitte and Touche audit of the health system as a "key milestone in the development of mental health services" which influenced policy through the 1990s.

[59] *Proposals for Plan 1984–1987*, pp. 308–312.

[60] Briefing note to Desmond from Departmental officials, Desmond's private papers.

[61] *OECD Health Data 2002* records that in 1986 Ireland had 3.9 acute beds per 1,000 people compared to an EU average of 5.2. The 2002 *Acute Hospital Bed Capacity* review quotes 4.8 acute hospital beds per 1,000 in Ireland in 1986. The Department's count of acute hospital beds in 1986 was 19,080, the OECD's count was 14,680 and the Department's 2002 count for 1986 was 16,878, reflecting differences in definition.

[62] Leader, *The Irish Times*, February 7th 1986.

[63] Garret FitzGerald, p. 622; Desmond, p. 315.

[64] Fine Gael's John Boland briefly added Health to his Environment portfolio, following Labour's withdrawal.

[65] Nolan, 1991, pp. 148–152.

[66] *The Irish Catholic*, August 16th 2001.

[67] *Draft Green Paper on the Health Services*, Chapter 8, pp. 13–14.

[68] *The Irish Times*, July 3rd 1985, and Department of Health briefing note for Desmond, undated, Desmond's private papers.

[69] *Irish Medical News*, May 31st 1984.

[70] Barry Desmond interview, February 2002.

[71] See p. 292.

[72] Jimmy Sheehan interview, March 2002.

[73] Ibid.

[74] This 44:56 split in the ordinary shareholding pertained from 1985, BUPA has confirmed.

[75] Maurice Neligan interview, May 2002.

[76] Report by Paul Tansey, *The Sunday Tribune*, April 20th 1986.

[77] *Irish Medical News*, May 31st 1984; Desmond's private papers.

[78] *Report of the Working Group on Public/Private Mix*, Department of Health, July 2001, FOI.

[79] Garret FitzGerald, pp. 377–379.

[80] Health (Family Planning) (Amendment) Act 1985.

[81] *The Irish Times*, October 20th 1986.

[82] Küng, p. 83.

[83] Hug, p. 116.

[84] Küng, p. 84.

[85] *The Irish Times*, February 8th 1985.

[86] Inglis, p. 81.

[87] Dáil Debates, February 20th 1985.

[88] *The Irish Times*, Letter from the Minister, August 22nd 1985.

[89] At its 1985 AGM.

[90] *The Irish Times*, Arminta Wallace, February 7th 1986.

[91] Garret FitzGerald, p. 631 and Jack Jones, *In Your Opinion*, TownHouse, 2001, p. 80.

92 The amendment stated: "The State acknowledges the right to life of the unborn and, with due regard to the equal right to life of the mother, guarantees in its laws to respect and, as far as is practicable, by its laws to defend and vindicate that right."

93 The proposed substitute stated: "Nothing in this Constitution shall be invoked to invalidate any provision of a law on the grounds that it prohibits abortion."

5. The era of the cuts

1 *Programme for National Recovery (PNR)*, October 1987.

2 See Table A.2, p. 372.

3 Nolan, 1991, Table 2.4, p. 24. Includes capital spending.

4 See Table A.2, p. 372.

5 See Tim Pat Coogan, *Michael Collins*, Arrow, 1991, p. 159.

6 Dáil Debates, Volume 395, February 6th 1990.

7 Brendan Howlin, ibid.

8 See Table A.4, p. 375.

9 *Value for Money Audit of the Irish Health System*, Deloitte and Touche in conjunction with the York Health Economics Consortium, on behalf of the Department of Health and Children, Deloitte and Touche Dublin, 2001, p. 61.

10 *OECD Health Data 2002*.

11 Dáil Debates, Volume 395, February 6th 1990.

12 See Table A.4, p. 375.

13 Dáil Debates, Volume 395, February 6th 1990.

14 Under a 1986 agreement, restored after the strike, junior doctors worked a maximum of 86 hours weekly.

15 *The Irish Times*, June 22nd 1987.

16 *The Irish Times*, June 25th 1987.

17 Eithne FitzGerald, *The Irish Times*, December 31st 1988.

18 National Economic and Social Forum, *Equity of Access to Hospital Care*, Forum Report No. 25, Government Publication Sales Office, 2002, pp. 44–45.

19 *Report of the Commission on Health Funding*, Stationary Office Dublin, 1989, p. 45.

20 Nolan, 1991, pp. 147–157.

21 As reported in the CSO's quarterly national household survey for the third quarter of 2001. Also, see Table A.4, p. 375.

22 *The Irish Times*, February 8th 1990.

23 A. Dale Tussing, *Irish Medical Care Resources: an economic analysis*, ESRI, 1985, pp. 285–288.

24 *The Irish Times*, September 18th 1987.

25 *Irish Medical Journal*, December 1987, pp. 342–345.

26 Tussing, 1985, pp. 273–274.

27 Letter to the Editor, *The Irish Times*, December 19th 1988.

28 *Primary (Health and Social Services) Care*. An unpublished draft of the 2001 government strategy for primary care.

29 See Chapter 7.

30 Jones, pp. 97–100.

31 On RTÉ Radio One's *Pat Kenny Show*, as reported in *The Irish Times*, June 10th 1989.

32 *The Irish Times*, January 8th 1990.

33 *The Irish Times*, June 23rd 1988.

34 Central Statistics Office. When female earnings are included, the average wage dropped to £11,000.

[35] *The Irish Times,* July 4th 1988.
[36] Ibid., December 31st 1988.
[37] Ibid., May 20th 1988
[38] VHI statement, March 1st 1991.
[39] *The Irish Times,* May 23rd 1996.
[40] A compilation of his colleagues' views.
[41] *Irish Medical News,* January 21st 2002.
[42] *The Irish Times,* October 24th 1988.
[43] *The Irish Times,* September 16th 1997.
[44] Finbarr Fitzpatrick at the IHCA's annual general meeting, *The Irish Times,* October 16th 2000.
[45] Finbarr Fitzpatrick interview, October 2002.
[46] The first meetings were held in 1988, while its formal establishment was in March 1989.
[47] *The Irish Times,* October 24th 1988.
[48] Brendan Howlin interview, June 2002.
[49] *Report of the Commission on Health Funding,* pp. 238–240.
[50] Ibid., p. 267.
[51] Miriam Hederman O'Brien interview, March 2002.
[52] *Report of the Commission on Health Funding,* p. 128.
[53] Ibid., pp. 109–110; 238–244.
[54] Ibid., p. 237.
[55] Ibid., p. 221.
[56] Ibid., p. 269–270.
[57] Ibid., p. 156.
[58] Ibid., p. 153.
[59] *The Irish Times,* October 12th 1989.
[60] Miriam Hederman O'Brien interview, March 2002.
[61] Dáil Debates, Volume 391, July 20th 1989.
[62] *The Irish Times,* October 31st 1990.
[63] Dáil Debates, Volume 395, February 7th 1990.
[64] *The Irish Times,* May 15th 1989.
[65] Dáil Debates, Volume 378, June 19th 1987.
[66] *The People's Health Service – proposals to meet the crisis in health care,* The Labour Party, June 8th 1989.
[67] Dáil Debates, Volume 391, July 20th 1989
[68] *Submission to the Commission on Health Funding,* Council for Social Welfare, September 1987.
[69] *Proposals for the Future of the Health Services,* Report of Executive Council 1987–88, ICTU.
[70] *The Irish Times,* October 9th and 12th 1987.
[71] *The Fianna Fáil–Progressive Democrats Programme for Government 1989–1993 in the National Interest,* Government Information Service, p. 9.
[72] "The Major Issues in Health Care Funding", Gerry McCartney, health policy conference, Beaumont Hospital, Dublin, October 20th–21st 1987.
[73] Dáil Debates, Volume 391, July 20th 1989.
[74] *Report of the Commission on Health Funding,* pp. 396–397.
[75] *Submission to the Commission on Health Funding.*
[76] *Report of the Commission on Health Funding,* p. 140.
[77] *Health Care – let's look again,* Joint Health Care Commission, July 1989, *passim.*

78 *The People's Health Service.*

79 *A Better Health Service,* Fine Gael Press Office, June 1988.

80 Dáil Debates, Volume 409, May 28th 1991.

81 *Programme for Economic and Social Progress (PESP),* Stationery Office Dublin, January 1991, pp. 24–30.

82 Tussing, 1985, p. 281; *Confronting the Jobs Crisis,* ICTU, September 1984.

83 *PESP,* p. 28.

84 As described in *Report of Executive Council 1988–89,* ICTU.

85 Dáil Debates, Volume 409, May 30th 1991.

86 Dáil Debates, Volume 409, May 29th 1991.

87 Tussing, 1985, p. 266.

88 *Medical Manpower in Acute Hospitals – a discussion document,* Department of Health, Comhairle na nOspidéal and Postgraduate Medical and Dental Board, June 1993.

89 National Economic and Social Council, *A Strategy for the Nineties,* NESC 1990, Chapter 9.

90 Dáil Debates, Volume 409, May 30th 1991.

91 Health (Amendment) Act 1991, Sections 5 and 6. Intent explained by Rory O'Hanlon, Dáil Debates, Volume 409, May 28th 1991.

92 Brian Nolan and Miriam Wiley, *Private Practice in Irish Public Hospitals,* Oaktree Press and ESRI, 2000, pp. 16–17.

93 Figures for April 2002, Department of Health, FOI.

94 See Chapter 9, pp. 169–174.

95 *Report of the Commission on Health Funding,* pp. 109, 240.

96 Rory O'Hanlon interview, July 2002.

97 Dáil Debates, Volume 409, May 28th 1991.

98 Dáil Debates, Volume 409, May 30th 1991.

99 Dáil Debates, Volume 409, May 28th 1991.

100 Dáil Debates, Volume 409, May 30th 1991.

101 *Draft Green Paper on the Health Services,* May and July 1984, Barry Desmond's private papers, Chapter 11, p. 11.

102 *Report No. 36 to the Minister for Finance on Hospital Consultants,* Review Body on Higher Remuneration in the Public Sector, Stationery Office Dublin, 1996, pp. 34–35.

103 In an interview in October 2002.

104 *Report No. 32 to the Minister for Finance on Hospital Consultants,* Review Body on Higher Remuneration in the Public Sector, Stationery Office Dublin, 1990, pp. 38–41.

105 Ibid., pp. 6–10.

106 *Common Contract for Consultant Medical Staff,* 1981, Clause 7.4.

107 *Consultants' Contract Documents,* 1991, Memorandum of Agreement, Paragraph 6.6.4.

108 Ibid., Appendix H, Outline Practice Plan.

109 *The Irish Times,* April 6th 1991.

110 Ibid.

111 Cormac MacNamara interview, March 2002.

112 Finbarr Fitzpatrick interview, October 2002.

113 Cormac MacNamara interview, March 2002.

114 *Report No. 36,* p. 12.

115 Rory O'Hanlon interview, July 2002.

116 George MacNeice interview, October 2002.

117 *Report No. 32,* pp. 6–10.

118 *Report No. 36,* p. 19.

[119] Dáil Debates, Volume 409, May 29th 1991.
[120] Dáil Debates, Volume 409, May 30th 1991.

6. No beds in the boom

[1] GNP per capita. Source: *OECD Health Data 2002* and Department of Finance.
[2] 2002 Census of Population.
[3] Cormac Ó Gráda, "Is the Celtic Tiger a Paper Tiger?", *Quarterly Economic Commentary*, ESRI, Spring 2002.
[4] See Table A.2, p. 372.
[5] Review of O'Connell's career by Pádraig Yeates in *The Irish Times*, August 11th 1992.
[6] Reports of the Central Bank of Ireland, Winter 1992 and Summer 1993.
[7] *Irish Times/MRBI* poll, November 1992.
[8] *Democratic Left Election Manifesto 1992*.
[9] *Making Ireland Work: justice into economics*, The Labour Party, 1992.
[10] *The Sunday Tribune*, May 9th, 1993.
[11] *Shaping a Healthier Future – a strategy for effective healthcare in the 1990s*, Department of Health, Stationery Office Dublin, 1994, p. 36.
[12] Ibid., p.64.
[13] Ibid., p. 36.
[14] The 1994 Health Insurance Act provided for community rating (charging the same premium regardless of age or health) and risk equalisation (subsidy from insurers with healthier members to those with less favourable risk).
[15] *Fianna Fáil and Labour Programme for a Partnership Government 1993–1997*, Government Information Service.
[16] Brendan Howlin interview, June 2002.
[17] Ibid.
[18] Wiley, *Critique of Shaping a Healthier Future*, pp. 8–9.
[19] *A Government of Renewal: a policy agreement between Fine Gael, The Labour Party and Democratic Left*, Government Information Service, December 1994, p. 67.
[20] Dáil Debates, Volume 391, July 12th 1989.
[21] Michael Noonan interview, June 2002.
[22] See Chapter 9, p. 174.
[23] *Towards a Better Quality of Life*, Fine Gael General Election Manifesto 2002.
[24] *The Irish Times*, April 1st 1997.
[25] Michael Noonan interview, June 2002.
[26] *White Paper Private Health Insurance*, Stationery Office Dublin, 1999, p.13.
[27] Ibid.
[28] Ibid., p.18.
[29] Ibid., pp. 24–26.
[30] Ibid., p. 89.
[31] *Irish Times/MRBI* poll, March 1997.
[32] Summary of parties' manifestos in *The Irish Times*, June 5th 1997.
[33] *Making the Vital Difference*, 1997 Labour Party general election manifesto.
[34] *An Action Programme for the Millennium*, Fianna Fáil and the Progressive Democrats.
[35] *People before Politics*, Fianna Fáil Manifesto, 1997.
[36] *The Irish Times*, November 25th 1998.
[37] Dáil Debates, Volume 496, November 18th 1998.
[38] The voluntary hospitals had formerly been directly funded by the Department of Health,

even though the health boards were legally responsible for running the health service.

39 *Shaping a Healthier Future*, p. 30.

40 *Report No. 36*, p. 19.

41 Ibid., p. 36.

42 *The Irish Times*, June 23rd 1997.

43 *The Irish Times*, December 16th 1996.

44 *The Irish Times*, September 16th 1997.

45 *The Irish Times*, February 18th 1997.

46 *The Irish Times*, February 18th 1997.

47 *Revised Contract for Consultant Medical Staff*, 1997, paragraph 5.2 and attached *Memorandum of Agreement*, 2.9.3.

48 *Programme for Competitiveness and Work*, Stationery Office, Dublin, 1994.

49 *Report of Proceedings*, ICTU Conference, Galway 1993.

50 *Report of Proceedings*, ICTU Conference, Tralee 1995.

51 Interview, March 2002.

52 *The Irish Times*, June 17th 1998.

53 *A Blueprint for the Future*, Report of the Commission on Nursing, Stationery Office Dublin, 1998.

54 *Partnership 2000*, Stationery Office Dublin, 1996.

55 NESC, *A Strategy for Competitiveness, Growth and Employment*, November 1993, pp. 513, 517.

56 *Programme for Prosperity and Fairness*, Stationery Office, Dublin, 2000.

57 Peter Cassells interview, June 2002.

58 *Value for Money Audit*, p. 62.

59 NESC, *Strategy for the Nineties*, 1990, Chapter 9.

60 When adjusted for inflation in public expenditure on goods and services. See Table A.2, p. 372.

61 See Table A.2.1, p. 373.

62 Employment growth did not exceed 3 per cent per annum from 1990 to 1998 but in the three years to 2001, employment grew by a cumulative 33 per cent. Department of Health personnel census. See Table A.3, 374.

63 See *Interim Report of the Steering Group*, Nursing and Midwifery Resource, Department of Health and Children, 2000, p. 41.

64 See Table A.2, p. 372.

65 See Table A.3, p. 374.

66 See Table A.3, p. 374.

67 *Shaping A Healthier Future*, p. 31.

68 The Health Amendment Act 1996 required health boards to submit annual service plans to be delivered within budget.

69 *The Irish Times*, November 14th 1998.

70 *The Irish Times*, November 10th 1998.

71 *The Irish Times*, November 12th 1998.

72 *Interim Report of the Steering Group*, pp. 39–48.

73 Ibid., p. 80; *Towards Workforce Planning*, final report of the steering group, The Nursing and Midwifery Resource, Department of Health and Children, 2002, p. 75.

74 *Report of the Review Group on the Waiting List Initiative*, Stationery Office Dublin, 1998.

75 ERHA Bed Capacity Review, January 25th 2001.

76 *The Irish Times*, January 15th 1999.

77 *The Irish Times*, January 12th 2000.

[78] *The Irish Times*, January 16th 2003.
[79] Answers to a survey conducted by *The Irish Times* library.
[80] John McManus, *The Case for Socialist Medical Care*, Repsol Publications, 1977.
[81] Liz McManus, *Proposals for a National Health Strategy*, Democratic Left Health, January 1994.
[82] Liz McManus, *Quality and Equality: a discussion document on the need for change in our acute hospital services*, Democratic Left, February 1998.
[83] Dáil Debates, Volume 513, February 1st, 2000.

7. The politics of blood

[1] Women whose blood is rhesus negative but who are pregnant with rhesus positive babies may develop antibodies to the baby's blood. They receive transfusions of Anti-D either after childbirth or during a subsequent pregnancy to prevent their antibodies from harming their next baby.
[2] *The Irish Times*, April 1st 1997.
[3] Michael Noonan interview, June 2002.
[4] In a letter from the BTSB's solicitors to the family's solicitors, September 20th 1996. *The Irish Times,* October 9th 1996.
[5] "Report by the Minister for Health and Children, Mr Brian Cowen, on the legal strategy adopted by the defence in the case of the late Mrs Bridget McCole", *The Irish Times*, August 2nd 1997.
[6] Ibid.
[7] Statement from Michael Noonan, *The Irish Times,* August 6th 1997.
[8] Report to the Minister for Health by Fidelma Macken S.C., July 30th 1997, p. 5.
[9] Dáil Debates, Volume 469, October 3rd 1996.
[10] Dáil Debates, Volume 470, October 16th 1996.
[11] *The Irish Times*, October 17th 1996.
[12] Dáil Debates, Volume 470, October 17th 1996.
[13] "How close to the truth is Michael Noonan's TV villain?" *The Sunday Tribune*, February 10th 2002.
[14] *The Irish Times*, January 29th 2002.
[15] *Report of the Tribunal of Inquiry into the Blood Transfusion Service Board*, Stationery Office Dublin, 1997. Conclusion for Chapter 13, nos 1 and 13.
[16] Ibid., Conclusion for Chapter 13, no. 12.
[17] "Tribunal removes cloud over Ministers' handling of 'worst public health scandal in State's history'", Denis Coghlan in *The Irish Times*, March 12th 1997.
[18] *Report of the Tribunal of Inquiry*, 1997, p. 147.
[19] Ibid., p. 148.
[20] Ibid., p. 147–149, Chapter 4 *passim*.
[21] Ibid., p. 138.
[22] Ibid., p. 151.
[23] Ibid., p. 151.
[24] Ibid., p. 149.
[25] *The Irish Times*, May 12th 1997.
[26] *The Irish Times*, May 15th 1997.
[27] *Report of the Tribunal of Inquiry into the Infection with HIV and Hepatitis C of Persons with Haemophilia and Related Matters*, Stationery Office Dublin, 2002, p. 230.
[28] *The Irish Times*, March 13th 1991
[29] *Report of the Tribunal of Inquiry*, 2002, p. 41.

30 *The Irish Times*, September 27th 1999.

31 "Stories of private suffering and official insensitivity dominated an emotionally charged week at the haemophilia tribunal", Kathy Sheridan in *The Irish Times*, May 13th 2000; "'Regret' at lag of 5 years in telling mother of sons' illness", *The Irish Times*, February 24th 2001; *Report of the Tribunal of Inquiry*, 2002, put the delay at four years, p. 185.

32 Quoted by Kathy Sheridan, *The Irish Times*, May 13th 2000.

33 *Report of the Tribunal of Inquiry*, 2002, p. 89.

34 "Document on compensation contained inaccuracies", *The Irish Times*, May 19th 2001; *Report of the Tribunal of Inquiry*, 2002, p. 232.

35 *The Irish Times*, May 25th 2001; *Report of the Tribunal of Inquiry*, 2002, p. 233.

36 *Report of the Tribunal of Inquiry*, 2002, p. 232.

37 Ibid., pp. 79–81.

38 *The Irish Times*, May 24th 2001.

39 *Report of the Tribunal of Inquiry*, 2002, p 233.

40 Rosemary Daly, administrator of the Irish Haemophilia Society, *Sunday Business Post*, September 8th 2002.

41 Ibid., pp. 224–229.

42 Ibid., pp. 120, 224.

43 Ibid., p. 122.

44 Joe Humphreys, *The Irish Times*, September 14th 2002.

45 *Report of the Tribunal of Inquiry*, 2002, p. 140.

46 Ibid., pp. 111–117.

47 *The Irish Times*, September 6th 2002.

48 *Report of the Tribunal of Inquiry*, 2002, p. 159.

49 Ibid., p. 165.

50 Ibid., pp. 166–167.

51 Ibid., p. 174.

52 Ibid., p. 168.

53 Ibid., p. 182.

54 Ibid., p. 148.

55 *The Irish Times*, November 13th 2002; Dáil Debates, Volume 556, November 6th 2002.

56 *The Irish Times*, March 13th 2002.

57 Dáil Debates, Volume 541, October 3rd 2001, written answers.

58 The Supreme Court, however, limited victims' ability to appeal tribunal awards in March 2003.

59 *The Irish Times*, June 14th 2002; *The Sunday Tribune*, June 16th 2002.

60 The case was subsequently appealed.

61 *The Irish Times*, November 16th 2002.

62 Reports of Dolores Moran's High Court action, *The Irish Times*, November and December 1998.

63 *Nursing Home Subventions: an investigation by the Ombudsman of complaints regarding payment of nursing home subventions by health boards*, Office of the Ombudsman, January 2001, p. 60.

64 Ibid., p. 52.

65 *Observations by the Department of Health and Children on Draft Report of the Ombudsman in Relation to Nursing Homes Subvention Scheme*, October 27th 2000, p. 6; *Nursing Home Subventions*, p. 14.

66 *Observations by the Department of Health*, p. 30; *Nursing Home Subventions*, p. 61.

67 *Nursing Home Subventions*, pp. 60–62.

68 Ibid., p. 69.

69 *Submission by the Ombudsman in Relation to Quality Customer Service in the Healthcare Sector*, presentation to the Oireachtas Joint Committee on the Strategic Management Initiative, June 26th 2001.
70 *Value for Money Audit*, p. 184.
71 *Report of the Tribunal of Inquiry*, 2002, p. 177.
72 "Health Inflation: cost pressures within the health services", paper prepared for the Public Accounts Committee, Department of Health, March 8th 1999.

8. Ethics, ownership and the Catholic Church

1 Patsy McGarry, *The Irish Times*, September 20th 2002.
2 Tony Fahey, "Is Atheism Increasing?" in Eoin Cassidy (ed.), *Measuring Ireland: discerning values and beliefs*, Veritas, 2002.
3 Tony Fahey, "The Catholic Church and Social Policy" in Healy and Reynolds.
4 Survey conducted for the Conference of Religious in Ireland (CORI), *The Irish Times*, October 22nd 2001.
5 John Walshe, *Irish Independent*, November 12th 2002.
6 76 per cent said Connell should resign in a telephone poll, *Sunday Independent*, October 20th 2002.
7 Marie Collins' account was published in *The Irish Times*, April 4th 2002.
8 Andy Pollak, *The Irish Times*, March 16th 1991.
9 *The Irish Times*, December 10th 1988.
10 *The Irish Times*, March 6th 1991.
11 Dermot Keogh, *Twentieth-Century Ireland: nation and state*, Gill and Macmillan, 1994, p. 380.
12 Hug, p. 123.
13 Health (Family Planning) Amendment Act 1992.
14 Health (Family Planning) (Amendment) Act 1993.
15 Hug, pp. 129–130.
16 Minister for Education, Noel Dempsey, in response to a Dáil question, December 10th 2002.
17 Report by the child-care unit of the MWHB, Department of Health, March 2001. FOI.
18 UCC study of teenage pregnancy, presented to the SEHB, *The Irish Times*, October 12th 2002.
19 Noted in the *Report of the Second Commission on the Status of Women*, Stationery Office Dublin, 1993, p. 345.
20 Confirmed by Helena O'Donoghue, provincial leader of the Sisters of Mercy, April 2002.
21 *Ethical Policy of the Mater Misericordiae Hospital*, September 1998, supplied by the hospital, August 2002.
22 *Philosophy and Ethical Code*, Religious Sisters of Charity, Health Service.
23 Declan Keane, Master of Holles Street, interview, 2002.
24 Donal O'Shea interview, March 2002.
25 Fergus O'Ferrall, director of the Adelaide Hospital Society, *Citizenship and Public Service*, Adelaide Hospital Society and Dundealgan Press, 2000.
26 Arminta Wallace, *The Irish Times*, February 7th 1986.
27 O'Ferrall, pp. 172–173.
28 *Charter of the Adelaide and Meath Hospital*, August 1st 1996, p. 16.
29 *Shaping a Healthier Future*, p. 56.
30 Wiley, *Critique of Shaping A Healthier Future*.
31 In a letter from John Cooney, CEO of the SEHB, to the Department of Health, April 25th 2001.
32 *The Irish Times*, March 24th 1995.
33 *The Irish Times*, April 10th 1997.

34 *The Irish Times*, April 19th 2002.

35 Trinity College Dublin, Department of Community Health and General Practice, *People Living in Tallaght and their Health*, Adelaide Hospital Society, 2002.

36 *The Irish Times*, December 27th 2001.

37 This proposed amendment read: "It shall be unlawful to terminate the life of an unborn unless such termination is necessary to save the life, as distinct from the health, of the mother where there is an illness or disorder of the mother giving rise to a real and substantial risk to her life, not being a risk of self-destruction."

38 Hug, p. 185.

39 *Fianna Fáil and Labour Programme for a Partnership Government 1993–1997*, p. 29.

40 Brendan Howlin interview, June 2002.

41 Medical Council, *A Guide to Ethical Conduct and Behaviour and to Fitness to Practise*, 4th edn, 1994, 39.03.

42 Regulation of Information (Services Outside the State for Termination of Pregnancies) Act, 1995.

43 Report commissioned by Noonan and published by Micheál Martin, *The Irish Times*, March 13th 1998.

44 Irish Times/MRBI poll, *The Irish Times*, December 11th 1997.

45 Medical Council, 5th edn, 1998.

46 Medical Council, 5th edn, 2001, Amendment No. 1.

47 *The Irish Times*, September 13th and 15th 2001.

48 Mark Brennock, *The Irish Times*, February 18th 2002.

49 *The Irish Times*, February 28th 2002.

50 *The Irish Times*, February 28th and March 5th 2002.

51 *The Irish Times*, February 11th 2002.

52 Letters to the Editor, *The Irish Times*, February 25th 2002.

53 *The Irish Times*, February 23rd 2002

54 *The Irish Times*, February 25th 2002

55 *The Irish Times*, March 1st 2002

56 *The Irish Times*, December 13th 2001.

57 *The Irish Times*, March 6th 2002.

58 *Sunday Independent*, March 10th, 2002.

59 Press release from the Minister for Health, December 18th 2001.

60 Announced by the Minister for Health, June 7th 2001.

61 Helena O'Donoghue interview, April 2002.

62 Confirmed by spokeswoman for the NEHB.

63 As explained by a spokesman for the Department of Health.

64 Helena O'Donoghue interview, April 2002.

65 As explained by Helena O'Donoghue.

66 The diocesan role was recollected by a former civil servant. The Department produced draft guidelines in 1986.

67 *Quality and Fairness*, p. 80.

68 Office of the Ombudsman, *Annual Report of the Ombudsman 2001*, 2002.

69 *Work is the Key – towards an economy that needs everyone*, Bishops' Pastoral, Veritas, 1992.

70 *Re-righting the Constitution*, Irish Commission for Justice and Peace, 1998.

71 Concluding observations, UN Committee on Economic, Social and Cultural Rights, 28th session 2002.

72 Fahey, 1998, p. 424.

73 CMRS Pre-Budget submissions, 1988 and 1989; CORI socio-economic review, 1996.

[74] Inglis, p. 222; Fahey, 1998, p. 426.

[75] Whyte, 1980, pp. 255–257.

9. Two-tier hospital care

[1] Letter to the Editor, *The Irish Times*, November 1st 2000.

[2] Reports of the High Court proceedings, *The Irish Times*, June 26th and 28th 2001.

[3] Society of St Vincent de Paul, *Health Inequalities and Poverty*, April 2001.

[4] First recounted on RTÉ One Television's *Prime Time*, "Unfair Care: Ireland's two-tier hospitals", January 31st 2001. The 1997–2002 government targeted cardiac surgery waiting lists with some success. In December 1996, there were 1,030 adults on the waiting list and by September 2002 this had dropped to 241 people, of whom 79 had been on the list for over 12 months. Discrimination remained between public and private cardiac patients.

[5] A consumer survey in 2000 found that, among patients who had visited an outpatient clinic, 2 per cent of uninsured patients without medical cards had waited over a year for an outpatients' appointment, whereas no private patients had waited over a year. Dorothy Watson and James Williams, *Perceptions of the Quality of Health Care in the Public and Private Sectors in Ireland*, Report to the Centre for Insurance Studies, University College Dublin, ESRI, 2001, Table 4.6, p. 32. Only very small numbers of people in the survey had visited outpatients in the preceding year. A larger sample would be required to gain a more representative picture. Similar reservations apply to the findings of *Experiences and Expectations of Health Services 2002*, ERHA, 2002, p. 38, which recorded that 3 per cent of patients waited over a year for outpatients' appointments. There is ample anecdotal evidence of long waits for outpatients by public patients.

[6] *The Irish Times*, June 25th 2001.

[7] *The Irish Times*, July 4th 2001.

[8] Killarney, Co. Kerry, May 2001.

[9] Professor Ray Kinsella, *Waiting Lists: analysis, evaluation and recommendations*, Centre for Insurance Studies, UCD, August 2001.

[10] *Quality and Fairness*, p. 105.

[11] "New patient data system 'on hold'", Kevin Moore, *The Sunday Independent*, August 25th 2002.

[12] Interview, September 2002.

[13] Finbarr Fitzpatrick interview, October 2002.

[14] As recounted by a hospital manager who was seeking their cooperation with the Fund.

[15] From the National Treatment Purchase Fund's principles of operation.

[16] Maureen Lynott interview, February 2003.

[17] Kinsella.

[18] An understanding volunteered by an experienced hospital manager in an off-the-record interview, September 2002.

[19] Day cases were 68 per cent of elective treatments in 2000. *Acute Hospital Bed Capacity: a national review*, Department of Health and Children, Stationery Office Dublin, 2002, p. 9.

[20] 19,236 public patients were waiting for elective inpatient surgery and 9,938 were waiting for day surgery in September 2002. There were then 8,655 designated inpatient beds for public patients. In targeted specialties, 6,273 adult patients had waited for inpatient treatment for over 12 months and 1,201 children had waited for over 6 months. At least 1,947 adults had waited over 12 months for day surgery, while 411 children had waited over 6 months and the waiting times of 3,512 day patients were unspecified.

[21] If children who waited more than six months were assumed to wait over a year, the Irish figure would be 25 per 10,000.

[22] While it might be argued that in September 2002 the number of inpatients waiting, at 19,236, had dropped below the 1994 level of 24,778, the increased significance of day procedures in the 1990s requires the inclusion of the day patient waiting list to get a true picture for 2002, when the total waiting then rises to 29,174. See Table A.3 p. 374.

[23] First highlighted in National Economic and Social Forum, *Equity of Access to Hospital Care*, Forum Report No. 25, Government Publication Sales Office, 2002. 2002 percentages my own calculations.

[24] *People Living in Tallaght and their Health*, Trinity College Dublin, 2002.

[25] Brian Nolan and Miriam Wiley, *Private Practice in Irish Public Hospitals*, Oaktree Press and the ESRI, 2000, p. 105.

[26] Watson and Williams, p. 33. This survey also reported that, among those who had been hospitalised in the preceding 12 months, 9 per cent of medical card patients had waited over 6 months, compared to 2 per cent of the insured. Of the insured, 1 per cent had waited over a year – a single individual and statistically insignificant result. "Waiting" was open to the respondent's interpretation, which might explain this patient's abnormal experience. See also note 5 above re sample size.

[27] *Experiences and Expectations of Health Services*, ERHA, 2002, p. 21.

[28] Watson and Williams, pp. 45–46.

[29] Department of Health, quoted in *Equity of Access to Hospital Care*, p. 21. Also see Table A.4, p. ???

[30] Watson and Williams, p. 18.

[31] Nolan and Wiley, p. 74.

[32] Watson and Williams, p. 59.

[33] *Quality and Fairness*, p. 74.

[34] National Economic and Social Forum, *Equity of Access to Hospital Care*, p. 84.

[35] *Report of the Working Group on Public/Private Mix*, July 25th 2001, p. 2. FOI.

[36] In a letter inviting participants to the group's first meeting on May 18th 2000.

[37] The papers and final report of the group were released to the author under FOI in June 2002 and had not been published at the time of going to print.

[38] *Draft report by sub-group on public-private mix: organisation/management incentives*, June 5th 2001.

[39] *Draft report by sub-group on public-private mix: organisation/management incentives*, May 30th 2001.

[40] *Activity in Acute Public Hospitals in Ireland 1990–1999*, ESRI, March 2002, Table 2.1, p. 32.

[41] Quoted in *Irish Medical Care Resources: an economic analysis*, A. Dale Tussing, ESRI, 1985, p. 266.

[42] *Medical Manpower in Acute Hospitals – a discussion document*, Department of Health, Comhairle na nOspidéal and Postgraduate Medical and Dental Board, June 1993.

[43] *Report of the Forum on Medical Manpower*, Department of Health and Children, January 2001, p. 19.

[44] *Annual Report of the Ombudsman 2001*, p. 12.

[45] Detailed account from Ombudsman's investigation report.

[46] *Annual Report of the Ombudsman 2001*.

[47] Ombudsman's investigation report.

[48] *Annual Report of the Ombudsman 2001*.

[49] Ibid.

[50] Ombudsman's investigation report.

[51] Joseph Robins (ed.), *Reflections on Health: commemorating fifty years of the Department of Health 1947–1997*, Department of Health, 1997.

[52] On RTÉ One Television's *Prime Time*, "Unfair Care: Ireland's two-tier hospitals", January 31st 2001.

[53] *Consultant Staffing*, Comhairle na nOspidéal, January 2003.

[54] *Revised Contract for Consultant Medical Staff*, Memorandum of Agreement, 1997, 2.11.4–2.11.6.

[55] *Revised Contract for Consultant Medical Staff*, Paragraph 5.2.

[56] *Report of the Working Group on Public/Private Mix*, p. 5.

[57] *Draft report by sub-group on public-private mix: organisation/management incentives*, pp. 3–4.

[58] Cormac MacNamara interview, March 2002.

[59] *Value for Money Audit*, p. 180.

[60] *National Patient Perception of the Quality of Healthcare 2002*, Irish Society for Quality and Safety in Healthcare, 2003.

[61] *Consultant Staffing*.

[62] Muiris FitzGerald, "Without medical manpower reform hospital 'crises' will persist", *Journal of Health Gain*, January 1999.

[63] Study by John McManus in his Bray practice, reported at *The Irish Times*/Royal Academy of Medicine lecture, October 23rd 2001.

[64] Recounted by a nurse at a workshop at the 2001 INO annual conference.

[65] *Report of the Forum on Medical Manpower*, Department of Health and Children, January 2001.

[66] *Report of the Forum on Medical Manpower*, p. 21.

[67] Post-graduate medical and dental board survey of NCHD staffing, October 1st 2002; *Consultant Staffing*.

[68] Muiris FitzGerald, Doolin memorial lecture delivered at the invitation of the IMO, December 1997.

[69] Post-graduate medical and dental board survey of NCHD staffing.

[70] Muiris FitzGerald, Doolin lecture.

[71] Ibid.

[72] *Report of the Committee on Accident and Emergency Services*, Comhairle na nOspidéal, February 2002, p. 22. While dated February, the report was published in April.

[73] Muiris FitzGerald, *Journal of Health Gain*.

[74] *Report of the Review Group on the Waiting List Initiative*, June 1998, pp. 18–19.

[75] *Quality and Fairness*, p. 106.

[76] Report of coroner's inquest, *The Irish Times*, July 20th 2001.

[77] *The Irish Times*, October 5th 2000.

[78] Muiris FitzGerald, Doolin lecture.

[79] Peter Kelly, *The Irish Times*, October 20th 2000. The reference to "many consultants who disagree with the IHCA" was not FitzGerald's.

[80] National Economic and Social Forum plenary session on Equity of Access to Hospital Care, October 2nd 2001.

[81] In an interview in *The Irish Times*, October 5th 2000.

[82] *Report of the Working Group on Public/Private Mix*, p. 4.

[83] Ibid., p. 5.

[84] *Value for Money Audit*, pp. 179–183.

[85] "Summary of immediate initiatives required to address overcrowding in A & E departments", INO, February 21st 2002.

[86] In a letter from Donal Duffy, assistant secretary-general of the IHCA, to Gerard Barry, chief executive officer of the Health Service Employers Agency, March 6th 2002.

[87] Comhairle na nOspidéal, 2002, p. 84.

[88] *Report of the Working Group on Public/Private Mix*, p. 11.

[89] *Report No. 38 to the Minister for Finance on the Levels of Remuneration Appropriate to Higher Posts in the Public Sector*, Review Body on Higher Remuneration in the Public Sector, Stationery Office Dublin 2000, p. 84.

[90] *Value for Money Audit*, p. 181.

[91] Robins (ed.), p. 60.

[92] *The Irish Times*, January 31st 2001.

[93] *Report of the Review Group on the Waiting List Initiative*, p. 7.

[94] *A Comparative Analysis of Waiting Lists for Acute Hospital Treatment in EU Countries*, Rapporteur: Liz McManus TD, Joint Oireachtas Committee on Health and Children, Houses of the Oireachtas, January 2001.

[95] Peter Kelly, *The Irish Hospital Health Service – a consultant's view*, delivered at the Colmcille Winter School, February 24th 2001.

[96] In an off-the-record interview, October 2002.

[97] See *Report No. 38*, p. 85.

[98] In an off-the-record interview, September 2002.

[99] In an off-the-record interview, October 2002.

[100] Unpublished draft report of the Commission on Financial Management and Control Systems in the Hospital Service, 2003.

[101] Ibid., Department of Health estimate.

[102] In 2002 there were 1,731 public consultants, of whom 1,585 engaged in private practice. When consultants who earn very little from private practice – psychiatrists, geriatricians, paediatricians – are excluded, some 1,173 consultants remain. If the 198 in exclusively private practice are assumed to earn an average of €200,000 each from private insurers, the remaining consultants engaged in public and private practice earned an average of €130,000 from the insurers on top of their state salaries.

[103] Carol Coulter, *The Irish Times*, October 2nd 2002.

[104] According to sources within the profession.

[105] *National Task Force on Medical Staffing: first report*, draft copy, 2003.

[106] All exchange rates as at December 31st of the stated year.

[107] See pp. 331–332.

[108] *Financial Times*, November 2nd/3rd 2002.

[109] Danish County Council's Association.

[110] New Zealand Association of Salaried Medical Specialists.

[111] New Zealand Medical Association.

[112] École Nationale de la Santé Publique.

[113] Canadian Institute for Health Information.

[114] Medscape, 2002 Physician Compensation and Production Survey. Median income is the income which falls in the middle of the distribution.

[115] If 1700 consultants earn €151,000 on average, this adds up to €257 million, 3 per cent of the €8.2 billion health budget in 2002.

[116] *National Task Force on Medical Staffing: first report*.

[117] As calculated by *Report of the Working Group on Public/Private Mix*, p. 4

[118] Emergency admissions were 71.2 per cent of total in 2000. *Acute Hospital Bed Capacity*, p. 32.

[119] *Quality and Fairness*, p. 100.

[120] *Report of the Working Group on Public/Private Mix*, pp. 3–4.

121 Department of Health Hospital Inpatient Enquiry data. FOI.

122 Nolan and Wiley, pp. 53–54.

123 Hospital bed designations released by the Department of Health under FOI, November 2002.

124 Nolan and Wiley, Table 2.2, p. 17.

125 Limerick regional had 24 day beds in 2002, of which 12 were private. Cork Regional had 10 day beds, of which 4 were private. Public hospitals had 562 day beds in total, of which 184 were private.

126 *Draft report by sub-group on public-private mix: organisation/management incentives*, p. 2.

127 Department of Health.

128 *Acute Hospital Bed Capacity*, p. 9.

129 Percentages for insurance cover, Central Statistics Office quarterly national household survey for the third quarter of 2001, to which a health module was attached. Further data on health, age and income status of the insured: Nolan and Wiley, Chapter 5.

130 The number of days on which beds are occupied, computed from length of stay data for each inpatient.

131 Nolan and Wiley, Chapter 3.

132 *Acute Hospital Bed Capacity*, p. 75.

133 *Report of the Working Group on Public/Private Mix*, p. 7

134 National Economic and Social Forum, *Equity of Access to Hospital Care*, pp. 44–45.

135 Nolan and Wiley, pp. 16–17.

136 In an off-the-record interview, September 2002.

137 As explained by a spokesperson for the VHI, October 2002.

138 In an off-the-record interview.

139 *Report of the Working Group on Public/Private Mix*, p. 11.

140 Revenue Commissioners' estimate. The relief was progressively reduced between 1994 and 1996 until it applied at the standard rate of tax rather than at the taxpayer's marginal rate, which lessened its value for higher earners.

141 Stated by the Minister for Health, when he announced increased charges on July 17th 2002. Nolan and Wiley, p. xiv, earlier analysed that in 1996, although private patients were one-fifth of patients treated in public hospitals, they accounted for a quarter of the overall cost to the state of providing hospital inpatient care, of which about a half was recovered from charges.

142 Statement from the VHI, July 17th 2002.

143 Figures quoted in *White Paper Private Health Insurance*, p. 11.

144 *The Irish Times*, October 5th 2000.

145 *Report of the Working Group on Public/Private Mix*, p. 4.

10. The potent politics of hospital location

1 *Outline of the Future Hospital System*, Report of the Consultative Council on the General Hospital Services, Stationery Office Dublin, 1968, p. 126.

2 *An Agreed Programme for Government between Fianna Fáil and the Progressive Democrats*, June 2002, p. 22.

3 *National Task Force on Medical Staffing: first report 2003*, draft copy as of February 6th 2003.

4 *Annual Report of the Chief Medical Officer 1999*, Department of Health and Children. Based on data from 1995 to 1997.

5 *Report of the Forum on Medical Manpower*, pp. 63–4. Based on data from 1997.

6 *Report of the Committee on Accident and Emergency Services*, Comhairle na nOspidéal, February 2002, p. 31.

7 Ibid., p. 96.

[8] Niall O'Higgins interview, July 2002.

[9] For a discussion of this see *Value for Money Audit*, pp. 244–245.

[10] In conversation, September 2000.

[11] *Outline of the Future Hospital System*, Report of the Consultative Council on the General Hospital Services, Stationery Office Dublin, 1968, *passim*.

[12] *Medical Manpower in Acute Hospitals*.

[13] *Shaping A Healthier Future*, pp. 62–63.

[14] *The Irish Times*, October 5th 2000.

[15] *Medical Manpower in Acute Hospitals*.

[16] *Report of the Forum on Medical Manpower*, p. 37.

[17] Gerard Bury interview, July 2002.

[18] Medical Practitioners (Amendment Act) 2002, Section 5.

[19] Medical Practitioners (Amendment Act) 2000.

[20] *The Irish Times*, May 20th 2002.

[21] *The Irish Times*, March 23rd 2002.

[22] 1999 statistics supplied by the Department of Health.

[23] A & E data from Comhairle na nOspidéal, 2002.

[24] *Report of the Independent Review Panel to the Minister for Health and Children Concerning the Birth of Baby Bronagh Livingstone on 11 December 2002*, Department of Health and Children, 2002, p. 20.

[25] Ibid., p. 24.

[26] Ibid., p. 12.

[27] Dáil Debates, Volume 286, December 3rd 1975.

[28] Dáil Debates, Volume 310, December 14th 1978.

[29] Dáil Debates, Volume 310, December 5th 1978.

[30] Barry Desmond interview, July 2002.

[31] Court report, *The Irish Times*, December 19th 1984.

[32] Barry Desmond interview, July 2002.

[33] Mick Molloy in conversation, September 2000.

[34] *The Report of the National Joint Steering Group on the Working Hours of Non-Consultant Hospital Doctors*, January 2001.

[35] *The Irish Times*, September 26th 2000.

[36] *Report of the Independent Review Panel Concerning the Birth of Baby Bronagh Livingstone*, p. 4.

[37] Condon report. See *Report of the Independent Review Panel Concerning the Birth of Baby Bronagh Livingstone*, p. 3.

[38] Evidenced in a study by Alf Nicholson, consultant paediatrician at Our Lady of Lourdes Hospital in Drogheda, where the majority of sick newborns from Monaghan were transferred.

[39] Kinder report. See *Report of the Independent Review Panel Concerning the Birth of Baby Bronagh Livingstone*, p. 4.

[40] As recounted by Gerard Bury, President of the Council, interview, July 2002.

[41] As recounted by Bury.

[42] As recounted by a spokesman for the Board.

[43] This argument is presented in detail in Comhairle na nOspidéal, *Report of the Committee on Accident and Emergency Services*, pp. 97–113.

[44] *The Irish Times*, July 4th 2002.

[45] *The Irish Times*, July 5th 2002.

[46] Interviewed on RTÉ Radio One's *Five Seven Live*, July 17th 2002.

[47] Confirmed by NEHB, July 29th 2002.
[48] As explained by health board sources.
[49] Confirmed by NEHB.
[50] *A Review of a Clinical Adverse Event in December 2002*, North-Eastern Health Board, Department of Health and Children, 2002, p. 13.
[51] *Report of the Independent Review Panel Concerning the Birth of Baby Bronagh Livingstone*, p. 33.
[52] Ibid., pp. 18–20.
[53] *A Review of a Clinical Adverse Event in December 2002*, p. 11.
[54] *Report of the Independent Review Panel Concerning the Birth of Baby Bronagh Livingstone*, p. 16.
[55] Ibid., p. 25.
[56] "Nurses act over 'diabolical' crowding", The Irish Times, June 13th 2002.
[57] As described by Martin Wall in *The Sunday Tribune*, April 5th 2002.
[58] In 1998 Ireland had 29.2 deaths per 100,000 women compared to an EU average of 24.9. In 1995 France diagnosed 80 cases of the disease per 100,000 women, of whom 25 died. In 1998 Ireland diagnosed 70 cases of the disease per 100,000 women, of whom 29 died. Source: *OECD Health Data 2002*.
[59] *Development of Services for Symptomatic Breast Disease*, Report of the Sub-Group of the National Cancer Forum, Department of Health and Children, March 2000.
[60] Letter to the Editor, *The Irish Times*, November 15th 2000.
[61] Niall O'Higgins interview, July 2002.
[62] Ibid.
[63] Speaking to RTÉ Radio One's *Morning Ireland*, April 30th 2002.
[64] *Acute Hospital Elective Bed Usage in the Eastern Region*, Report to the Board of the ERHA from Donal O'Shea, chief executive, June 11th 2001.
[65] Ibid.
[66] The east lost 29 per cent of beds in the late 1980s compared to 19 per cent nationally.
[67] *ERHA Bed Capacity Review*, January 25th 2001.
[68] *OECD Health Data 2002*
[69] Stated by Michael Kelly, secretary-general of the Department of Health, at cabinet meeting, Ballymascanlon, 2001.
[70] Described by a health administrator.
[71] ERHA analysis for the first five months of 2002 revealed that among patients from the East, 21 per cent were private, while among patients from outside the East, 26 per cent were private.
[72] Speech to the Colmcille Winter School, February 24th 2001.
[73] Charles Haughey told the Dáil on October 19th 1978, "It seems to be generally agreed now that the regional hospital boards are unnecessary and should be abolished." Dáil Debates, Volume 308.
[74] 1996 Health (Amendment) Act No. 3, Section 16.
[75] Ruth Barrington, *Health, Medicine and Politics 1900–1970*, Institute of Public Administration, 1987, p. 275.
[76] Ruth Barrington, "Governance in the Health Services" in a forthcoming book of essays, edited by Donal de Buitleir, to honour the contribution to public life of Miriam Hederman O'Brien.
[77] *The Irish Times*, October 3rd 2001.
[78] Brendan Drumm interview, June 2002.
[79] *Report of the Commission on Health Funding*, Stationery Office Dublin, 1989, p. 156.
[80] *Value for Money Audit*, p. 169.
[81] Ibid., p. 190.

82 Ibid., p. 171.

83 *National Task Force on Medical Staffing: first report 2003*, draft copy as of February 6th 2003.

84 At a press conference on the Health Strategy, November 26th 2001.

85 *Quality and Fairness*, pp. 103, 127.

86 *Audit of the Structure and Functions of the Irish Healthcare System*, Prospectus and Watson Wyatt, draft copy, Department of Health, 2003.

87 An insight from an informed source.

88 *Report of the Commission on Financial Management and Control Systems in the Health Service*, draft copy, 2003.

89 As related by an informed source.

11. When the doctor costs too much

1 *The Irish Times*, November 24th 2000.

2 *Your Views About Health – report on consultation*, Department of Health and Children, 2001, p. 36.

3 In 2003, individuals without medical cards must pay the first €70 in monthly expenditure on medication, after which their costs were met by the state. The threshold had risen 24 per cent in 12 months.

4 The income eligibility level for a medical card in 2002 was €132 weekly for an individual. On incomes above that an individual would have to pay GP fees of typically between €40 and €45 per visit.

5 GPs deliver a national vaccination programme with mixed uptake.

6 The World Health Organisation has promoted primary health care as the "central function" of a country's health system since the Declaration of Alma Ata in 1978.

7 *Primary Care – a new direction*, Department of Health and Children, Stationery Office Dublin, 2001.

8 The first definition appeared in *Primary (Health and Personal Social Services) Care – a vision*, an early draft written in 2001 by the informal working group on primary care, established by the Department of Health to work on the preparation of its primary care strategy. The second definition appeared in *Primary Care – a new direction*, p. 15.

9 Launch of the primary care strategy, November 28th 2001.

10 Tom O'Dowd interview, *The Irish Times*, November 29th 2001.

11 Reported in *The Irish Times* in the days following the launch of the primary care strategy on November 28th 2001.

12 In an interview with Muiris Houston, *The Irish Times*, December 1st 2001.

13 At the Adelaide Health Debate, October 5th 2002.

14 This unpublished study was conducted in 1999 and 2000 as part of an ongoing men's health research programme.

15 Income guidelines for medical cards are drawn up by health board chief executive officers, who are responsible for determining eligibility under the 1970 Health Act, and are revised annually in line with the consumer price index. These guidelines are not statutorily binding so CEOs have discretion to award cards on "hardship" grounds.

16 The unpublished study was conducted by Alan Kelly, Hamish Sinclair and Conor Teljeur of the TCD Department of Community Health and General Practice.

17 *Primary (Health and Personal Social Services) Care – a vision*, see note 8 above.

18 Stated by the IMO, June 2002.

19 Capitation rates vary depending on gender and distance from surgery.

[20] Capitation rates from GMS Payments Board.

[21] See p. 79.

[22] In a lecture to the Adelaide Hospital Society's Annual Public Conference, October 13th 2001.

[23] Ibid.

[24] *The Health of Our Children*, 2000 Annual Report of the Chief Medical Officer, Department of Health and Children, 2001.

[25] *Primary (Health and Personal Social Services) Care – a vision.*

[26] *Report of the Working Group on Eligibility*, Department of Health, June 2001. FOI.

[27] Department of Health presentation to the Cabinet, Ballymascanlon, May 2001.

[28] See Table A.6, p. 377.

[29] Richard Brennan, chairman of the ICGP, interview, October 2002.

[30] Department of Health presentation, Ballymascanlon, May 2001.

[31] *Turning Vision into Reality*, IMO benchmark study, October 2000.

[32] Department of Health presentation, Ballymascanlon, May 2001.

[33] Richard Brennan interview, October 2002.

[34] *Primary Care – a new direction.*

[35] *National Task Force on Medical Staffing: first report 2003*, draft copy as of February 6th 2003.

[36] *Audit of the Structures and Functions of the Irish Healthcare System*, draft copy.

[37] Thresholds are indexed to the Consumer Price Index.

[38] Figures from the reports of the GMS Payments Board. See Table A.4, p. 375.

[39] *Primary Care: balancing health needs, services and technology*, Barbara Starfield, OUP, 1998.

[40] *Value for Money Audit*, p. 259.

[41] *Primary (Health and Personal Social Services) Care – a vision.*

[42] See Chapter 1, note 50, for membership of panel.

[43] Summaries of the proceedings at meetings between the international panel and the steering group and project team for the 2001 health strategy, May 23rd 2001, Department of Health. FOI.

[44] *Irish Medical Times*, October 27th 2000.

[45] The debate took place in Killarney on April 6th 2002. This account is based on a later analysis by the author in *The Irish Times* on April 15th. The defeated motion stated: "That this IMO AGM calls on the incoming government to introduce a national whole population GP service, exchequer or insurance based and seamless in its delivery of primary care to the poor and the rich."

[46] Cormac MacNamara interview, March 2002.

[47] George MacNeice interview, October 2002.

[48] Ibid.

[49] According to a Department of Health source.

[50] *ICGP/IMO – a vision of general practice 2001–2006*, January 2001.

[51] Cormac MacNamara interview, March 2002.

[52] Michael Boland and Richard Brennan, *The Irish Times*, August 8th 2001.

[53] Off-the-record interview, October 2002.

[54] See p. 328.

[55] At his press conference, November 28th 2001.

[56] Richard Brennan interview, October 2002.

[57] Press release from Department of Health, April 1st 2002.

[58] *The Irish Times*, October 24th 2002.

[59] *Primary (Health and Personal Social Services) Care – a vision*, p. 15 and *passim*.

60 Muiris Houston, *The Irish Times*, July 28th 2001.

61 At his press conference, November 28th 2001.

62 George MacNeice interview, October 2002.

63 Tom O'Dowd interview, October 2002.

64 Cormac MacNamara interview, October 2002.

65 *The Irish Times*, March 30th 2002.

66 See p. 330 and Figure A.1, p. 378.

12. Health spending and the black hole

1 ESRI survey of July and August 2000 in Watson and Williams.

2 *Irish Times*/MRBI poll, May 15th 2001.

3 *Curing Our Ills: Labour Party proposals for hospital and GP care in a new century, A Discussion Document*, April 2000.

4 *Restoring Trust – a health plan for the nation*, Fine Gael's policy proposals on health, November 2000.

5 2002 Census of Population.

6 *The Irish Times*, November 12th 1998.

7 See Table A.2, p. 372. This was a 66 per cent increase after price inflation.

8 *The Sunday Times*, November 17th 2002.

9 €7.85 billion in current spending and €507 million in capital. A wider measure of current spending is used in tables A.2 and A.5 in the appendix. 2003 Revised Estimates for Public Services and Public Capital Programme.

10 23 per cent of gross current expenditure in 2002.

11 The measure of national income used for Ireland in these comparisons is GNP (Department of Finance 2002 estimate), whereas GDP is used for the EU and other states. This is considered a valid comparison because Irish GDP is an overstated measure of national income, as it includes the repatriated profits of multinational companies. In this comparison, Irish public health spending has been reduced by 10 per cent to remove the cost of personal social services, which are not considered health spending in other states. Total health spending has been estimated by assuming that private health spending will account for 25 per cent of the total. These assumptions follow Department of Health practice.

12 See Table A.6, p. 377.

13 Department of Health presentation, Ballymascanlon, May 2001. Content reported in *The Irish Times*, May 24th.

14 See Table A.6, p. 377.

15 See Table A.6, p. 377.

16 *Value for Money Audit*, pp. 277–284.

17 Ibid., p. 274.

18 Ibid., p. 268.

19 *Quality and Fairness*, p. 161.

20 The analysis appeared in *The Irish Times*, April 24th 2002, and was produced by Professor John FitzGerald of the ESRI, in collaboration with the author, by applying the growth forecasts of the ESRI's medium-term review to a detailed breakdown of the health strategy by programme and year supplied by the Department of Health under FOI. The forecast assumed that the economy would remain on a favourable growth path of 4.5 per cent average volume growth in GNP over ten years to 2011 and that inflation would gradually fall towards the EU rate. Private health spending was assumed to fall to 16 per cent of the

total, reflecting planned extension of eligibility for medical cards and increased demand for improved public services. Public health spending was reduced by 10 per cent to exclude spending on social services. If the health strategy were to be implemented by 2011 at the pace envisaged by the Department of Health, the analysis revealed that this would require current health spending to increase by some 20 per cent in 2003 and capital spending to double from €497 to €942. The Department envisaged heavier increases in the early years of the strategy so that current spending increases would gradually reduce to annual increases of 7 per cent in the final three years of the strategy. Capital spending would further increase in the mid-years of the strategy.

[21] *The Irish Times*, November 3rd 2001.

[22] Letter to the Editor, *The Irish Times*, July 8th 2000.

[23] See Table A.4, p. 375.

[24] *Quality and Fairness*, p. 102.

[25] *Acute Hospital Bed Capacity: a national review*, Department of Health and Children, Stationery Office Dublin, 2002.

[26] *Quality and Fairness*, p. 82.

[27] See Table A.4, p. 375.

[28] An estimate of 3.1 in 2000 in *Acute Hospital Bed Capacity*, p. 20, predated the 2002 census of population, which showed greater than forecast population growth.

[29] *Acute Hospital Bed Capacity*, p. 54.

[30] See Table A.6, p. 377.

[31] *Value for Money Audit*, pp. 267–271.

[32] November data supplied by Department of Health.

[33] *An Agreed Programme for Government between Fianna Fáil and the Progressive Democrats*, June 2002.

[34] *The Irish Times*, November 15th 2002.

[35] *Quality and Fairness*, pp. 117–118.

[36] *Towards Workforce Planning*, Final report of the steering group, The Nursing and Midwifery Resource, Department of Health and Children, 2002, p. 221.

[37] *The Irish Times*, December 4th 2002

[38] *Quality and Fairness*, pp. 145–147.

[39] *Towards Workforce Planning*, p. 189.

[40] Kate Ganter interview, September 2002.

[41] "Half of homeless people mentally ill – Simon", *The Irish Times*, May 30th 2001; "Some 40 per cent of homeless have mental illness", report in *Cornerstone*, magazine of the Homeless Agency, *The Irish Times*, April 16th 2002.

[42] *Acute Hospital Bed Capacity*.

[43] See Table A.3, p. 374.

[44] *Medical Manpower in Acute Hospitals; Consultant Staffing*, Comhairle na nOspidéal, 2003; Post-graduate medical and dental board survey of NCHD staffing, 2002.

[45] Department of Health personnel census. Refers to whole-time equivalent employment.

[46] Calculated from *Towards Workforce Planning*, pp. 71–76, and Department of Health 2001 personnel census.

[47] Department of Health presentation, Ballymascanlon, *The Irish Times*, May 24th 2001

[48] *Health Inflation: Cost Pressures within the Health Services*. Paper prepared for the Public Accounts Committee, Department of Health, March 8th 1999.

[49] *Audit of the Structures and Functions of the Irish Healthcare System*, draft copy. Also see Table A.4, p. 375.

50 *Acute Hospital Bed Capacity.*
51 *Health Inflation: cost pressures within the Health Services.*
52 After adjusting for price inflation in public expenditure on goods and services. See Table A.2, p. 372.
53 *Value for Money Audit,* p. 22.
54 Ibid.
55 See Table A.5, p. 376.
56 See Table A.1, pp. 370–371, for list of ministers and their briefs.
57 When comparing Irish health spending with the EU average in the government's health strategy (2001), the Department of Health excluded spending on personal social services. The OECD has traditionally excluded programmes funded from the European Social Fund in computing Irish health spending. As Ireland's ESF funding has reduced, the OECD has excluded fewer programmes, so in its international comparisons, the Irish health spend is probably overstated.
58 Statement from the Minister for Children, Mary Hanafin, junior minister at the Department of Health and Children, December 17th 2001
59 Statement to an ERHA meeting, *The Irish Times,* July 12th 2000.
60 *Value for Money Audit,* p. 262.
61 *Quality and Fairness,* p. 45; *The Irish Times,* May 24th 2001.
62 *Value for Money Audit,* p. 17.
63 Ibid., p. 225.
64 Ibid., p. 10.
65 Ibid., p. 61.
66 Ibid., p. 230.
67 Ibid., p. 162.
68 *Report of the Commission on Financial Management and Control Systems in the Health Service,* draft copy, 2003.
69 *Value for Money Audit,* p. 100.
70 *Report of the Commission on Financial Management and Control Systems in the Health Service,* draft copy, 2003.
71 *Value for Money Audit,* p. 145.
72 *Report of the Commission on Financial Management and Control Systems in the Health Service,* draft copy, 2003.
73 *OECD Health Data 2002.* See Table A.6, p. 377.
74 *Value for Money Audit,* p. 25.
75 Ibid., p. 47.
76 Ibid., p. 239.
77 Miriam M. Wiley, "Reform and Renewal of the Irish Health Care System", *Budget Perspectives,* ESRI, 2001. See Table A.3, p. 374.
78 *The Irish Times,* July 19th 2002.
79 Hospital Watch column, *The Irish Times,* August 28th 2001
80 *Quality and Fairness,* p. 41; and more detailed breakdown from the Department of Health.
81 *Value for Money Audit,* p. 185.
82 Ibid., p. 132.
83 *Report of the Independent Estimates Review Committee to the Minister for Finance,* Department of Finance, 2002, p. 9.
84 *Audit of the Structure and Functions of the Irish Healthcare System,* draft copy, 2003, p. 140.
85 *National Task Force on Medical Staffing: first report,* draft copy, p. 59, analysed average

registrar's pay including overtime as €116,624.

[86] National Economic and Social Forum, *Equity of Access to Hospital* Care, p. 88.

[87] Wiley in *Budget Perspectives*, p. 80.

[88] *Value for Money Audit*, p. 124.

[89] Ibid., pp. 226–7.

[90] Department of Health presentation, Ballymascanlon, *The Irish Times*, May 24th 2001.

[91] Deflator for new construction in the health sector, *Construction Industry Review and Outlook*, Department of the Environment.

[92] *Report of Commission on Financial Management and Control Systems in the Health Service*, draft copy, 2003.

[93] PricewaterhouseCoopers report to Forfas, *Comparative Consumer Prices in the Eurozone and Consumer Price Inflation in the Changeover Period*, Forfas, June 2002.

[94] See p. 215.

[95] VHI statement, July 17th 2002.

[96] Minister for Health statement, July 17th 2002.

[97] *Central Bank Quarterly Bulletin*, Summer 2002, p. 8.

[98] In an IMS poll conducted for the Independent newspaper group on May 13th 2002, days before the election, 59 per cent of voters said the health service should be the top priority of the incoming government. No other issue rivalled it in importance.

[99] Minister for Finance, Charlie McCreevy, launch of the Fianna Fáil health manifesto, May 6th 2002.

[100] Implemented between August and December 2002.

[101] The income eligibility level for the medical card in 2002 was €132 weekly for an individual living alone and €238.50 for a couple with two children. An individual on €135 per week was not eligible for a medical card and must pay up to €65 monthly for prescribed drugs and typically between €40 and €45 for each GP visit.

[102] The charge was increased by 26 per cent to €40.

[103] The statutory inpatients' charge was increased by €3 to €36 per overnight or day case subject to a maximum of €360 in any year.

[104] In private conversation with the author.

[105] 2003 Revised Estimates for Public Services, also see Table A.1, p. 372.

[106] *The Irish Times*, November 15th 2002.

[107] Refers to spending under the public capital programme, which had been €532 in 2002. Exchequer-financed investment was planned to rise from €507 million to €514 million. Source: *2003 Public Capital Programme*.

[108] See note 20 above.

[109] Refers to whole-time equivalent employment not numbers employed.

[110] 2002 end-year census of employment not available at time of writing but the Central Statistics Office recorded an increase of 11,700 in health sector employment in the year to November 2002, which while not comparable to the Department of Health's count of whole-time equivalent posts and not restricted to the public sector, indicated that health employment had continued to grow strongly.

[111] *The Irish Times*, January 24th and 22nd, February 27th, March 27th, April 5th 2003.

[112] *The Irish Times*, November 16th 2002, January 15th 2003.

[113] *The Irish Times*, March 17th 2003.

[114] *Sunday Independent*, December 8th 2002.

[115] 2003 Revised Estimates for Public Services.

[116] *Financial Times*, April 18th 2002.

117 Pre-Budget report speech, reported in the *Financial Times*, November 28th 2001.

118 "Labour wants to return to the tax-and-spend policies which brought this country to the brink of ruin in the 1980s", Mary Harney, *The Irish Times*, November 11th 2000.

119 *The Irish Times*, July 31st 2001.

120 *The Irish Times*, July 31st 2001.

121 *Irish Independent*, June 4th 1997.

122 *Sunday Independent*, August 26th 2001.

123 At a meeting of the American Bar Association in the Law Society of Ireland, Friday July 21st 2000.

124 John FitzGerald, *Understanding Ireland's Economic Success*, ESRI Working Paper No. 111, July 1999.

125 *Just Economics: Fine Gael's economic framework for Ireland 2002–2006*, Fine Gael, March 2002.

126 *The Irish Times*, November 16th 2001.

127 George Lee of RTÉ interview, April 6th 2000.

128 European Commission – Autumn 2002 Economic Forecasts, statistical annex.

129 Letter to the Editor from Dermot Ryan, Department of Finance press officer, *The Irish Times*, February 3rd 2003.

130 Dáil Debates, June 22nd 2002.

131 *The Irish Times*, November 16th 2001.

132 *The Sunday Business Post*, May 13th 2001.

133 *The Irish Times*, May 15th 2001.

134 *The Irish Times*, May 15th 2002.

135 *Sunday Tribune*, May 20th 2001.

136 Letter from Minister for Finance, Charlie McCreevy, to Minister for Health, Micheál Martin, November 14th 2001. Released by Department of Health under FOI.

137 *The Irish Times*, May 14th and 15th 2002.

138 D. Wanless, *Securing our Future Health: taking a long-term view – final report*, HM Treasury, 2002.

13. Reform without equity

1 At a debate hosted by the Royal Academy of Medicine at the Royal College of Physicians, Dublin, February 15th 2001.

2 Opinion page, *The Irish Times*, October 20th 2000.

3 Letters to the Editor, *The Irish Times*, November 27th 2000.

4 Letters to the Editor, *The Irish Times*, October 25th 2000.

5 Letters to the Editor, *The Irish Times*, October 19th 2000.

6 *Value for Money Audit*, p. 238.

7 *Report of the Working Group on the Public/Private Mix*, July 2001, pp. 14–15. FOI.

8 *Quality and Fairness*, p. 108.

9 *Sunday Independent*, December 2nd 2001.

10 *Report of the Working Group on the Public/Private Mix*, p. 12.

11 *Quality and Fairness*, p. 101. The strategy document also refers to "what should ideally be an 80/20 division" (p. 100) and makes a commitment that the designated ratio should be "maintained"(p. 107). That the ratio to be maintained would be other than 80/20 was not clear and was only clarified in the Minister's subsequent aside.

12 At a press conference in the Mansion House, Dublin, November 26th 2001.

13 *Quality and Fairness*, pp. 107–108.

14 Discussion Outline from chair of working group on public/private mix to aid discussion at group's first meeting. FOI.

[15] *The Irish Times*, November 27th 2001.

[16] On RTÉ Radio One's *Five Seven Live*, November 27th 2001.

[17] "Why private patients are feeling sick", *Magill*, January 2002.

[18] "Middle class the scapegoat in health farce", *Sunday Independent*, December 2nd 2001.

[19] *Sunday Independent*, December 2nd 2001.

[20] National Economic and Social Forum, *Equity of Access to Hospital Care*, July 2002, pp. 87–93.

[21] George MacNeice interview, October 2002.

[22] Finbarr Fitzpatrick interview, October 2002.

[23] *Quality and Fairness*, p. 100.

[24] *Report of the Working Group on the Public/Private Mix*, p. 13.

[25] *The Irish Times*, September 26th 2001.

[26] *The Irish Times*, September 27th 2001.

[27] E-mail from Tánaiste's political advisor, Oliver O'Connor, to the Department of Health, October 30th 2001, refers to the Department's desire that the Progressive Democrats should drop their "fee per item" proposal. FOI.

[28] Ibid.

[29] E-mail from David Brennan, Department of Finance, to Michael Kelly, secretary-general of the Department of Health, November 9th 2001. FOI.

[30] Department of Health document, apparently prepared in response to Finance query above, undated. FOI.

[31] *The Irish Times*, September 29th 2001.

[32] *The Irish Times*, October 27th 2001.

[33] *Quality and Fairness*, p. 104.

[34] Statement from Minister for Health, July 3rd 2002.

[35] Statement from Minister for Health, January 9th 2003.

[36] *The Irish Times*, September 26th 2001.

[37] Oliver O'Connor e-mail, see note 27 above

[38] *Quality and Fairness*, p. 107.

[39] *Report of the Working Group on Public/Private Mix*, pp. 5–6.

[40] *Draft Report by Sub-group on Public-Private Mix: organisation/management incentives*, May 2001, p. 3.

[41] *Report of the Working Group on Public/Private Mix*, p. 11.

[42] Ibid., pp. 10–11.

[43] IMO Submission on the New Health Strategy, May 2001, and *Consultant Staffing*, Comhairle na nOspidéal, 2003.

[44] Kate Ganter interview, September 2002.

[45] George MacNeice interview, October 2002.

[46] Finbarr Fitzpatrick interview, October 2002.

[47] *Audit of the Structure and Functions of the Irish Healthcare System*, draft copy, 2003, p. 119.

[48] National Economic and Social Forum, *Equity of Access to Hospital Care*, pp. 37–40.

[49] *Quality and Fairness*, p. 117.

[50] Written Government decision of April 3rd 2001. FOI.

[51] On RTÉ Radio's "The Truth About the Health Service" series, March 11th 2002; again at IMO AGM, Killarney, April 6th 2002.

[52] Letter to David Doyle, second secretary, Department of Finance, January 24th 2002. FOI.

[53] *Medical Manpower in Acute Hospitals*.

[54] *National Task Force on Medical Staffing: first report*, draft copy, February 2003.

[55] Muiris FitzGerald, *Journal of Health Gain*, January 1999.

[56] *Report of the Forum on Medical Manpower*, p. 26.

[57] Peter Kelly, chairman IHCA manpower committee, Letter to the Editor, October 26th 2000; and opinion page article, October 20th 2000, *The Irish Times*.

[58] Opinion page article, *The Irish Times*, October 20th 2000.

[59] Finbarr Fitzpatrick interview, October 2002.

[60] *The Irish Times*, October 5th 2000.

[61] Survey results published in a letter to *The Irish Medical Journal*, July/August 2000.

[62] *Report of the Forum on Medical Manpower*, p. 32.

[63] Ibid., pp. 53–54.

[64] *National Task Force on Medical Staffing: first report*, draft copy, February 2003.

[65] Ibid.

14. Private sector solutions

[1] At the publication of the estimates for public spending in November 2001, McCreevy said that he welcomed private provision of health care.

[2] *Consultant Staffing*, Comhairle na nOspidéal, 2003.

[3] Letter to the Editor, *The Irish Times*, November 1st 2000.

[4] *A Comparative Analysis of Waiting Lists for Acute Hospitals Treatment in EU Countries*.

[5] In an off-the-record interview.

[6] As described by the Minister for Finance, Seanad Debates, Volume 165, March 28th 2001.

[7] Seanad Debates, Volume 165, March 28th 2001.

[8] The Department of Health's Working Group on the Public-Private Mix observed that a small reduction in bed numbers in the private sector had increased demand on public hospitals. FOI.

[9] *Irish Medical News*, January 13th 2003.

[10] Explained by Sheehan, February 2003.

[11] Briefing Note for the Minister for Finance from Liam Murphy, principal officer, February 22nd 2001. FOI.

[12] Sheehan later estimated the value of the tax subsidy at €13 million, reducing the cost of beds to €650,000.

[13] *Audit of the Structure and Functions of the Irish Healthcare System*, draft copy, p. 39.

[14] Released by the Departments of Health and Finance under FOI.

[15] Letter to the Minister for Finance, dated November 21st 2000. FOI.

[16] Note from Dermot Smyth, assistant secretary in Health, to Paul Barron, assistant secretary in Health, February 5th 2001. FOI.

[17] E-mail from Fred Foster, assistant principal in Finance, to Paul Barron, February 13th 2001. FOI.

[18] Letter from Fred Foster to Dermot Smyth, October 5th 2000. FOI.

[19] Letter from Dermot Smyth to Fred Foster, undated, November 2000. FOI.

[20] Briefing Note for the Minister for Finance from Liam Murphy, principal officer, undated, February 2001. FOI.

[21] Letter from Joseph Cregan, principal officer, Health, to Jim McCaffrey, assistant secretary, Finance, March 1st 2001. FOI.

[22] Letter from Charlie McCreevy to Micheál Martin, March 2nd 2001. FOI.

[23] If the 101 beds in Sheehan's Galway hospital liberated for public patients an equal number of private beds in public hospitals, the state would have gained these beds at an average cost of €129,000 to €200,000, depending on the value of Sheehan's tax subsidy,

which Finance originally estimated at €20 million and Sheehan later at €13 million.

[24] Unsigned letter from Micheál Martin to Charlie McCreevy, undated, March 2001. FOI.

[25] Note dated April 5th 2001. FOI.

[26] Seanad Debate on the Committee Stage of the Finance Bill, Volume 165, March 28th 2001.

[27] *Report of the Working Group on the Public/Private Mix*, pp. 7, 13. FOI.

[28] *Quality and Fairness*, pp. 102–103.

[29] Finance Act 2002, enacted March 25th 2002.

[30] Letter from Michael Heavey to Micheál Martin, April 9th 2001. FOI.

[31] Memo from Paul Barron to Minister's private secretary, re the Independent Hospital Association of Ireland's request for a meeting, May 5th 2001. FOI.

[32] Letter from Vera McManamon, private secretary to the Minister for Health, May 17th 2001. FOI.

[33] Memo to the Minister for Finance from Liam Murphy, principal officer, November 21st 2001. FOI.

[34] "McCreevy wants private patients out of public hospitals", Shane Coleman and Martin Wall, *The Sunday Tribune*, May 20th 2001.

[35] *The Irish Catholic*, August 16th 2001.

[36] Sister Helena O'Donoghue interview, April 2002.

[37] Letter from IHAI to Department of Health, January 18th 2002. FOI.

[38] Letter from Paul Barron, assistant secretary, Department of Health, to IHAI, January 25th 2002. FOI.

[39] PricewaterhouseCoopers for the VHI, *Report on Private Bed Requirements*, VHI, June 2002, executive summary.

[40] In a letter to the Minister for Health, June 27th 2002. FOI.

[41] In a letter to the secretary-general of the Department of Health, Michael Kelly, July 10th 2002. FOI.

[42] In a letter to Vincent Sheridan, July 11th 2002. FOI.

[43] In a letter to the secretary-general of the Department of Health, Michael Kelly, July 10th 2002. FOI.

[44] In a letter to Dermot Smyth, assistant secretary of the Department of Health, June 13th 2002. FOI.

[45] Letter of July 10th 2002 to Michael Kelly. FOI.

[46] *White Paper on Private Health Insurance*.

[47] Neither the government nor the VHI's advice was published. It was deemed too commercially sensitive for release under FOI. This account has been assembled from informed sources.

[48] Letter from the Health Insurance Unit of the Department of Health, refusing access to some material in the state's financial interests, August 15th 2002.

[49] According to informed sources.

[50] According to documentation from the Department of Health. FOI.

[51] *2002 Business Plan of the Department of Health*, www.doh.ie, p. 271.

[52] Described as Public Private Partnerships (PPP) in Ireland and Private Finance Initiative (PFI) in the UK.

15. Changing the system

[1] Surveys of international systems from an Irish perspective were published in *Value for Money Audit* and National Economic and Social Forum, *Equity of Access to Hospital Care*. See also Chapter 16.

[2] Liz McManus interview, September 2002.

[3] *Quality and Equality: a discussion document on the need for change in our acute hospital services*, Liz McManus, Democratic Left, February 1998.

[4] Liz McManus interview, September 2002.

[5] *Our Good Health*, The Labour Party, Autumn 2001, p. 23.

[6] Ibid., p. 24.

[7] *The Rainbow's Record and Policies*, Fianna Fáil briefing document, May 9th 2002.

[8] This passage draws on an interview with Mitchell, September 2002, from other Fine Gael sources and from observation of Mitchell's advocacy.

[9] *Restoring Trust – a health plan for the nation*, Fine Gael's policy proposals on health, November 2000, p. 7.

[10] Ibid., p. 8.

[11] Ibid., p. 28.

[12] *Towards a Better Quality of Life*, Fine Gael General Election Manifesto, April 2002, pp. 20–21; *A Different Kind of Ireland*, FG programme for government, May 5th 2002, pp. 19–21.

[13] *Our Good Health*, p. 10.

[14] *Restoring trust*, p. 28.

[15] *The Irish Times*, October 6th 2000.

[16] Liz McManus interview, September 2002.

[17] *Curing our Ills*, Labour discussion document, April 2000, p. 4.

[18] As explained by Mitchell, September 2002.

[19] *Restoring Trust*, p. 51.

[20] Publicly stated at a Fine Gael health policy conference in Ennis, Co. Clare, November 2001.

[21] Elias Mossialos, Martin McKee, et al., *The Influence of EU Law on the Social Character of Health Care Systems in the European Union*, report submitted to the Belgian Presidency of the European Union, Brussels, November 19th 2001, subsequently published in Mossialos and McKee, *EU Law and the Social Character of Health Care*, Work and Society No. 38, PIE-Peter Lang, 2002.

[22] *Our Good Health*, p. 2.

[23] *Manifesto 2002*, Progressive Democrats, p. 65.

[24] *A lot Done, More to do: Fianna Fáil manifesto 2002–2007*, April 2002, p. 54. Percentages author's calculations.

[25] *Manifesto 2002*, Progressive Democrats, p. 67.

[26] The Eastern Regional Health Authority was established in 1999 as a purely commissioning body, which enters provider agreements with health boards and voluntary hospitals, a commissioner-provider split without the competitive internal market of the UK's managed competition.

[27] *Curing our Ills*, pp. 12–13.

[28] *The Irish Times*, April 15th 2000.

[29] Letters to the Editor, *The Irish Times*, May 26th 2000.

[30] A. Dale Tussing, *Confronting the Hard Issues: the way forward to reform*, paper delivered at the Adelaide Hospital Society annual public conference, October 13th 2001.

[31] *Our Good Health*, pp. 27–29.

[32] *The Rainbow's Record and Policies*.

[33] *Our Good Health*, p. 27.

[34] For a discussion of HMOs, see pp. 351–352.

[35] In RTÉ radio's series *The Truth About the Health Service*, March 4th 2002.

[36] *Restoring Trust*, pp. 29–30, 52–53.

[37] *Restoring Trust*, p. 28.

[38] *Curing our Ills*, p. 23.

[39] *Our Good Health, passim.*

[40] Elaborated by Gay Mitchell, September 2002.

[41] *Restoring Trust*, pp. 25–26.

[42] *Restoring Trust*, p. 35.

[43] Fitzpatrick's objections were later described to the author by Mitchell.

[44] *Curing our Ills*, p. 14.

[45] *Our Good Health*, p. 24.

[46] Information Pack provided by the Labour Party, April 26th 2002.

[47] Bradford Kirkman-Liff, "The United States" in Chris Ham (ed.), *Health Care Reform: learning from international experience*, Open University Press, 1997, p. 33.

[48] Labour leader, Ruairí Quinn, stated that mutualisation (ownership by its members) of the VHI was "the best option" at a party press conference on April 26th 2002. *Our Good Health*, p. 26, suggested that the VHI might become a statutory trust.

[49] Mossialos, McKee, et al., generally informs this discussion.

[50] *The Irish Times*, January 31st 2001.

[51] Tussing, *Confronting the Hard Issues*, 2001.

[52] *The Irish Times*, January 31st 2001.

[53] Tussing, *Confronting the Hard Issues*, 2001.

[54] *The Irish Times*, December 29th 2000.

[55] In RTÉ radio's series *The Truth About the Health Service*, March 4th 2002.

[56] Department of Health presentation, Ballymascanlon, *The Irish Times*, May 24th 2001.

[57] *Value for Money Audit*, pp. 76–106.

[58] Office of the Ombudsman, *Nursing Home Subventions*, January 2001, p. 70.

[59] In an aside when delivering a paper, *Private Health Insurance: what are the implications of moving from a tax-based to an insurance-based system*, to the Society of Actuaries in Ireland, September 27th 2001.

[60] Jimmy Sheehan interview, March 2002.

[61] *The Irish Times*, January 9th 2002.

[62] *Irish Medical News*, October 23rd 2000.

[63] *The Irish Times*, January 9th 2002.

[64] Donal Duffy, assistant secretary-general, IHCA, Letter to the Editor, *The Irish Times*, March 19th 2002.

[65] Finbarr Fitzpatrick interview, October 2002.

[66] Although some analysts argue that Canada's system should be defined as tax-based, since it is now primarily tax-funded, it evolved from an insurance system in which a publicly owned insurance body purchased care on insurance principles. See p. 337.

[67] *Audit of the Structure and Functions of the Irish Healthcare System*, draft copy, p. 83.

16. Lessons from abroad

[1] Romanow, Roy J., *Building on Values: the future of health care in Canada*, Commission on the Future of Health Care in Canada, November 2002.

[2] Brian Abel-Smith, *The Hospitals 1800–1948*, Heinemann, 1964, p. 480.

[3] Paul Barker (ed.), *Founders of the Welfare State*, Heinemann, 1984, p. 107.

[4] John Campbell, *Nye Bevan: a biography*, Hodder and Stoughton, 1994, p. 179.

[5] Ibid., p. 166.

[6] Michael Foot, *Aneurin Bevan: volume II 1945–1960*, Davis-Poynter, 1973, p. 180.

[7] Campbell, p. 175.

[8] Ibid.

[9] Foot, p. 161.

[10] Campbell, p. 174.

[11] Foot, p. 130.

[12] Ibid., p. 146.

[13] Campbell, p. 168.

[14] Foot, pp. 188–189

[15] Campbell, p. 177.

[16] Foot, p. 213.

[17] Ibid., p. 138.

[18] Barker (ed.), p. 112.

[19] European Observatory on Health Care Systems, *Health Care Systems in Transition: UK*, 1999, p. 107.

[20] 2002 UK Budget, *Financial Times*, April 18th 2002. National income refers here to GDP.

[21] Derek Wanless, *Securing our Future Health: taking a long-term view – final report*, HM Treasury, 2002. Known as the Wanless Report, after Derek Wanless, chairman of the review group and former group chief executive of National Westminster Bank.

[22] See Table A.6, p. 377 and Figure A.1, p. 378.

[23] *Financial Times*, December 12th 2001.

[24] See Figure A.1, p. 378.

[25] *Delivering the NHS Plan*, as outlined to the House of Commons by Health Secretary Alan Milburn, April 18th 2002.

[26] Anna Dixon and Elias Mossialos (eds), *Health Care Systems in Eight Countries: trends and challenges*, European Observatory on Health Care Systems, London School of Economics and Political Science, 2002, p. 113.

[27] Northern Ireland Department of Health.

[28] See Table A.6, p. 377.

[29] European Observatory on Health Care Systems, 1999, p. 92.

[30] British Medical Association.

[31] Discussed in National Economic and Social Forum, *Equity of Access to Hospital Care*, pp. 37–38.

[32] Ibid.

[33] Dixon and Mossialos (eds), p. 111.

[34] British Medical Association and *Health Care Systems in Transition: UK*, pp. 92–93.

[35] Peter R. Hatcher, "United Kingdom" in Marshall W. Raffel (ed.), *Healthcare and Reform in Industrialised Countries*, The Pennsylvania State University Press, 1997, p. 244.

[36] UK Department of Health, *The NHS Plan*, Secretary of State for Health, HMSO, 2000.

[37] *Financial Times*, November 2nd/3rd 2002.

[38] British Medical Association.

[39] European Observatory on Health Care Systems, 1999, pp. 90–93.

[40] See Table A.6, p. 377.

[41] European Observatory on Health Care Systems, 1999, pp. 52–53.

[42] Ibid., p. 19.

[43] UK Department of Health, *The NHS Plan*.

[44] Scottish Executive Health Department, *Partnership for Care: Scotland's Health White Paper*, 2003.

[45] UK Department of Health, April 1st 2002.

[46] Public speech, UK Department of Health, January 15th 2002.

[47] Nicholas Timmins in the *Financial Times*, January 21st 2002.

[48] *BMJ*, March 1st 2003.

[49] See Table A.6, p. 377.

50 World Health Organisation, *Health Care Systems in Transition: Canada*, Copenhagen, 1996, p. 2.

51 M. G. Taylor, *Health Insurance and Canadian Public Policy – the seven decisions that created the Canadian health insurance system and their outcomes*, 2nd edn, The Institute of Public Administration of Canada/McGill-Queen's University Press, 1987. Professor M. G. Taylor's history is the source for my account of this period.

52 Ibid.

53 World Health Organisation, 1996, pp. 3, 5.

54 2003 First Ministers' Accord on Health Care Renewal.

55 Romanow, p. 60.

56 Ibid., p. 64.

57 World Health Organisation, 1996, p. 14.

58 *Value for Money Audit*, p.78.

59 World Health Organisation, 1996, p. 6.

60 Ibid., p. 7.

61 Romanow, pp. 60–61.

62 Thomas A. Rathwell, *Private Medical Insurance in Canada: panacea or Pandora's box?* Dalhousie University, Halifax, Nova Scotia. Paper presented to the Fourth International Conference on the Scientific Basis of Health Services, Sydney, Australia, September 2001.

63 World Health Organisation, 1996, p. 41. Also Table A.6, p. 377.

64 *Value for Money Audit*, p. 313.

65 *Waiting your Turn: hospital waiting lists in Canada*, The Fraser Institute, Vancouver, 2001. Other studies argued that this conservative think-tank had overstated waits.

66 *Average Payment per Physician Report: Canada 1999/2000 and 2000/2001*, Canadian Institute for Health Information, 2003. These are averages of incomes for physicians paid by FFS and earning at least $60,000.

67 Canadian Institute for Health Information, an independent, not-for-profit organisation, *Health Care in Canada 2001*, 2001, pp. 77–78.

68 Canadian Institute for Health Information, *Health Care in Canada 2002*, 2002, p. 31.

69 Robert G. Evans et al., "Phantoms in the snow: Canadians' use of health care services in the United States", *Health Affairs*, May/June 2002, 21:3, pp. 19–31.

70 See Figure A.1, p. 370.

71 An approximate calculation based on trends in German and Irish health spending suggests that in 2002 Irish per capita public health spending was at 90–95 per cent of the German level. Comparable international data are only available to 1998.

72 European Observatory on Health Care Systems, *Health Care Systems in Transition: Germany*, 2000, p. 8.

73 In 2000, the average person's health insurance contribution was 6.75 per cent of pre-tax income up to an income ceiling. This was matched by the employer. Low-income employees paid nothing and their employer a greater contribution.

74 European Observatory on Health Care Systems, 2000, p. 39.

75 Friedrich Wilhelm Schwartz and Reinhard Busse, "Germany", in Ham (ed.), p. 104.

76 European Observatory on Health Care Systems, 2000, p. 62.

77 Ibid., pp. 103–104, 12.

78 Ibid., p. 105.

79 Markus Worz and Reinhard Busse, "Structural reforms for Germany's health care system", *Euro Observer – Newsletter of the European Observatory on Health Care Systems*, Winter 2002.

80 European Observatory on Health Care Systems, 2000, pp. 46–49, 114–116.

81 Mathias Perleth and Reinhard Busse, Department of Epidemiology and Social Medicine, Hanover Medical School, paper delivered to the Institute of Public Administration, Dublin, April 1998.

[82] European Observatory on Health Care Systems, 2000, pp. 45–46

[83] Worz and Busse, *Euro Observer*, 2002.

[84] See Table A.6, p. 377.

[85] WHO,*The World Health Report 2000*, 2000.

[86] See Table A.6, p. 377.

[87] See Table A.6, p. 377.

[88] Dixon and Mossialos (eds), p. 41.

[89] *The Changing Health System in France*, OECD Economics Department Working Papers No. 269, 2000, p. 2.

[90] Dixon and Mossialos (eds), p. 41.

[91] *A Comparative Analysis of Waiting Lists for Acute Hospital Treatment in EU Countries.*

[92] Christophe Segouin and Christine Thayer, "The French Prescription for Health Care Reform", *International Journal of Health Planning and Management*, 14, 1999, p. 315.

[93] Ibid., p. 318.

[94] *The Changing Health System in France*, p. 9.

[95] Ibid., pp. 9–15.

[96] Ibid., p. 28.

[97] Segouin and Thayer, p. 323.

[98] *The Changing Health System in France*, p. 10.

[99] Ibid., p. 24.

[100] As reported by Lara Marlowe, *The Irish Times*, October 23rd 2001.

[101] Dixon and Mossialos (eds), pp. 37–38.

[102] *The Changing Health System in France*, p. 24.

[103] See Table A.6, p. 377.

[104] See Table A.6, p. 377.

[105] Segouin and Thayer, p. 320.

[106] *The Changing Health System in France*, p. 27.

[107] Segouin and Thayer, p. 316; *The Changing Health System in France*, p. 17.

[108] Segouin and Thayer, pp. 313–314.

[109] *The Changing Health System in France*, pp. 18, 33.

[110] Dixon and Mossialos (eds), p. 43.

[111] *The Changing Health System in France*, p. 20.

[112] Dixon and Mossialos (eds), p. 34.

[113] Ibid., p. 12.

[114] In conversation prior to the publication of the health strategy in November 2001.

[115] See Table A.6, p. 377.

[116] WHO, *The World Health Report 2000*, 2000.

[117] Dixon and Mossialos (eds), p. 25.

[118] Signild Vallgarda, "The Danish health care system: a commentary", *Euro Observer – Newsletter of the European Observatory on Health Care Systems*, 4:2, summer 2002.

[119] European Observatory on Health Care Systems, *Health Care Systems in Transition: Denmark*, 2001, p. 72.

[120] Ibid., p. 10.

[121] Ibid., p. 53.

[122] Ibid., pp. 30, 53.

[123] Danish Ministry of Health.

[124] Rates for 2002 supplied by the Danish County Councils' Association.

[125] European Observatory on Health Care Systems, 2001, p. 72.

[126] Ibid., p. 23.

[127] Vallgarda, *Euro Observer*.

[128] Ibid.

[129] Danish Ministry of Health.

[130] European Observatory on Health Care Systems, 2001, p. 40.

[131] Vallgarda, *Euro Observer*.

[132] Claudia Scott, "Reform of the Health System of New Zealand", in Marcus Raffel (ed.).

[133] Beverly Sibthorpe, "Models of Primary Health Care: the New Zealand experience", *New Doctor*, Issue No 74. Based on a paper presented in October 2000.

[134] *OECD Health Data 2002*.

[135] D. Ritchie, "Management of health system reform: a view of changes within New Zealand", *Health Services Management Research 11*, 1998.

[136] Helen Rodenburg, president of the Royal New Zealand College of General Practitioners, *The Irish Times*, November 25th 2002.

[137] Bradford Kirkman-Liff, School of Health Administration, Arizona State University, *Options for the Irish Health Care System*, paper delivered to the Society of Actuaries in Ireland, September 27th 2001.

[138] Dixon and Mossialos (eds), p. 87.

[139] New Zealand Ministry of Health, *The New Zealand Health Strategy*, 2000, p. 3.

[140] Dixon and Mossialos (eds), p. 84.

[141] New Zealand Ministry of Health.

[142] New Zealand Association of Salaried Medical Specialists.

[143] Information supplied by New Zealand Medical Association.

[144] See Table A.6, p. 377.

[145] Information supplied by A. Dale Tussing, Syracuse University.

[146] Bradford Kirkman-Liff, "The United States", in Ham (ed.), p. 30.

[147] Ibid., p. 36.

[148] Ibid., pp. 22–23.

[149] Ibid., pp. 24–27.

[150] A. Dale Tussing, "The Healthcare System of the USA", lecture delivered in Syracuse University, New York, 2001.

[151] Kirkman-Liff in Ham (ed.), p. 28.

[152] Ibid.

[153] Diverse sources: Kirkman-Liff, Tussing and Raffel.

[154] Kirkman-Liff in Ham (ed.), p. 40.

[155] Tussing, "The Healthcare System of the USA".

[156] Kirkman-Liff in Ham (ed.), p. 33.

[157] Observation by A. Dale Tussing.

[158] Marshall W. Raffel and Norma K. Raffel, "United States" in Raffel (ed.), p. 277.

[159] Ibid., p. 268.

[160] Medscape, 2002 Physician Compensation and Production Survey. Median income is the income which falls in the middle of the distribution.

[161] Kirkman-Liff in Ham (ed.), p. 42.

[162] European Observatory on Health Care Systems, 1999, p. 35.

[163] National Economic and Social Forum, *Equity of Access to Hospital Care*, pp. 37–40, and earlier discussion of France.

17. A healthier state

[1] Foot, p. 104.

2 Deeny, p. 311.
3 Ibid., p. 107.
4 See Mair in Coakley and Gallagher (eds), pp. 127–131.

SELECT BIBLIOGRAPHY

Books

Abel-Smith, Brian, *The Hospitals 1800–1948*, Heinemann, 1964.

Allen, Kieran, *Fianna Fáil and Irish Labour: 1926 to the Present*, Pluto Press, 1997.

Barker, Paul (ed.), *Founders of the Welfare State*, Heinemann, 1984.

Barrington, Ruth, *Health, Medicine and Politics in Ireland 1900–1970*, Institute of Public Administration, 1987.

Browne, Noel, *Against the Tide*, Gill and Macmillan, 1986.

Campbell, John, *Nye Bevan: a biography*, Hodder and Stoughton, 1994.

Cassidy, Eoin (ed.), *Measuring Ireland: discerning values and beliefs*, Veritas, 2002.

Cleary and Treacy (eds), *The Sociology of Health and Illness in Ireland*, University College Dublin Press, 1997.

Coakley and Gallagher (eds), *Politics in the Republic of Ireland*, 3rd edn, Routledge, 1999.

Coogan, Tim Pat, *Michael Collins*, Arrow, 1991.

Cooney, John, *John Charles McQuaid – ruler of Catholic Ireland*, The O'Brien Press, 1999.

Daly, Mary E., *Social and Economic History of Ireland*, The Educational Company, 1981.

Deeny, James, *To Cure & To Care – memoirs of a Chief Medical Officer*, The Glendale Press, 1989.

Desmond, Barry, *Finally and in Conclusion: a political memoir*, New Island, 2000.

Dixon, Anna and Mossialos, Elias (eds), *Health Care Systems in Eight Countries: trends and challenges*, European Observatory on Health Care Systems, London School of Economics and Political Science, 2002.

European Observatory on Health Care Systems, *Health Care Systems in Transition: Denmark*, 2001.

European Observatory on Health Care Systems, *Health Care Systems in Transition: Germany*, 2000.

European Observatory on Health Care Systems, *Health Care Systems in Transition: UK*, 1999.

Farmar, Tony, *Holles Street 1894–1994: the National Maternity Hospital – a centenary history*, A & A Farmar, 1994.

FitzGerald, Garret, *All in a Life – an autobiography*, Gill and Macmillan, 1991.

Foot, Michael, *Aneurin Bevan: Volume II 1945–1960*, Davis-Poynter, 1973.

Ham, Chris (ed.), *Health Care Reform: learning from international experience*, Open University Press, 1997.

Bibliography

Hannon and Gallagher (eds), *Taking the Long View: 70 years of Fianna Fáil*, Blackwater Press, 1996.

Healy, Seán and Reynolds, Brigid (eds), *Social Policy in Ireland*, Oaktree Press, 1998.

Hensey, Brendan, *The Health Services of Ireland*, 4th edn, Institute of Public Administration, 1988.

Horgan, John, *Noel Browne – passionate outsider*, Gill and Macmillan, 2000.

Horgan, John, *Seán Lemass – the enigmatic patriot*, Gill and Macmillan, 1997.

Hug, Chrystel, *The Politics of Sexual Morality in Ireland*, Macmillan, 1999.

Inglis, Tom, *Moral Monopoly: the rise and fall of the Catholic Church in modern Ireland,* 2nd edn, University College Dublin Press, 1998.

Jones, Jack, *In Your Opinion*, TownHouse Dublin, 2001.

Kennedy, Kieran A. (ed.), *Ireland in Transition*, Mercier Press in collaboration with RTÉ, 1986.

Keogh, Dermot, *Twentieth-Century Ireland: nation and state*, Gill and Macmillan, 1994.

Kirby, Peadar, *Is Irish Catholicism Dying?*, Mercier Press, 1984.

Küng, Hans, *Church and Change*, Gill and Macmillan, 1986.

Lee, J. J., *Ireland 1912-1985*, Cambridge University Press, 1989.

Manning, Maurice, *James Dillon: a biography*, Wolfhound Press, 1999.

Mossialos, Elias and McKee, Martin, *EU Law and the Social Character of Health Care*, Work and Society No. 38, PIE-Peter Lang, 2002.

Nolan, Brian, *The Utilisation and Financing of Health Services in Ireland*, Economic and Social Research Institute, 1991.

Nolan, Brian and Wiley, Miriam, *Private Practice in Irish Public Hospitals*, Oaktree Press and ESRI, 2000.

OECD, *Economic Surveys 1996–1997: Ireland*, OECD, Paris, 1997.

O'Ferrall, Fergus, *Citizenship and Public Service*, Adelaide Hospital Society and Dundealgan Press, 2000.

O'Reilly, Emily, *Masterminds of the Right*, Attic Press, 1988.

Raffel, Marshall W. (ed), *Healthcare and Reform in Industrialised Countries*, The Pennsylvania State University Press, 1997.

Reidy, Maurice (ed.), *Ethical Issues in Reproductive Medicine*, Gill and Macmillan, 1982.

Robins, Joseph, *Custom House People*, Institute of Public Administration, 1993.

Robins, Joseph (ed.), *Reflections on Health: commemorating fifty years of the Department of Health 1947-1997*, Department of Health, 1997.

Starfield, Barbara, *Primary Care: balancing health needs, services and technology*, OUP, 1998.

Taylor, M.G., *Health Insurance and Canadian Public Policy – the seven decisions that created the Canadian health insurance system and their outcomes*, 2nd edn, The Institute of Public Administration of Canada/McGill-Queen's University Press, 1987.

Tussing, A. Dale, *Irish Medical Care Resources: an economic analysis*, ESRI, 1985.

Walsh, Dick, *The Party - inside Fianna Fáil*, Gill and Macmillan, 1986.

Whyte, J. H., *Church and State in Modern Ireland 1923-1970*, 1st edn, Gill and Macmillan, 1971.

Whyte, J. H., *Church and State in Modern Ireland 1923-1979*, 2nd edn, Gill and Macmillan, 1980.

World Health Organisation, *Health Care Systems in Transition: Canada*, Copenhagen, 1996.

World Health Organisation, *The World Health Report 2000*, 2000.

Irish official reports

Consultants' pay:

Report No. 32 to the Minister for Finance on Hospital Consultants, Review Body on Higher Remuneration in the Public Sector, Stationery Office Dublin, 1990. (Gleeson Report.)

Report No. 36 to the Minister for Finance on Hospital Consultants, Review Body on Higher Remuneration in the Public Sector, Stationery Office Dublin, 1996. (Buckley Report.)

Report No. 38 to the Minister for Finance on the Levels of Remuneration Appropriate to Higher Posts in the Public Sector, Review Body on Higher Remuneration in the Public Sector, Stationery Office Dublin, 2000.

Health spending:

Acute Hospital Bed Capacity: a national review, Department of Health and Children, Stationery Office Dublin, 2002.

Proposals for Plan 1984–87, National Planning Board, 1984.

Report of the Commission on Health Funding, Stationery Office Dublin, 1989.

Report of the Independent Estimates Review Committee to the Minister for Finance, Department of Finance, 2002.

Value for Money Audit of the Irish Health System, Deloitte and Touche in conjunction with the York Health Economics Consortium, on behalf of the Department of Health and Children, Deloitte and Touche Dublin, 2001.

White Paper Private Health Insurance, Department of Health and Children, Stationery Office Dublin, 1999.

Health strategies:

Health – the wider dimensions, Department of Health, December 1986.

Outline of the Future Hospital System, Report of the Consultative Council on the General Hospital Services, Stationery Office Dublin, 1968. (FitzGerald Report.)

Primary Care – a new direction, Department of Health and Children, Stationery Office Dublin, 2001.

Quality and Fairness – a health system for you, Department of Health and Children, Stationery Office Dublin, 2001.

Shaping a Healthier Future – a strategy for effective healthcare in the 1990s, Department of Health, Stationery Office Dublin, 1994.

The Health Services and their Further Development, laid by the Government before each House of the Oireachtas, January 1966, Stationery Office Dublin, 1966.

Your Views About Health – report on consultation, Department of Health and Children, 2001.

Medical manpower:

Medical Manpower in Acute Hospitals – a discussion document, Department of Health, Comhairle na nOspidéal and Postgraduate Medical and Dental Board, June 1993. (Tierney Report.)

Report of the Forum on Medical Manpower, Department of Health and Children, January 2001.

Report of the National Joint Steering Group on the Working Hours of Non Consultant Hospital

Doctors, January 2001. (Formerly known as the Hanly Report but superceded by later Hanly Report on medical staffing: see draft reports below.)

Nursing:

A Blueprint for the Future, Report of the Commission on Nursing, Stationery Office Dublin, 1998.

Interim Report of the Steering Group, Nursing and Midwifery Resource, Department of Health and Children, 2000.

Towards Workforce Planning, Final report of the steering group, Nursing and Midwifery Resource, Department of Health and Children, 2002.

Tribunals:

Report of the Tribunal of Inquiry into the Blood Transfusion Service Board, Stationery Office Dublin, 1997. (Finlay Tribunal.)

Report of the Tribunal of Inquiry into the Infection with HIV and Hepatitis C of Persons with Haemophilia and Related Matters, Stationery Office Dublin, 2002. (Lindsay Tribunal.)

Waiting lists:

A Comparative Analysis of Waiting Lists for Acute Hospital Treatment in EU Countries, Rapporteur: Liz McManus TD, Joint Oireachtas Committee on Health and Children, Houses of the Oireachtas, January 2001.

Report of the Review Group on the Waiting List Initiative, Stationery Office Dublin, 1998.

Other:

A Review of a Clinical Adverse Event in December 2002, North Eastern Health Board, Department of Health and Children, 2002.

Annual Report of the Chief Medical Officer 1999, Department of Health and Children, 1999.

Development of Services for Symptomatic Breast Disease, Report of the Sub-Group of the National Cancer Forum, Department of Health and Children, 2000.

Report of the Second Commission on the Status of Women, Stationery Office Dublin, 1993.

Report of the Independent Review Panel to the Minister for Health and Children Concerning the Birth of Baby Bronagh Livingstone on 11 December 2002, Department of Health and Children, 2002.

Strategic Task Force on Alcohol Interim Report May 2002, Department of Health and Children, 2002.

The Health of Our Children, 2000 Annual Report of the Chief Medical Officer, Department of Health and Children, 2001.

The National Health and Lifestyle Surveys, Centre for Health Promotion Studies, National University of Ireland Galway, 2003 and 1999.

Other reports and papers

Canadian Government, *2003 First Ministers' Accord on Health Care Renewal*, 2003.

Canadian Institute for Health Information, *Health Care in Canada 2001*, 2001.

Canadian Institute for Health Information, *Health Care in Canada 2002*, 2002.

Cardiovascular Health Strategy Group, *Building Healthier Hearts*, Stationery Office Dublin, 1999.

Central Bank of Ireland quarterly bulletins.

Comhairle na nOspidéal, *Report of the Committee on Accident and Emergency Services*, 2002.

Durkan, Joe, director, Health Economics Centre, UCD, *"Private Health Insurance: what are the implications of moving from a tax-based to an insurance-based system"*, paper delivered to the Society of Actuaries in Ireland, September 27th 2001.

Eastern Health Board, Health Promotion Department, *Towards Health for All: reducing inequalities in Ireland*, proceedings from seminar of April 21st 1999.

ESRI quarterly economic commentaries.

FitzGerald, John, *Understanding Ireland's Economic Success*, ESRI Working Paper No.111, July 1999.

Kinsella, Ray, *Waiting Lists: analysis, evaluation and recommendations*, Centre for Insurance Studies, UCD, August 2001.

Kirkman-Liff, Bradford, School of Health Administration, Arizona State University, *Options for the Irish Health Care System*, paper delivered to the Society of Actuaries in Ireland, September 27th 2001.

Marmot, Michael and Wilkinson, Richard G., *"Psychosocial and material pathways in the relation between income and health: a response to Lynch et al"*, *BMJ* , May 19th 2001.

Medical Council, *A Guide to Ethical Conduct and Behaviour and to Fitness to Practise*, 4th edn, 1994; 5th edn, 1998; Amendment to 5th edn, 2001.

Mossialos, Elias, McKee, Martin et al., *The Influence of EU Law on the Social Character of Health Care Systems in the European Union*, report submitted to the Belgian Presidency of the European Union, Brussels, November 19th 2001, subsequently published in Mossialos and McKee, *EU Law and the Social Character of Health Care*, Work and Society No. 38, PIE-Peter Lang, 2002.

National Cancer Registry Board, *Cancer in Ireland 1994-1998*, 2001.

National Economic and Social Council, *A Strategy for Competitiveness, Growth and Employment*, NESC, 1993.

National Economic and Social Council, *A Strategy for Development*, NESC, 1986.

National Economic and Social Council, *A Strategy for the Nineties*, NESC, 1990.

National Economic and Social Council, *Strategy into the 21st century*, NESC, 1996.

National Economic and Social Council, *Opportunities, Challenges and Capacities for Choice*, NESC, 1999.

National Economic and Social Forum, *Equity of Access to Hospital Care*, Forum Report No. 25, Government Publication Sales Office, 2002.

New Zealand Ministry of Health, *The New Zealand Health Strategy*, 2000.

Nolan, Brian, *Income Inequality During Ireland's Boom*, unpublished article to appear in *Studies*, summer 2003.

Nolan, Brian et al., *Monitoring Poverty Trends in Ireland*, Results from the 2000 Living in Ireland Survey, ESRI, 2002.

OECD, *OECD Health Data 2002: a comparative analysis of 30 countries, CD-ROM*, Paris, OECD and Credes, 2002.

Office of the Ombudsman, *Annual report of the Ombudsman 2001*, 2002.

Office of the Ombudsman, *Nursing Home Subventions: an investigation by the Ombudsman of* complaints regarding payment of nursing home subventions by health boards, a report to the Dáil and Seanad, 2001.

O'Keane, Veronica, Jeffers, Anne, Moloney, Eamon and Barry, Siobhain, *The Stark Facts – the need for a national mental health strategy*, Irish Psychiatric Association, 2003.

PricewaterhouseCoopers report to Forfas, *Comparative Consumer Prices in the Eurozone and Consumer Price Inflation in the Changeover Period*, Forfas, June 2002.

PricewaterhouseCoopers for the VHI, *Report on Private Bed Requirements*, VHI, June 2002, executive summary

Rathwell, Thomas A., *Private Medical Insurance in Canada: panacea or Pandora's box?*, Dalhousie University, Halifax, Nova Scotia. Paper presented to the Fourth International Conference on the Scientific Basis of Health Services, Sydney, Australia, September 2001.

Romanow, Roy J., *Building on Values: the future of health care in Canada*, Commission on the Future of Health Care in Canada, November 2002. (Romanow Commission.)

Scottish Executive Health Department, *Partnership for Care: Scotland's Health White Paper*, February 2003.

Society of St Vincent de Paul, *Health Inequalities and Poverty*, April 2001.

The Institute of Public Health in Ireland, *Inequalities in Mortality 1989–1998: a report on all-Ireland mortality data*, 2001.

The Vincentian Partnership for Social Justice, *"One Long Struggle"– a study of low income families*, 2001.

Trinity College Dublin, Department of Community Health and General Practice, *Inequalities in Health in Ireland – hard facts*, TCD, 2001.

Trinity College Dublin, Department of Community Health and General Practice, *People Living in Tallaght and their Health*, Adelaide Hospital Society, 2002.

Tussing, A. Dale, *Confronting the Hard Issues: the way forward to reform*, paper delivered at the Adelaide Hospital Society annual public conference, October 13th 2001.

UK Department of Health, *The NHS Plan*, Secretary of State for Health, HMSO, 2000.

Wanless, D., *Securing our Future Health: taking a long-term view – final report*, HM Treasury, 2002.

Watson, Dorothy and Williams, James, *Perceptions of the Quality of Health Care in the Public and Private Sectors in Ireland*, Report to the Centre for Insurance Studies, University College Dublin, ESRI, 2001.

Wiley, Miriam, *Critique of Shaping a Healthier Future*, ESRI, 2001.

Wiley, Miriam, *"Reform and Renewal of the Irish Health Care System"*, *Budget Perspectives*, ESRI, 2001.

Released under Freedom of Information and other unpublished documents

Correspondence:

Correspondence between chief executive of the VHI and the Department of Health on the role of private hospitals. FOI.

Correspondence between Departments of Health and Finance on establishing a Treatment

Purchase Fund, on the Medical Manpower task force and on tax reliefs for private hospitals. FOI.

Correspondence between Ministers for Finance and Health on cost of the 2001 health strategy and on tax reliefs for private hospitals. FOI.

Correspondence between promoters of private hospitals and government departments. FOI.

Papers:

Department of Finance papers on tax reliefs for private hospitals. FOI.

Proceedings at meetings between international advisory panel and health strategy steering group and project team, 2001. FOI.

Reports and related papers of Department of Health strategy working groups and sub-groups on eligibility, 2001, and the public/private mix, 2001. FOI

Draft reports:

Audit of the Structure and Functions of the Irish Healthcare System, draft copy, Prospectus and Watson Wyatt, Department of Health, 2003. (Prospectus Report.)

Draft Green Paper on the Health Services, May and July 1984, Barry Desmond's private papers.

National Task Force on Medical Staffing: first report, draft copy, 2003. (Hanly Report.)

Primary (Health and Social Services) Care, an unpublished draft of the 2001 Government strategy for primary care.

Report of Commission on Financial Management and Control Systems in the Health Service, draft copy, 2003. (Brennan Commission.)

Newspapers, magazines, journals, television and radio

British Medical Journal (BMJ)

Euro Observer – Newsletter of the European Observatory on Health Care Systems

Financial Times

Health Affairs

Health Services Management Research

International Journal of Health Planning and Management

Irish Independent

Irish Medical News

Irish Medical Times

Journal of the Irish Medical Association

Magill

New Doctor

RTÉ One television's *Prime Time*

RTÉ Radio One's *Five Seven Live*

RTÉ Radio One's *The Truth About the Health Services* series, 2002

Sunday Independent

The Irish Catholic

Bibliography

The Irish Medical Journal
The Irish Times
The Journal of Health Gain
The Sunday Business Post
The Sunday Times
The Sunday Tribune

Other sources include Dáil debates, Programmes for Government, Social Partnership programmes, manifestos and policy publications of the political parties, the hospital consultants' common contract in its 1981, 1991 and 1997 versions, and Catholic Church publications including Papal encyclicals, bishops' pastorals and publications of the Council for Social Welfare and CORI.

INDEX